The Solution Lies Within

THE SOLUTION LIES WITHIN

Towards a New Medicine of Body and Mind

Thierry Janssen

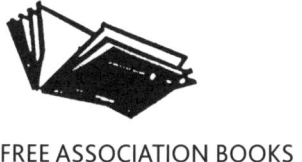

FREE ASSOCIATION BOOKS

First published in Great Britain in 2010 by
FREE ASSOCIATION BOOKS
One Angel Cottages, Milespit Hill, London NW7 1RD

First published in French by Librairie Arthème Fayard 2006

Copyright © Thierry Janssen, 2010

The right of Thierry Janssen to be identified as the author of this work has been asserted by him in accordance with the Copyright, Designs and Patents Act 1988

A CIP record for this book is available from the British Library

ISBN 978-1-85343-206-4 pbk

This book is made from paper suitable for recycling and made from fully managed and sustained forest sources. Logging, pulping and manufacturing processes are expected to conform to the environmental standards of the country of origin.

10   9   8   7   6   5   4   3   2   1

Produced for Free Association Books by Chase Publishing Services Ltd
Printed and bound in the European Union by
CPI Antony Rowe, Chippenham and Eastbourne

*To the memory of Denis Mahy.
For all who seek to understand.*

Disclaimer

The points of view, comments and information presented in this book have as their sole purposes to inform the reader, to present a better understanding of the human animal and to open a discussion about the evolution of contemporary medicine. In no way do these views, comments and information constitute a recommendation of any treatment, and should not be considered as such.

The ideas portrayed in the following pages are founded on scientifically established facts published in the medical literature. The reader who seeks to increase his knowledge and gain support for his thinking will find the necessary sources listed in the notes and bibliography at the end of the text.

The clinical cases described come from my practice, the scientific literature, or the experiences of practitioners I have met. Names and any information that would permit identification of these persons have been changed. Their histories have often been shortened to facilitate understanding.

CONTENTS

INTRODUCTION: The start of a medical revolution   1

PART 1   A MEDICINE OF THE MIND TO HEAL THE BODY

1   Embarrassing: The placebo effect   13
2   Clarifying: Psycho-neuro-immunology   24
3   Disturbing: The dangers of stress   39
4   Reassuring: The power of the mind   52

PART 2   A MEDICINE OF THE BODY TO HEAL THE MIND

5   Observing the body that suffers   81
6   Interrogating the body that remembers   90
7   Touching the body that relaxes   111
8   Aligning the body that balances itself   120

PART 3   A MEDICINE OF ENERGY TO HEAL BODY AND MIND

9   Behind the Chinese theories   137
10   Behind the Indian traditions   154
11   Behind the beliefs of the 'New Age'   169

CONCLUSION: A medicine of the human potential for life in the 21st century   187

Acknowledgements   203
Notes   204
Bibliography   234
Index   240

The ambition of a true search is to open the way to new questions.

Henry Corbin

INTRODUCTION
THE START OF A MEDICAL REVOLUTION

At the time that I worked in a hospital, the future of medicine seemed to me to be essentially in the fields of genetics, neurosciences and robotic surgery. At that time I was absorbed in long days passed in the operating theatre, in the training of young doctors in urological surgery, and in research on the influence of hormonal and other factors involved in the development of prostate cancer. Overloaded with work like most of my colleagues, I lived in a closed universe: I had no idea that outside my world many patients consulted therapists who had not trained at a university. What they met at the hands of these 'alternative' or 'complementary' therapists had nothing to do with the sophisticated technology of contemporary medicine. It seemed, above all, to be a question of quality of human contact: a different way of listening, common sense, and, above all, the awakening of a potential for healing that is dormant in all of us.

A survey carried out by the United States government in 2002, showed that 36% of the population had had recourse to alternative and complementary therapies.[1] This represents several billions of dollars which these sufferers did not hesitate to spend without any possibility of reimbursement. This tendency is not limited to the United States. In Canada, for example, the number of patients consulting alternative practitioners has more than doubled in ten years.[2] In Quebec alone, between 1989 and 2000, the amount paid out by private insurances for alternative medicines rose from 20 million to 250 million dollars.[3] In Europe, one study estimated that the proportion of users of alternative or complementary medicines varied from 20% to 50%, according to the country concerned.[4] In Australia, the number is estimated at 45%,[5] and in Japan, 65%.[6] France has followed the same trend, since 75% of the population have had recourse at least once to alternative or complementary medicine, principally for problems of anxiety, depression or back pain.[7]

It was not until after I left my post as surgeon at the University of Brussels that I discovered the importance of this current phenomenon. It was unexpected, since at the outset my intention had not been to undertake research in other care systems, but above all to understand the nature of the links connecting body and mind. To that end, I was led to study Indian and Chinese systems of medicine, to meet chiropractors and osteopaths, to experiment with massage and *shiatsu*, to practice meditation, yoga and *qigong*, and to be trained in various bodywork psychotherapies as well as hypnosis, and even – especially disconcerting for a surgeon – to be initiated into certain shamanistic practices at the hands of traditional healers. These experiences were fascinating and brought insight into my understanding of illness and healing. Nonetheless, although conditioned as I had been by a scientific education, I was convinced that this therapeutic universe which I had explored lay parallel to our own and never integrated with conventional medicine.

Since then, my opinions have changed. Several periods in the United States made me recognise that, in response to the behaviour of its population, the pragmatism of American society has stimulated a process which, over time, was able to transform the medical landscape. Thus, in 1992, the American Congress voted for the creation of a National Center for Complementary and Alternative Medicine: a new department of the National Institutes of Health (an organisation responsible for medical research in the United States), endowed with a budget of more than 100 million dollars, and devoted entirely to the scientific study of traditional remedies based on plants, alternative approaches such as meditation, yoga, acupuncture, osteopathy and chiropractic, and even controversial approaches such as shamanism, Therapeutic Touch or *reiki*.[8] Ideas have therefore evolved. This evolution produced a revolution: currently in the United States more than 80 faculties of medicine include certain alternative and complementary approaches in their training programmes.[9] Amongst these schools are prestigious universities such as Harvard, Columbia, Duke and Stanford, the universities of Arizona, Maryland and Pennsylvania, the Georgetown University School of Medicine and several university centres in California.[10]

A DIFFERENT PHILOSOPHY

This interest in other systems of medicine appears altogether justified when one realises that, according to the World Health Organisation (WHO), 80% of treatments the world over include traditional medicines.[11] In fact, the greater part of alternative and complementary therapies are direct descendants of traditional medicines. Some of the latter are very old. The WHO defines them as 'A collection of practices where the patient is considered as a whole within the context of his ecological system.'[12]

In other words, the alternative and complementary therapies take account of all the different dimensions of the human being – physical (body and movement), emotional (sensations and emotions), intellectual (the brain and its cognitive capacities) and spiritual (awareness of the self, the world and the transcendent aspects of life) – in close relation to the environment. From their point of view, good health is defined as a state of equilibrium, a harmonious relationship between the body, the emotions and the thoughts of an individual, separate and isolated from each other. They advocate, therefore, a fluid communication between these three aspects of the person and intelligent relationships between an individual, his fellows and the milieu in which he lives.

This approach is wide, global, 'holistic'. It is very different from the attitudes to which the Western mentality is accustomed, and with reason: in the West, since the time of Aristotle, the world has been regarded as a set of separate and isolated individuals. Further, since René Descartes it has been considered impossible to study anything but that which is visible, perceptible, physical and material, the immaterial being left to the good care of the religions. In establishing this dichotomy, Descartes, and later the philosophers of the Enlightenment, favoured the development of a divided image of the human being. On one side was the body; on the other, the mind. Reduced to its material dimension, the body is described as a precise mechanism, logical and sequential. Its constituents are objectified, categorised and analysed in their most minute details. The natural world and the entire universe being treated in the same way, cartesianism, reductionism and materialism formed the basis of the greatest discoveries of Western science.

In medicine, reductionism has allowed immense progress, while at the same time being the roots of a major crisis. Through regarding the body as an object, medical science forgot that the human being has also thoughts, beliefs, feelings and emotions. Consequently, many patients complain that they are being reduced to a list of the results of analyses; they regret not being able to express their sensations and intuitions and when faced with being dehumanised, even brutally treated, by technological medicine, they turn towards 'gentler' medicine. At the same time, physicians, impregnated with materialist science, have a tendency to focus only on a particular problem, an abnormal parameter, and in doing this they neglect the repercussions their treatment will have on the rest of the organism and ignore the consequences for the environment. This lack of vision of the whole commonly involves an over-use of examinations and treatments. Consequently, the pharmaceutical industry prospers and grows, the costs of health care grow in all provisions, and one may well ask how much longer the social services and insurers can continue to meet such expense.

Alternative and complementary approaches could perhaps be capable of finding solutions that may counter this escalation of medical consumption. In effect, by favouring an overall or global view of the human being, these systems insist on the inner potential of every individual: they encourage and preserve the fragile equilibrium of the body and the mind and endeavour to mobilise the self-healing capacities of the organism. Their concern to *prevent* the illness rather than cure it is without doubt more intelligent, more responsible, cheaper and less polluting, and endeavours to do so in a perfect harmony with the logic of an ecological awareness, respectful of both the human and the planet.

Andrew Weil, pioneer in the field and originator of a training programme in alternative and complementary medicines at the University of Arizona, said: 'Allopathic medicine is necessary for the treatment of 10% to 20% of health problems. For the other 80% to 90%, when there is no urgency, or any necessity of setting up fast-acting treatment, one has the time to experiment with other methods: treatments commonly cheaper, less dangerous, and eventually more effective because they work in concert with the healing mechanisms of the body instead of weakening them.'[13]

The logic which sets conventional medicine in opposition to alternative therapies is no longer topical. We are now concerned above all with evaluating the efficacy and the role of every approach to form an 'integrated medicine'. It is in this spirit that the WHO has recently recommended better collaboration between conventional doctors and alternative and complementary practitioners. A global consensus is emerging: we must press forward with reform of the health sector.

INSUFFICIENT INFORMATION

My journey between conventional or orthodox and science-based medicine, and the alternative and complementary therapies, as well as my research into the nature of the relationship between body and mind led me to create a psychotherapeutic approach adapted to accompany orthodox treatments of physical diseases. In my consultations I meet many patients who find that the help of alternative practitioners complements that of scientific medicine. Most of them do not dare to tell their doctor. Usually their justification is on the lines of 'He does not understand', 'He will shrug his shoulders and laugh', or even 'He will be angry'. In the United States, 62% of those who take alternative or complementary medicines hide the fact from their physician.[14] In Japan, the figure is 79%.[15] This is to be deplored: in the fifth century BC Hippocrates emphasised the importance of a *confident* relationship between doctor and patient as an essential element in healing.

The major danger in this lack of communication is that it opens the door to many charlatans. I have met many such in the course of my exploration of the world of 'parallel medicines'. I have also met many amongst those in white coats in the corridors of great university hospitals. These charlatans do not necessarily abuse people intentionally: they are at times inadequately trained or misinformed. Many act in good faith but are completely blinded by their beliefs and their superstitions. Thus the need to convince felt by certain alternative therapists and orthodox doctors can become a real danger to the health of patients.

Sometimes lack of openness of mind in either group causes them to deny or discredit certain approaches without having taken the trouble to check their effectiveness or to understand the mechanisms involved. This is a shame, because ignorance maintains the beliefs which block the opening of an objective debate capable of developing knowledge and responding to the anxieties of patients. Left to themselves, the ill then seek their information in popular works or websites where commercial motives and ideological influences are not always easy to detect. It therefore appears urgent that health professionals seriously seek to learn in order to be able to steer their patients honestly. The function of 'The Doctor' then takes on its proper dimension, since, etymologically, *docere* in Latin means 'to teach'.

It is patently clear that the sick wish to receive clear advice from their orthodox physician. A study carried out on patients suffering from rheumatoid arthritis showed that 69% wish their physician to recommend an alternative practitioner in addition to their treatment.[16] Happily, it seems that this wish is more and more frequently fulfilled nowadays: one American study showed that 40% of doctors questioned refer their patients to a chiropractor or an acupuncturist and that, in 50% of cases, they were satisfied with the results of the treatment.[17] Another study, in Canada this time, showed that 56% of family practitioners believed in the effectiveness of alternative therapies: 40% of them encouraged their patients to seek such help and 16% themselves practised one or another of non-conventional treatments.[18] One general practitioner in Quebec who had practised acupuncture for 17 years confided to me: 'I don't always understand how it works, but it works!'

A NEW SCIENCE

An inadequate understanding of how a treatment works is not a reason for doubting its effectiveness. It was thus that aspirin was prescribed well before the mechanism of its anti-inflammatory effect was understood. On the other hand, proof of the efficacy of a remedy must be rigorously provided. This is the weak point of alternative and complementary medicines.

Giving priority to clinical experience, improving methods and teaching new techniques is not enough. Nowadays, medicine demands proofs, an indispensable requirement for recommending recourse to a new therapy. Conscious of this necessity, research is being set up. Thus the International Society of Complementary Medicine Research was founded in London in November 2003. Elsewhere one finds increasingly specialised journals, the selection committees of which demand the same rigorous approaches as the classical medical journals. It is now no longer rare to find articles about alternative therapies in prestigious publications such as *Science*, *The Lancet*, the *Journal of the American Medical Association*, the *New England Journal of Medicine*, or the *British Medical Journal*. In 2002, *The Medical Clinics of North America* devoted the entire January issue to alternative and complementary medicines, going as far as the benefits of prayer and therapies identified as 'energetic', in the treatment of patients.[19] In 2004, Asian researchers founded *Evidence-Based Complementary and Alternative Medicine*, a journal published in London and available on-line.[20] This initiative constitutes a bridge between Asia and the West, where publications on alternative therapies were heavily influenced by American contexts and preoccupations.

Growing interest in the scientific community concerning unconventional medicines promises to transform our view of the nature of Man and to influence how we think of illness, health and therapy. In evidence, we should remind ourselves how each stage of scientific advance over the last three centuries has been the occasion for changing the concept of illness. This went from organic malfunction, cellular disorder, molecular disequilibrium, and, most recently, genetic anomalies. Nonetheless, an illness is not limited in this way. An illness is 'something' which causes an individual to suffer in his entirety. Lacking the means to objectify the multiple dimensions of the human being, reductionist medicine is incapable of quantifying or modelling the physical, emotional and intellectual suffering of the sick. The more it specialises and focuses on details, the less it is capable of understanding and providing relief for the *whole* of the individual. It is there that alternative practices have a role to play.

The need is, therefore, to translate the holistic concepts of alternative and complementary medicines into the terms of our modern scientific culture. This task is not easy. In effect, the methods of reductionist science are intended to evaluate the effects of a specific treatment on well-defined pathological features. However, in the case of numerous alternative and complementary treatments, the need is to evaluate the effectiveness of complex agents – for example, a plant composed of numerous chemicals, or the practice of *qigong*, which is made up of massages, movements, breathing exercises and meditation – on the entirety of the individual. Thus a reductionist analysis does not seem adequate for the study of unconventional therapies. Numerous specialists have claimed to be equal to the task of creating an 'epimedical science' capable of studying the effects of complex agents on the 'supersystem', which is the human being considered in all its dimensions.[21]

A BETTER UNDERSTANDING OF THE HUMAN BEING

In an attempt at clarification, the researchers of the National Center for Complementary and Alternative Medicine have classified the unconventional therapies into five fields:[22]

1. Alternative health systems founded on their own philosophy, theories and practices. Many of these systems appeared well before conventional medicine. We find here Chinese and *ayurvedic* medicines, homoeopathy and naturopathy.
2. Biological therapies that employ plants and natural substances, vitamins and food supplements at dosages that differ from those prescribed by conventional medicine.
3. The medicine of mind and body, which brings together a range of approaches allowing thought to influence physical symptoms and physiological processes. This group includes psychotherapy, meditation, visualisation, hypnosis and biofeedback.
4. Methods centred on the body, employing movements and physical manipulations such as massage, chiropractic, osteopathy, and the techniques of Alexander and Feldenkrais.
5. 'Energetic' therapies supposed to act on bioelectromagnetic fields – magnet therapy, therapeutic touch and *reiki*.

In studying certain of these disciplines, I had been impressed by the absence of any links between them. It seemed paradoxical that methods envisaging a global view of the individual should appear so isolated, even mutually antipathetic. However, in taking the time to penetrate the culture and background of these different systems of care, I found that the contradictions were not as important as they appeared. In fact, behind the codes and the metaphors belonging to each therapeutic approach, universally accepted physiological mechanisms were hidden. It is therefore appropriate to analyse the facts despite their appearances.

According to Leon Chaitow, naturopath and osteopath in charge of a teaching programme at the University of Westminster, London, if we wish to create 'integrated medicine clinics' we need to understand and assimilate the languages of others, place the patient at the centre of all attention and abandon all the problems of 'ego'.[23] The 'ego' is human; consequently, the ego is also a medical concern. This is as much true in alternative practices as in the conventional. The problem is not new since already in the 17th century Molière denounced it in the theatre: that often the interest of the patient is forgotten in pursuing the benefit of the interests of medicine or of physicians. Careful to avoid this pitfall, Leon Chaitow meets once a week with a multidisciplinary team to discuss specific cases and to assess as many different approaches as possible. Over 15 years, the therapists at his clinic have learned the theories and methods of their colleagues, developing a real co-operation in the service of their patients.

Alternative and complementary therapies have evolved over a long period within contexts of religious faith, superstition and esotericism. Human nature being what it is, this kind of environment has sometimes favoured the exploitation of the credulity of sufferers. It therefore seems important to free these practices of their folklore in order to establish a dialogue with 21st century medical science. At the same time, one cannot neglect the role that may be played by the cultural context of these therapies in the process of healing. Thus it is equally important that Western science avoids the traps of reductionist dogmatism. It was for these reasons that, at the time of the annual symposium held in 2004 at Exeter, in Britain, the American delegates declared that they wished to stimulate a much larger number of researchers to interest themselves in alternative and complementary medicines, while inviting the practitioners of these approaches to train in the methods of scientific research.

Certain intuitions in traditional cultures are now explained rationally by our scientific culture. Others remain completely strange to Western medical thought. This need not represent an obstacle to the study of alternative and complementary medicines. On the contrary, the truly scientific approach consists of observing the facts, attempting to reproduce them and endeavouring to understand the mechanisms involved. This understanding comes through the formulation of hypotheses which need to be tested *in vitro* – in the laboratory – or *in vivo* – on living organisms. Sometimes it will be necessary to invent new methods of observation in order to verify the validity of a hypothesis. It is of little importance whether it proves true or false: the true scientist always rejoices in either case since the result advances knowledge. To construct new hypotheses and devise new methods of observation, we need to be able to detach ourselves from concepts and beliefs that we think definitive. 'When the fact that what we have encountered does not fit in with the dominant theory, we must accept the fact and reject the theory', advised the celebrated physiologist Claude Bernard as early as the 19th century. This means we must change our paradigm.

Sometimes the desire to explain everything in erudite terms results in nonsense. In such situations, it would be better to admit the validity of certain metaphors while waiting to become able to translate them into the language of modern science. This is the more important since the speed at which scientific knowledge is growing is such that one can hope that we shall soon be able to bridge the gap between alternative and complementary medicines on the one hand and conventional medicine on the other. We are already beginning to accept the idea that states of mind work upon the body and that, in turn, the state of the body influences cognitive processes and emotional reactions. More advanced studies suggest that the oriental concept of energy is a physiological, biochemical and electrical reality, fundamental to the organisation of the living matter. Some researchers think that the electromagnetic field emitted by the body mediates a subtle and invisible communication between individuals. The laboratories of the larger universities are exploring the influence of love and the positive emotions on the good health of both body and mind. Concepts of fluidity and coherence are at the heart of scientific enquiry. New models are being invented to describe the human being.

Why does one fall ill? What is it that triggers healing? We have invented numerous medicines to relieve tensions and pain. How shall we discover links and build bridges between different approaches? We have medicines of the mind that work on the body and we have medicines of the body that work on the mind; and we have medicines of energy that treat the body and the mind. Understanding these varied therapeutic practices offers a unique opportunity to put the human being – as a creature at once physical, emotional and intellectual – back at the centre of the scientific debate. It is also an unhoped-for chance to invent solutions better adapted to the development of our societies confronted as we are with the task of preserving the planet on which we live. It is this which I suggest that we should explore together in this book.

I am deliberately not exploring homoeopathy, plant medicines and the influence of food. These fields are certainly important but I wish to focus on examining those practices in which the sole agent of healing is the human person. On reaching the end of our enquiry I hope that our ideas will be clearer and we will have new ways of developing the potentials we all possess.

Monsieur Tomès: Sir, we have discussed the illness of your daughter and, in my opinion, it arises from overheating of the blood; therefore I have decided that she must be bled as soon as possible.

Monsieur de Fonandres: But I think that the malady is a rotting of the humours caused by over-eating, I therefore consider giving her an emetic.

Monsieur Tomès: I maintain that that will kill her.

Monsieur de Fonandres: And I maintain that bleeding will kill her.

Monsieur Tomès: You show yourself a cunning man.

Monsieur de Fonandres: Yes, and I think you fall into the trap of every kind of erudition.

Monsieur Tomès: Do you remember the man you caused to burst a few days ago?

Monsieur de Fonandres: Do you remember the woman whom you sent to another world three days ago?

Monsieur Tomès: I have told you my opinion.

Monsieur de Fonandres: I have told you what I think.

Monsieur Tomès: If you do not bleed this girl now, we shall have a dead body.

Monsieur de Fonandres: If you bleed her, she will not be alive in a quarter of an hour.

Sganarelle: Which of these two shall I believe, and what decision shall I take about these opposite opinions? Gentlemen, I beg you to make me decide, and to tell me without passion what you believe to be the right way to relieve my daughter.

Molière, *L'Amour médecin*, 1665

PART ONE
A MEDICINE OF THE MIND TO HEAL THE BODY

1
EMBARRASSING: THE PLACEBO EFFECT

THE POWER OF THE IMAGINATION

Life is full of strange facts and bizarre stories, but sometimes the curiosity of certain scientists penetrates the mysterious.

Walter Cannon, professor at the University of Harvard between the two world wars, had this kind of mind: always ready to question and to create. We owe to him, together with others, our understanding of the working of the autonomic nervous system in response to outside stimuli, the concept of self-regulation of biological systems (homoeostasis) and the idea of 'flight or fight'.

Intrigued by all unusual phenomena, Cannon corresponded with a Doctor Lambert, a physician who worked with the indigenous people of Australia. The two accounts that I have chosen from this correspondence illustrate the enormous challenge presented to Western science by traditional societies.[1]

Rob lived in northern Australia, on the land of his ancestors. One evening, not long after he had converted to Christianity, he met on his way home Nebo, the witch-doctor of his clan. The old man resented Rob's repudiation of the ancestral traditions. With an angry look he pointed an animal bone at him. Immediately, Rob felt a profound discomfort. When Dr Lambert examined him he could find neither pain nor fever. All the same, Rob felt ill. His state deteriorated very quickly. The following day, he could not get out of bed. He was convinced he was going to die because no one had ever escaped from the spells of Nebo. In despair, Dr Lambert went in search of Nebo and threatened to drive him away from the territory if anything happened to Rob. Alarmed by the doctor's menaces, Nebo ended by agreeing to visit the sick man to explain it was all a misunderstanding. Rob's relief was almost immediate. The same evening he took up his work again, happy and in good shape.

Some time later, a native of New Caledonia who worked in a sugar cane plantation consulted Dr Clarke, a colleague of Dr Lambert. In a state of panic, he claimed that he was going to die because a witch-doctor had put a spell on him. After a thorough examination, including urine and faeces, had proved completely normal, Clarke attempted to reassure the patient. Nonetheless, the latter weakened quickly. Clarke then asked the New Caledonian foreman to comfort the worker. This failed; the foreman confirmed that the man would die. There was no uncertainty, and there was no hope of escaping the witch-doctor's sentence. The next day, the man died despite anything the doctor could do.

I happened to relate these two stories to a group of medical students. Inevitably their first reactions were of the kind that is expressed by: 'These stories of witch-doctors are all in the mind', or 'Primitive people are easily influenced by suggestion'. I drew their attention to the fact that the curse had passed through the mind, but that it was the bodies of the victims of sorcery that died or were cured. Sometimes some students would frown. One day, one of them said to me: 'If the body can be influenced by the mind, how can we know what is really involved in healing the sick?' All doctors and therapists need to ask themselves that question.

In Walter Cannon's view, death through voodoo bewitchment would be the result of intense and prolonged exposure to an emotional stress. A psychological cause (the fact of believing one is condemned to die, victim of a curse) could involve a physiological effect (excessive arousal of the sympathetic system, massive cardiovascular changes and the disturbance and exhaustion of the whole organism).

What actually happens seems that the bewitched individual wishes to 'please' the bewitching agent by showing the signs foretold by the spell that had been cast on him. We shall see that this kind of event is not confined to people we call 'primitive'. One meets them daily in medical practice when a patient reacts to a treatment which, in principle, should have no effect. We call this mysterious phenomenon 'the placebo' – that is to say 'I shall please' in Latin.

THE MEANING EFFECT

A study published in 1955 in the *Journal of the American Medical Association* by Henry Beecher of the University of Harvard, showed that among 35% of patients, pain was relieved by taking a tablet of sugar or an injection of physiological serum.[2] A critical attitude would raise doubts as to the reality of the suffering. Nevertheless, numerous patients in this study showed serious postoperative pain. The placebo effect is not limited to '*maladies imaginaires*', but involves real symptoms.

At the University of Turin, Italy, Fabrizio Benedetti showed that the analgesic effect produced by a placebo is suppressed by giving naloxone to the patient – a substance that blocks the cortical receptors for morphine and the natural opiates produced *by the body*. It is therefore clear that placebo analgesia works in a specific way on the neurological circuits relevant to pain.[3] A Scandinavian study carried out with a tomographic positron scanner (PETscan) has moreover shown that a placebo analgesic stimulates the same cortical areas as are affected by opiate analgesia.[4] According to an American study carried out under functional Magnetic Resonance Imaging (fMRI) in 2004, published in *Science*, a placebo acts simultaneously on the sensitive component involved and on the subjective component of pain.[5]

The placebo effect has, therefore a physical basis: it is real. It can affect blood pressure, reduce oedema, decrease stomach acidity, lower the level of cholesterol, change the number of red and white blood cells, and even improve cardiac rhythms as monitored by cardiogram.[6] The most recent studies re-evaluate the incidence of the placebo effect as rising. Estimates range from 70% to 100%.[7] Some workers suggest that any and every therapeutic act brings with it an effect which does not depend specifically upon the treatment, but simply on factors inherent in the relationship between the therapist and the patient.

We now know that the reputation of the practitioner and confidence in his capacities are involved in the appearance of the placebo effect. A kindly therapist, friendly and capable of empathy, will arouse an even more pronounced effect. However, something that works in one cultural context does not necessarily work in another. The magical formulae of an African witch-doctor would probably have little effect on a patient in New York or Paris. On the other hand, in the Western therapeutic milieu, the number of pills prescribed, their size and colour, influence the result produced. For example, it has been observed that taking two pills of a placebo is more effective than a single pill. The same placebo is shown to be more powerful if administered by intravenous injection. This last observation applies in the United States, but not in Europe, where this method of administration does not have the same significance. On the other hand, capsules are perceived as more beneficial than pills. White, blue and green pills are calming; yellow, red and orange are stimulant. Medication is all the more effective if the pills are large, with the exception of small red or yellow pills which seem to be the most active.[8]

The causative mechanisms therefore appear to embrace both the suggestion provided by the therapist and the expectations of the patient. A study carried out in 1975 on patients with asthma proved it. Herbert Benson, a pioneer in the field of the interaction of mind and body, proposed to his patients that they inhale a highly active allergen. The intention was to aggravate their respiratory symptoms in order to test the efficacy of a new medication contained in a second inhaler. Having taken two breaths from the first inhaler, half the patients developed acute respiratory difficulties. As soon as they inhaled from the second, the symptoms rapidly diminished: their breathing eased and blood tests showed that the blood oxygen levels returned to normal. One can imagine the surprise of the patients tested when, at the end of the experiment, Benson revealed that the two bottles contained neither an allergen nor any medicament – but solely a saline solution.[9]

Daniel Moerman, an anthropologist at the University of Michigan, preferred to describe the placebo effect as the 'meaning effect':[10] the significant factor is the *information* carried by the medication or the therapeutic procedure. Thus the novelty of a treatment appears to exert a positive influence on its efficacy. Let us take the example of cimetidine, a molecule capable of inhibiting acidic stomach secretions. In the 1970s, its marketing under the name of Tagamet® was considered a major revolution in the treatment of gastro-duodenal ulcers. Scientific researches published at that time showed the therapeutic efficacy of cimetidine of around 72%. These good results declined to 64% after 1981, the date at which ranitidine, a new and 'better' antacid was launched on the market under the name of Zantac®. With a rating of 75%, the efficacy of ranitidine was close to that of cimetidine at the time that it was in fashion and gained from the enthusiasm of its prescribers.[11]

The conviction of the *therapist* is therefore a basic factor in achieving a therapeutic result. A study carried out in several hospitals illustrated this well. The intention was to test the efficacy of a new treatment for hypertension. In one, the medical staff were convinced of the superiority of the new molecule over former treatments. They obtained excellent results: blood pressure was reduced in their patients by significant amounts. In the other hospitals, there was no indication of superiority of the treatment over a placebo. Doubts arose and the researchers lost interest. Nevertheless, it was decided to continue the study, and, to general surprise, no further positive results were recorded, even in the centre where the first tests had shown its efficacy. The only thing that had changed was the conviction of the researchers, one which they could not communicate to the patients.[12]

A remarkable study carried out in England clearly confirmed the impact of the reputation of a treatment on its efficacy. More than 800 women suffering from migraine were divided randomly into four groups, without the investigators being aware of the treatment proposed. The first group received a sugar pill (placebo) labelled 'analgesic'. The second were given the same pill which had been labelled with the name of a well-known form of aspirin (proprietary placebo). The third were given an aspirin tablet marked 'analgesic', and the last group a tablet of aspirin labelled with a well-known marque. The results were unequivocal: the well-known aspirin appeared more effective than the aspirin labelled 'analgesic', and the 'proprietary' placebo showed itself more effective than the simple placebo.[13]

DOCTOR OR WITCH-DOCTOR?

It seems then that the belief that the patient holds of the efficacy of a treatment influences the process of healing. It is curious that modern medicine seems to fear this aspect of therapeutic practice. When I was working at a university, I took part in numerous clinical studies aimed at evaluating the effectiveness of certain medicines or technologies. Each time it was necessary to exclude the placebo effect, as though that were an enemy, a spoilsport of peaceful practice.

The explanation for this must stem from the value attributed to power in our culture. The physician must prove his technical competence, and therefore roles are clearly divided: the patient submits, the doctor treats and heals. Active participation by the patient in the healing process puts in question the effectiveness and utility of the doctor. In a similar way, the pharmaceutical industry seeks to minimise the placebo effect in order to demonstrate the necessity of the medication they propose and produce. To believe that the sufferer possesses in himself a potential for healing threatens the omnipotence of modern science.

Several years ago, I questioned around a hundred medical students about the motivations that had led them onto the course. Apart from personal reasons rooted in their own histories, the majority seemed to fear illness and death. This fear, not always fully conscious, perhaps explains why many doctors withdraw when an illness evades treatment and death wins the battle. In reducing illness, the body and the sufferer to predictable mechanisms, science offers the doctor a very reassuring promise of control. One can, therefore, suppose that the potential for self-healing represents something unknown that is too powerful to include in the therapeutic strategies. As the philosopher of science Isabelle Stengers and the ethnopsychiatrist Tobie Nathan underline, the placebo effect is a real 'narcissistic wound' for the physician.[14]

However, instead of eliminating the placebo effect, we could regard it in all conscience as a major therapeutic tool and reinforce it, even foster its appearance. Whether or not they are aware of what they are doing, the witch-doctors whom I have met have recourse without hesitation to dramatisations which impress the sick. These 'sacred tricks'[15] are an integral part of their therapy. They appear to mobilise the psychic forces of the patient and release the potential for healing which exists in everyone. The images, symbols, metaphors and the explanations used are not important as long as the imagination of the patient is stimulated in a positive direction and sets in motion the physiological reactions which work towards the recovery of health. Employing this natural healing process can bring about miracles. Claude Lévi-Strauss relates how Quesalid, an Indian *kwakiult* on the island of Vancouver, had obtained initiation by the shamans of his tribe in order to expose their tricks.[16] Their technique was simple: it was enough to keep a small piece of fabric in a corner of the mouth, to bite one's tongue to soak the cloth in blood, and, at the right moment, brandish it as a pathological object removed from the patient's entrails. Just when he was at the point of denouncing his teachers, the apprentice witch-doctor was called to the bedside of an invalid. Having no other way of helping him, Quesalid had recourse to the shamans' trickery. Astonished by the efficacy of the technique, he abandoned the idea of exposing the secret he had received. On the contrary: he followed a long and brilliant career as a healer.

As a surgeon, I had condemned for a long time the practices of traditional healers. They appeared to me to be simple manipulations of the mind. For all that, observing shamans at work forced me to admit that they induced real physiological effects in their patients. I undertook training in certain of their methods and this brought me to regard the surgical approach from a different angle. In effect, besides a purely mechanical effect, surgical interventions seemed to provoke a 'meaning effect', the influence of which on the therapeutic results was by no means negligible.

Let us take the example of ligaturing the internal mammary artery, a procedure practised in the 1950s to relieve chest pains from cardiac problems. The explanatory mechanism invoked was that the operation produced an increase of the blood flow in the arteries feeding the heart – the coronary arteries – by the device of creating a natural connection between them and the network of the internal mammary arteries. This anatomical explanation being unproven, it seemed legitimate to eliminate a placebo effect. At random, and without saying anything to the patients, in half the cases the surgeons simply dissected the artery without making a ligature. The results were surprising: in the absence of this ligature the symptoms of the patients diminished, their use of medication reduced and the electrocardiograms taken showed improvements that persisted over at least six months.[17]

More recently, Bruce Mosely, orthopaedic surgeon at the University of Houston, obtained permission to study the placebo effect of endoscopic surgery in the treatment of arthritis of the knee. The 180 patients knew that they might undergo a 'blank' operation – a 'sham'. This was limited to small incisions in the skin of the knee without introducing the endoscope into the joint and therefore without removal of the damaged cartilage. The postoperative state was followed for two years during which period the patients were not informed as to which type of surgery had been applied to them. Astonishingly, there were no differences between the operated group and the placebo group, either in terms of pain or in terms of mobility of the knee.[18] These results stimulated a debate, the importance of which is highlighted by the fact that around 650,000 operations of this kind are carried out every year in the United States.

At the university of Denver, a number of neurosurgeons used the implantation of nervous tissue from human foetuses into the brains of people suffering from Parkinson's disease. This intervention raises the level of dopamine in brains damaged by this disease. Here too a 'sham' operation was evaluated. Twenty patients received a foetal cell graft under local anaesthesia, with radiographic control through the scalp and skull bones. Twenty other patients received simply an incision in the scalp while the surgical team mimicked the activities of a normal operation. Each patient knew the conditions of the experimental protocol but none of them knew whether they had had the real operation or the sham. The investigators responsible for evaluating the improvement of life experienced by the patients did not know which patient was in which group. Once again, the results were surprising. As expected, the level of dopamine in the patients who had received the graft had increased while it remained low in the placebo group. However, what determined the observed improvement of the symptoms of psychological depression, trembling, muscular rigidity and speech difficulties was the fact that the patients believed that they had benefitted from a graft whether this was true or not.[19]

It is essential for every human to see both meaning in his experiences and direction in his life. This is especially true in periods of illness. An ill person is suffering; illness is a period of doubt and uncertainty – a state of chaos. Healing consists above all in recovering an equilibrium, a state of stability. One who is suffering needs to be able to restructure his view of the world. The mythology and the rituals of traditional healers provide a framework for reordering the experienced chaos. In this sense they represent precious therapeutic tools. For example, the *tang-kis* healers in Taiwan spend much time explaining to patients the causes of their illness and the methods of treatment.[20] This is a rather different attitude from that of Western doctors, whose consultations have an average span of ten minutes.

Understanding the diagnosis of a disease and the principles of its treatment is a key factor in healing. The imagery used to explain is not important. The essential is that there *is* an explanation. The words and concepts employed are culturally based. Behind them, meaning seems universal. One day, Arnulfo Olivares, a Mexican healer who had just chased the evil spirits out of the body of a patient, turned to me and said: 'You have an air of doubt about you, doctor.' He was right: the patient had clearly appeared resuscitated, but I could not believe that a few passes of bare hands over his abdomen were enough to obtain such a good result. 'You, the doctor, said to me, the healer, that you remove tumours, you kill microbes, and you fight viruses. I? I chase the demons out, I calm the angry ancestors and I talk with evil spirits. We are in the same trade, only the words are different. Inside the heads of our patients are images. It is these images that heal the heart and body of man.'

THOU SHALT NOT INJURE

Western medicine too has its symbols and rituals. The diplomas hung on the wall of the consulting room and the books in the bookcases attest the expertise of the modern witch-doctor. The stern manner, the complicated language, the white jacket – all this belongs to the scenery. The lasers, the dopplers, and other sophisticated tools have an obvious magical function too. As for the scenery of the surgical theatre, one may imagine how much it impresses the spirit and mobilises the internal healing resources of the patient.

Unfortunately, the 'meaning effect' is not always positive: it can also provoke negative reactions. We call this the 'nocebo effect'. Recall the deaths through voodoo that were described at the beginning of this chapter. Without going as far as that, studies have shown that merely seeing the white coat of the physician can provoke hypertension or hyperglycaemia in patients.[21] Jerome Groopman, professor of medicine at Harvard, relates that every time he mentioned the possibility of side effects of a medication to one of his patients, a side effect unfailingly appeared. Once aware of this phenomenon, the patient would come to prefer not to know the list of possible side-effects of the medicine he needed to take.[22]

The power of autosuggestion is fascinating, even in connection with the arousal of disagreeable symptoms. This was found amongst the participants in a study, the character of which was worthy of Dr Frankenstein. The subjects were seated comfortably in an armchair and electrodes were attached on either side of the head. At a given moment, they were told that a low voltage current would be passed from one electrode to the other; naturally, there was no current and no possible source of a current. Nonetheless more than one third of the subjects reported having felt pain in their head following the passage of the fictitious current.[23]

We know how a smile, an open look, or a reassuring tone can exert a helpful influence on the process of healing. We are not surprised either to know that a shrug of the shoulders, a doubtful facial expression, or a touch of anxiety in the voice have an equal but negative effect. The words of the therapist are then a remedy – or a poison. Unaware of their power, the majority of doctors fail to take account of the fate they impose on the patient. This factor should be obvious to all health professionals, and, in a more general way, to all mankind, because suggestion and its influence are at the heart of all relationships.

In my practice, I meet patients suffering from cancer. From the appearance of their skin and the look in their eyes I can tell whether their oncologist had spoken hopefully or otherwise. I recall here Suzanne, a young women with cancer of the lung. Her oncologist had requested that she had a check scan. As agreed, Suzanne called the doctor two days later to ask the results of the examination. Unfortunately, the report was not yet available; she must await the following day. Both irritated and anguished, Suzanne decided that she must comfort herself. 'After all', she said, 'I'm not going to worry myself about a report I can't know to be good or bad.' She decided therefore to remain in the present: she was alive, she felt well and she had no wish to be overcome by fears which had no foundation.

The next day, she called the oncologist again. 'The results are good', he told her in a somewhat morose tone. Suzanne felt her body stiffen and the veins in her temple beat. 'Really good?' she asked, her throat choking. 'Good.' replied the doctor. Insisting forcefully, Suzanne eventually heard the verdict: the scan showed no tumour. The doctor added, 'But we must be careful, we cannot cry "victory" because a relapse is always possible.' Suzanne could not believe her ears. She had struggled against the disease for six months; she had endured the trials of surgery, of radiotherapy and chemotherapy, the tumour was no longer visible on the scanner – and all that her doctor could say was that we must fear a recurrence. At that moment, she was enraged, but dared not say anything other than to thank the doctor and hang up. Her rage made her want to kill, and at the same time her joy made her want to dance.

The following night she woke with a start: 'What if the gloomy tone of the doctor was hiding something', she wondered in anguish. And if he had tried to be tactful? Perhaps the scanner results were catastrophic. In having spoken of the possibility of a relapse, perhaps the oncologist had wanted to prepare her for the worst. Suzanne was no longer in the real world. Her imagination was tormented by fear. She did not close her eyes again that night. The next day she felt a pain in her throat. In the evening, she began to tremble, and she was seized with a marked fever. She was convinced she would die.

Several months later, I had occasion to talk about this episode with Suzanne's oncologist. He had never imagined that the tone of his voice could provoke such stress in his patient. He confided to me that he had lost his wife through cancer, and since then had himself had great difficulty in remaining optimistic in the face of this illness.

THE PROMISES OF OPTIMISM

Fear is an alarm signal that is vital for the survival of the individual. Without it, we would not adopt the strategies necessary to evade danger. Nonetheless, fear itself brings about dangers, of which the nocebo effect is the best example. We often experience irrational fears and create disturbances for ourselves for reasons which perhaps do not exist. Unconsciously, we transmit our fears to others, and fear can become a contagious curse that causes damage, even mortal damage.

A large part of my work with patients suffering from cancer or AIDS consists of teaching them to remain in the present to avoid their succumbing to useless fears. We will see later that this strategy is excellent for supporting good immunity functions and a return to health, because the power of beliefs about the health of the body is truly real.

An epidemiological study published in 1992 proves this. A number of women were followed regularly over 20 years and treated to suppress cardiovascular risk factors such as tobacco, raised cholesterol levels and high blood pressure. Amongst these women, the mortality rate due to infarcts were four times higher amongst those who believed they would die one day from cardiac problems.[24]

At the time of the beginning of the AIDS epidemic in San Francisco during the 1980s, a colleague told me that a deterioration in the health of young seropositive patients seemed to occur in an almost systematic way a precise number of weeks after the diagnosis of infection. One factor was shared by these patients: they had all read an article published in a gay magazine according to which the illness became fatal after an exact period of time. The official denial of this misinformation lifted the spell cast on these patients.

Phenomena such as this can constitute a major problem for public health. It is for this reason that the epidemiologist Robert Hahn expresses anxiety about the influence of the media on health. In a report published in 1997 he analysed the influence of an eventual nocebo effect in a number of diseases across the world. Numerous pathologies could, in particular cultural contexts, emerge following the diffusion of specific information. It is this that happens to young medical students when they become anxious and develop symptoms similar to those they are studying. Hahn concluded that since the nocebo effect on public health is not adequately studied, we need to encourage the media to take more care concerning the dissemination of information about the risks and causes of diseases and to generate more optimism in what is addressed to the public.[25]

If fear exerts a negative influence on health, optimism, on the other hand, is very helpful. During the 1940s, several hundred men were enrolled in the Harvard Study of Adult Development. They were rated by a questionnaire on a scale ranging from 'very pessimistic' to 'very optimistic'. Twenty years later, when the average age of these men was 45, it appeared that the quality of their health was closely related to their degree of optimism at the beginning of the study.[26] During the 1960s, the Department of Psychology at the Mayo Clinic began a similar study, designed to evaluate the effects of optimistic or pessimistic attitudes on health over a period of 30 years. The results were equally conclusive, since the optimists lived 19% longer than the pessimists, with physical capacities and a quality of life clearly better than the latter.[27] More recently, psychologists at the University of Kentucky conducted an enquiry amongst members of a religious group. Their results emphasised an overall difference between those believers who felt happy and content in their lives and those, on the other hand, who found little satisfaction in their daily lives. The life expectation of the optimists was ten years longer than that of the pessimists.[28]

Numerous studies support these conclusions. Optimism reduces the period of illness,[29] improves immune responses,[30] favours recovery from infarctions,[31] helps women with breast cancer to a better and longer life.[32] A positive attitude to life undeniably leads towards a positive future. Pessimists, it seems, should not be surprised to see their fears realised. However, *how* a state of mind can influence the state of the body remains to be explained.

2
CLARIFYING: PSYCHO-NEURO-IMMUNOLOGY

APPEARANCES CAN BE VERY DECEPTIVE

To understand how a voodoo sorcerer, a sugar pill or an optimistic attitude influences the health of the body is not possible unless one abandons the Cartesian concept of the separation of mind and body.

This need not present us with too much difficulty on condition that we pay attention to the manifestations of the influence of our thoughts on our bodies. Who has not known his cheeks flush at the thought of having to speak in public, one's hands becoming moist at the thought of an examination to pass? Good news, a compliment or a pleasant task to perform can be enough to make one feel light-hearted, full of energy and ready to move mountains. Others see us as lit-up, sparkling, in good form. But for all that, a fraction of a second later, a disagreeable telephone call, an argument or the prospect of an annoyance can cause us to tip from this profound well-being to an unbearable unease. We are then wiped out, psychologically and physically. We sink into a condition of stress, fatigue or depression. We become fragile, sensitive to pain, less resistant to infection. We know all this intuitively.

'The separation of psychology from the premises of biology is wholly artificial because the mind of man lives in an inextricable union with the body', stated Carl Gustav Jung.[1] While empirically obvious, this truth took time to become inscribed in the concepts of science. To collect the facts, verify their accuracy, construct hypotheses and seek proofs is a long and painstaking process. This slowness is to the credit of the scientific method. If one considers the sheer size of the task, the concept of the relationship between the body and the mind have developed really quickly over the last century. If we include the recent developments in the neurosciences, discovery even seems to accelerate. One of my friends, a researcher in a psychobiology laboratory, told me he felt as though he were a sailor at the side of Christopher Columbus, seeing ahead of him the shores of a new continent. This left me reflecting on what the future of the psychosomatic adventure would hold.

An article that appeared in 1895 in *The American Journal of Medical Science* described the case of an asthmatic crisis provoked by an artificial paper rose.² Similar phenomena had been observed by the writer Marcel Proust, who, himself allergic to roses, was suddenly seized with sneezing while assisting at a production of *Pelleas and Melisande* by Claude Debussy, at the very moment that Pelleas emerged from the grotto and breathed the scent of roses. At that time, there was no theory to explain such reactions. Incredulity and derision were more frequent responses than curiosity and reflection. Nonetheless, to the great profit of scientific progress, some researchers continued to publish their strange observations.

And so we come to Ivan Pavlov. In his laboratory in St Petersburg he had noticed that the ringing of a bell habitually rung at meal times was enough to trigger the secretion of saliva in his dogs. Pavlov had concluded that the animals associated the sound of the bell with the approach of food according to a 'conditioned reflex' under the control of a 'higher nervous function'. This discovery was recognised in 1904 by a Nobel Prize in medicine.

Pavlov's theory provided an explanation as to *why* sensitive subjects experienced a reaction to the sight of a paper rose or a photograph of a mown hayfield.³ Nonetheless, it said nothing about *how* such phenomena were produced.

A start on that explanation was made in the 1970s by Robert Ader and Nicholas Cohen, researchers in psychology, who studied conditioning in animals. In one of their experiments, rats were fed with sugar solution to which cyclophosphamide – an immunosuppressor with a very unpleasant taste – had been added. The hypothesis was that immunosuppression could be behaviourally conditioned as had appeared to be a possible explanation for illness-induced taste aversion that had been observed in some studies. The question was whether it was possible to develop a distaste for pure sugared water, i.e. without the added chemical. When fed again on pure sugared water, the researchers noted that the animals died. The greater the quantity of sweetened water that they consumed, the more the level of antibodies diminished and the faster they died. The evidence clearly pointed to the fact that the immunosuppressive effects of the cyclophosphamide were produced in the absence of that substance. The conditioning worked as though the rats had 'imagined' drinking the water mixed with this product. This observation led Ader and Cohen to postulate a link between the psyche and the immune system.⁴ However, they ignored the question of the process by which this link operated.

The answer came a few years later when David Felten showed a very rich innervation at the level of lymph tissues responsible for producing and storing the immune cells (the thymus, the spleen, the lymphatic ganglions, the bone marrow and the mucous membranes).⁵ The nervous system was thus revealed as the missing link in the psycho-immune system chain. The term 'psycho-neuro-immunology' was proposed by Ader to identify the science that had just emerged.

MIND–BODY UNITY

Until the publication of Ader and Felten's work, researchers, impregnated with reductionist beliefs, imagined that the nervous and the immune systems functioned separately, independent of each other.

It was believed that the communication at the heart of these two systems was mediated by specific molecules belonging to each: the neurotransmitters (for example, adrenaline, dopamine, serotonin, acetylcholine) or the neuropeptides (for example, the endorphins) in the case of the nervous system; the cytokines (for example, interleukin and interferon) in the immune system. Now the reality was revealed to be very much more complex – and this because some neurotransmitters and some cytokines are recognised simultaneously by both the nervous and the immune systems.

For example, some receptors for neurotransmitters produced by the brain are shown on the surface of immune cells, such as white blood cells or leucocytes. These cells secrete some neurotransmitters which in turn act on the brain. The connections between the brain and the immune system do not rely solely on nerves which reach the lymphoid organs. The leucocytes behave as real nervous cells working in the bloodstream. Some researchers come near to terming them a 'mobile brain'.

As far as the cytokines produced by immune cells are concerned, they exert a comparable and direct influence on the brain. For example, they trigger off fever, mood changes, sleep disturbance and changes in eating habits, of which we have experience every time we develop influenza, sweating in the depths of our bed, the appetite gone and morale at rock-bottom – withdrawal into oneself being a normal adaptation by the brain to that illness.

The border between the nervous and immune systems is therefore much less well defined than we had thought.[6] Candace Pert, professor at the University of Georgetown and co-discoverer of endorphins, has even shown that the neuropeptides which serve communication between neurones in the brain affect equally the transmissions between other cells in the body whether immune, digestive or vascular.[7]

These discoveries raise questions about the idea that mind is produced exclusively by the brain. Certainly, the brain is the site of cognitive processes involved in the elaboration of thoughts and exercises influence over the body. At the same time, in return, information arising in the body constantly influences the functioning of the brain and the elaboration of thoughts. Thus even the concept of a *link* between body and mind begins to appear too dualistic and is progressively being replaced by a more realistic definition: a 'body–mind unit.'

In the present state of our knowledge, we can identify certain key elements of this 'body–mind unit':

1. the brain – composed as it is of two hemispheres which perform different functions in the management of the emotions;
2. the autonomic nervous system – transmitting information between the brain and the rest of the body by means of stimulating nerves (sympathetic system) or soothing (parasympathetic system);
3. the immune system – connected to the brain by the autonomic nervous system and by a regulatory system known as the 'hypothalamic-pituitary-adrenal axis';
4. the hypothalamic-pituitary-adrenal axis drives a chain reaction of hormonal production in the brain (from the hypothalamus to the pituitary gland), then from the brain as far as the adrenal glands which secrete a hormone (cortisol) which is implicated in the immune reactions;
5. the endocrine system – made up of glands producing messenger-molecules (hormones) which control the functioning of the organism (growth, maturation, digestion, production and use of energy, sexuality and reproduction) as well as the emotions, and memory, learning and behaviour.

THINKING IN TERMS OF INFORMATION

A common denominator which links the different components of this unitary model is the information that circulates throughout. The concept of information represents a very subtle element in our understanding of living creatures

In science, everything begins with examining the material. Since the celebrated equation of Einstein: $E = mc^2$ (energy varies with the mass of the matter multiplied by the square of the velocity of light), we have understood that every particle of matter is condensed energy. Thus matter and energy are interchangeable. More recently, the theory of information has shown that the principal factor organising matter and/or energy is information. This can be expressed in the form of matter or that of energy.[8] Matter, energy and information are three different ways of expressing the natural world that have given birth to three major technological revolutions: mechanical, electronic and now computational.

Life has evolved in a hugely complex manner which allows the translation of material information into emotions and thoughts. Thoughts, in turn, can be expressed in the form of emotions, and emotions end in physical manifestations in the form of biological reactions or behaviours. This is, then, the pathway of information which we must follow in order to understand how the mind influences the body.

My psychobiologist friend was right: we have the opportunity to land on a new continent. Twenty years ago when I was a student, most physicians, and, *a fortiori*, the majority of patients, ignored this. Now we understand how the mind can make us ill or, contrariwise, help us heal. Since that understanding, we are no longer in the same position as before; we must now pay more attention to the ways in which we think. No doubt we shall avoid exposing ourselves to too much stress; our medical practice will be centred on prevention and we shall know how to profit from the advances of scientific knowledge.

The intimate mechanisms of body–mind communication described later will, perhaps, seem to you somewhat off-putting. If this is the case, you may move on to the next chapter without prejudice to your reading. Nonetheless, I would encourage you to endeavour to understand these processes, because they are amongst the most fascinating elements of current medical research and open a door onto the prodigious organisation of a living being.

THE MEANDERS OF THE BRAIN

Three layers

The human brain is the result of a long period of evolution. Information is handled there by three superimposed layers: the brain stem (sometimes called the reptilian brain), the limbic system (mammalian brain, often considered the seat of the emotions) and the neocortex (common to the large primates and man). The purpose of this network is the preservation of the equilibrium of the organism, that is to say its homoeostasis, the indispensable basis of survival. To achieve this end, physical stimuli arising in the environment or from the body are transformed into feelings and thoughts, which in turn may produce actions.

To take the example of a physical stimulus (such as heat, noise, pressure or pain), the information is first treated in the oldest part of the brain. There, automatic reactions and reflexes are triggered off to maintain homoeostasis. Then the information is translated into emotion within the limbic system, and in turn this emotion affects the body in stimulating physical responses (raising of the heart rate, reddening of the cheeks, moist hands, tension, or relaxation). The sensations involved indicate whether the actual experience is favourable or otherwise for maintaining homoeostasis. At the same time, the emotion can be analysed in the most evolved part of the brain, the neocortex. There it is experienced in the form of a feeling (for example fear, anger, pleasure or joy). Once decoded by the neocortex and compared with experiences stored in memory, the physical and emotional information gives rise to thought, which itself can be the source of feelings, emotions and therefore their bodily manifestations. Thus between the body and the brain, information circulates in both directions.

Two hemispheres

The sophistication of our cerebral equipment does not stop there. The brain is divided almost equally into two hemispheres, the right being a little larger than the left. In the 1950s, some neurosurgeons carried out sectioning of the connection between the hemispheres (the corpus callosum) in order to treat certain cases of epilepsy.[9] The results of this surgery were relatively satisfactory. Nevertheless, the patients who had undergone this operation did not have altogether the same behaviour post-operatively. It was supposed that there were differences in the ways of handling information at the core of each of the cerebral hemispheres.[10]

To listen to a symphony by Mahler while simultaneously analysing the score, stimulates the activity of the left hemisphere. To listen to that music whilst allowing the melody to lull the listener activates the right hemisphere.[11] The left hemisphere is directed towards the outside world, which it is continually deciphering. It specialises in analytic thought, logical reasoning – and words. The right hemisphere perceives information as metaphor and analogy. Its more global manner of thinking allows it an overall view. It plays an important part in the production of mental images, handles emotional impressions by giving them a meaning, and organises self-awareness. In summary: if the left hemisphere is a mathematician, the right is a poet.

The American psychologist Arthur Janov – who devised 'Primal Therapy', founded on the emergence of memories buried in the deepest layers of the brain – named the right hemisphere 'the hemisphere of love'. It is that which allows one to feel what others are feeling; it is also that hemisphere which gives us the possibility of deciding if others are sincere. The maturation of the right hemisphere is completed around the age of two years; that of the left hemisphere comes later. The young child is therefore before anything else an emotional creature. It is only in maturing that he begins to reason and to separate from his feelings. When the baby perceives his parents' emotions, it is the right hemisphere which becomes active. Unfortunately, the increase in production of cortisol following from the stress of lack of affection can cause him serious harm.[12] Thus, from that moment, certain people, profoundly traumatised in infancy in this way, relate their history, their faces frozen, without expression, with the detachment of a journalist who announces that day's death toll on the television news. Dominated by the influence of the left hemisphere, they are cut off from their pain. Their logical reasoning allows the suppression of frustration, but their emotional suffering is immense. They are no longer aware of this as though the right hemisphere were anaesthetised. Therefore they can commit monstrous acts without feeling the least empathy. On the contrary, they justify their attitude by a very elaborate explanation that comes from the left hemisphere which has become the heartless master of their thoughts.

Some emotions

Emotion, considered for a long time as a disturbing, even useless, phenomenon, is in fact an important source of information for maintaining homoeostasis. As indicated by its etymology – Latin *emovere* (move out, remove, agitate) – it is emotion that puts both thought and body into movement. Made visible by its bodily manifestations, emotion constitutes a form of communication that precedes verbal language. Thus a change of expression in appearance or a different intonation in the voice, informs others of our feelings. They are then enabled to adapt their behaviour appropriately.

A very ancient group of structures located in the middle of the brain – the limbic system – constitutes the centre of emotional information. Sensory stimuli arising in the body or the outside world are received in the hypothalamus. From there, they are sent, on the one hand towards a small structure called the amygdala, and on the other to those cortical areas responsible for conscious representation of visual, auditory, tactile, gustatory and olfactory information. The amygdala assigns an emotional value to the information, stores the emotional memory of what has happened (the contextual memory of which is stored in the neighbouring hippocampus) and sends alerting signals to the body by activating the autonomic system as well as the hypothalamic-pituitary-adrenal axis.

In recent years, much work has been carried out in an endeavour to understand the function of the emotions. From a biological point of view, it appears that negative emotions stimulate effective responses in order to survive when faced by a whole series of problems. Anger mobilises the energy required for attack or defence. Fear stimulates flight from danger. Disgust stimulates repulsion, or vomiting something toxic. The evolutionary advantages of negative emotions are clear.

Moreover, certain emotional reactions are deeply inscribed in the neuronal circuits of the brain and they arise even before we become conscious of them. For example, the neurobiologist Joseph LeDoux has shown that there are two neuronal circuits creating fear. One is conscious, the other not. The conscious circuit goes from the eye to the thalamus and the visual cortex (where the information captured by the eye is made conscious) before reaching the emotional centres of the limbic system. Fear is then aroused by a conscious representation. At the same time, the unconscious circuit leads directly from the thalamus to the amygdala without passing through the cortex. Thus the premature emotional reaction which follows, draws attention to a stimulus that threatens survival before it has been analysed with precision by the visual cortex. The advantage of the unconscious circuit is that we do not have to wait to understand the situation in detail before reacting. This is how we can jump over an elongated shape on the ground before recognising that it is not a snake but simply a branch. In the same way, we can recognise a disturbing expression on a face and feel a reaction before having identified the person in front of us.[13]

Negative emotions trigger physical reactions that are automatic or inbuilt, and designed to preserve our integrity and balance. But what is the function of positive emotions? Alice Eisen, psychologist at Cornell University, tested the creativity of subjects whom she had instructed to complete a series of words by one word that fitted. For example, the word 'black' could be followed by words such as 'night', 'market' and 'humour'. She established that her subjects did best when they were in a positive frame of mind. In another study, she examined the diagnostic skills of physicians in relation to their emotional state. The results were unequivocal: those physicians in a good mood summarised the facts more quickly, were less fixated on one idea and were much more prepared to give up premature conclusions.[14] Positive emotions, therefore, help to preserve an open mind. Barbara Fredrickson, director of a research laboratory concerned with positive emotions at the University of Michigan, showed that people in a distressed frame of mind concentrated more on details, while those in a good mood tended to take greater account of the overall picture, which indicates a more open and creative approach.[15] She concluded that our ancestors evolved thanks to their aptitude for happiness. It is true that negative reactions serve to solve immediate problems, an indispensable factor for our survival, but it is the recourse to positive emotions that favours the development of the personality and the creation of novel solutions in anticipation of times of greater difficulty. Further, to feel well within oneself reinforces social relationships; consequently, the 'positive' individual tolerates hard blows better and sees the future more hopefully. Joy, pleasure, gratitude, compassion and all the positive emotions are then major assets augmenting the capacities of imagination and strength when facing traumatising events. More than just permitting us to survive, they enable us to live.

To each hemisphere its own feelings

Richard Davidson, in his neuroscience laboratory at the University of Wisconsin, studied the role of the cerebral hemispheres in the management of the emotions. To do this, he showed images designed to evoke either positive or negative emotions in subjects whose cortical activity was recorded by means of electrodes attached to the scalp. When the images provoked positive emotions, the left hemisphere became active. On the other hand, when the images aroused negative emotions and stress, the recordings showed an increase in the activity of the right hemisphere.[16]

In continuing his investigations, Davidson and his team established that those people who were able to minimise disagreeable events in their daily life had a prominent level of left hemisphere activity, while those who tended to be sad or depressive presented a greater level of activity in the right hemisphere.[17]

Emotions and feelings seem, therefore, to be the result of a balance; their positive aspects are managed by the left hemisphere, while their more negative aspects depend upon the right hemisphere.[18] That explains why a trauma, a tumour or a surgical intervention involving the loss of function in the left hemisphere can be accompanied by weeping, anger and despair, while a lesion in the right hemisphere stimulates laughter, joy and a feeling of well-being.[19]

This lateralisation of the control of the emotions is related to an asymmetry of the neurotransmitters establishing the communication in the brain: dopamine, associated with reward and pleasure, is more concentrated in the left hemisphere, while noradrenaline and serotonin are found in greater quantities in the right. An excessive level of these last two substances is associated with states of distress, while a too low concentration is followed by depression. It is there that medications such as Prozac® work by augmenting the level of serotonin.[20]

The mechanisms of the emotions and thoughts stimulated by sensory perception are being continuously further explained. However, this does not explain how the emotions and cognitive processes can influence the health of the body. To do so, we must leave the brain and enter the defence system of the body.

THE RAMPARTS OF IMMUNITY

An army of cells

At every moment of life, without actually being aware of it, we need to re-define who we are, because there is the world around us. At all times, we are required to delineate our boundaries. We set what seems to us a good space between ourselves and others and to do so we learn to express our needs and assert refusal. Whilst this is happening, our immune system protects us at a microscopic level from possible intrusion. Thousands of white blood cells circulate without cease through every corner of our organism to hunt for invaders (bacteria) or to rid us of cells that are no longer considered part of us (cells which are infected by a virus or are cancerous). This organised and hierarchical army is the guarantee of our identity, and without it we cannot continue to exist. The sophistication of this defence system is the culmination of long evolution. Thus we possess a *natural immunity* that we share with markedly less developed organisms, and a *specific immunity* of more recent origin.

Natural immunity is innate, and is not especially specific but has the advantage of speedy action. The least wound or infection sets in motion an army of white blood cells (neutrophil granulocytes) which coagulate at the site of the lesion and release toxic substances in order to destroy the invading microbes. A cleansing service is provided by other white blood cells (macrophages) which digest the dead cells and damaged tissues. In the course of this battle, molecules of communication (cytokins) are released in large numbers. They stimulate fever, arouse inflammatory symptoms (reddening, swelling, pain) and promote the healing process of the wound by stimulating yet other immune system cells. In the event of a parasitic invasion or allergic reaction other granulocytes (eosinophils and mastocytes) are mobilised. Finally, and most recently, highly specialised cells have been identified: *natural killer cells* (NK cells). These recognise cells infected by a virus or that have become cancerous, and destroy them by sprinkling them with toxic substances. The NK cells, therefore, inhibit the development of cancerous cells and the development of metastases. In addition, they protect us at an early stage of viral infections until specific immune responses become effective.

The more recently evolved specific immune responses are aroused at the moment that various different infections attack the organism. They bring into play the white blood cells called lymphocytes. Their army is made up of three battalions: T-cytotoxic lymphocytes recognise specific proteins (antigens) which appear on the surface of cells infected with viruses and destroy them immediately, and act in the same way with cancerous cells. The T-helper lymphocytes produce some cytokins in order to support the action of other immune cells. Finally, the B-lymphocytes recognise foreign proteins (antigens) at the surface of bacteria, viruses, allergenic substances and cells that have been transfused or transplanted. They then produce antibodies or immunoglobulins (IgA, IgM, IgG, IgE and IgD) which become diffused in the blood, the saliva and other secretions, in order to neutralise bacterial toxins and to adhere to viruses to inhibit their entering into cells.

We are therefore doubly protected: if an intrusion escapes from the innate immunity it is immediately attacked by the acquired immunity system. In addition, this extraordinary defence network provides the possibility of intervention at two levels: either the NK cells and the T-cytotoxic lymphocytes attack the pathogens inside the cells – which we call *cellular immunity* – or the B-lymphocytes produce antibodies which attack the intruder when they are outside the cells – *humoral immunity*.

The supremacy of positive emotions

Richard Davidson and his team sought to discover whether the kind of immune response varied according to which cortical hemisphere was activated. The results of their work showed that cellular immunity was under the direction of the left hemisphere while, by contrast, humoral immunity was controlled by the right.[21] Now we already know that the left hemisphere preferentially governs the positive emotions, whilst the right is more in control of the negative. Thus maintenance of positive emotions reinforces cellular immunity. This is our first line of defence, indispensable for a quick reaction to kill the enemy hiding inside the cells. From this fact we understand better why a positive and sound attitude influences the course of an illness in a positive direction.

Numerous studies confirm this lateralisation of emotional and immune supervision. Adopting a negative attitude brings about a weakening of the immune response and lays one open to a greater risk of illness, while developing a positive attitude protects one well against problems.[22] To take the example of AIDS, we know that the progression of this disease is associated with a movement from cellular to humoral immunity.[23] At the University of Westminster, London, John Gruzelier recorded the cortical activity of patients infected with this virus, and showed that those patients whose cortical activity was greater in the left hemisphere had a better morale, retained their cellular immunity longer and experienced slower development of the disease.[24] This is why I encourage the patients I meet to fight their fear, to see their treatment in a positive light and to reinforce their immune defences by choosing to seek pleasures. Apropos pleasure, Angela Clow, psychologist at the University of Westminster studied the influence of odours on the secretion of immunoglobulin IgA, an antibody secreted on the surface of the mucosa to protect against possible invaders. We know that pleasant odours arouse the left hemisphere while nauseous smells activate the right. When the subjects smelled the pleasant odour of chocolate, the secretion of IgA increased, while the smell of putrefying meat reduced the level of IgA.[25] Thus even pleasant smells reinforce our immunity. I can never refuse the opportunity of communicating this information to those who believe that idea of seeking a little pleasure is culpable.

THE CHANNELS OF INFORMATION

Yin–yang neurology

Transmission of emotional information, both positive and negative, to the cellular or the humoral immune system and to the whole of the body is carried out along neural pathways organised, in the same way, into two different modes. For a long time it was believed that the activity controlled by these pathways was autonomic and out of the control of the will. Now we know that this is not so: the functioning of the 'autonomic nervous system' can in fact be modulated by our thoughts and feelings.

The whole autonomic system seems to be designed to allow a subtle balance between two opposed and complementary processes. One of these pathways, called *sympathetic*, arouses the organism to fight or flight. The other, called *parasympathetic*, stimulates, by contrast, a slowing of physiological processes in order to economise on energy and to allow the activation of reparatory processes. Thus the sympathetic system dominates the day and the parasympathetic the night. Nonetheless, our survival depends at all times on the capacity for adaptation of these two neural command systems.

Ideally, we ought to be able to preserve an equal balance between sympathetic tension and parasympathetic relaxation. The Chinese Taoists explain this in terms of energies: *yang*, when the thrust and activity of the sympathetic system is manifested; *yin* when the relaxation and passivity of the parasympathetic system is predominant. For them, good health is a balance between these opposed forces at a level as much psychological as physical. We shall see later how they have created a system of medicine of the body and the mind capable of ensuring such a neurological balance (Chapter 9, p. 137).

Occidental medicine has quite recently begun to interest itself in the psychological and physical interactions responsible for the balance of the autonomic nervous system. Thus it has been demonstrated that the left cerebral hemisphere preferentially activates the parasympathetic and the right influences principally the sympathetic.[26] We can then understand that thought and feeling influence the nervous system and hence the health of the body.

To take the case of positive thoughts and feelings arousing the parasympathetic system: the muscles relax, the cardiac rhythm slows, breathing is calmer, the blood vessels dilate, the skin warms, and the energy thus released is used for repairing wounds, and the body recovering from physical effort. At the same time, cellular immunity, itself under the control of the left hemisphere, provides an especially effective protection. The advantages of a serene emotional climate no longer needs to be demonstrated.

The stress hormones

We still have to understand how stress and negative feelings can damage health. To do so means we have to return to the meanders of the brain, more precisely to the level of the right hemisphere where negative emotions are generated. In effect, every time that we experience a negative emotion or conflictual feelings, the arousal of the right hemisphere triggers off what Hans Selye – the endocrinologist who first developed our understanding of the phenomenon – called 'the stress response'.[27] This is made up of two concomitant reactions: the first is neural, the second hormonal.

The neural reaction stimulates the sympathetic system. Automatically, the central part of the adrenal or suprarenal gland (which, as its name suggests is situated just above the kidney) – the *adrenal medulla* – secretes adrenaline: the cardiac rhythm accelerates, respiration increases, the peripheral blood vessels close, blood is preferentially directed to the muscles, salivary secretion is reduced, temperature rises and all energy is mobilised so that the muscles are readied for flight or fight.

The hormonal reaction itself initiates a chemical chain reaction involving the hypothalamus, the pituitary gland, and the periphery of the adrenal glands – the *adrenal cortex*. Following this, the hypothalamus secretes *corticotrophin releasing hormone* (CRH), the CRH stimulates the production of *adreno-cortico-trophic-hormone* (ACTH) by the pituitary gland, and once released into the bloodstream, the ACTH triggers off the production of cortisol in the adrenal glands. A real 'stress hormone', cortisol produces metabolic changes serving to supply sufficient energy for confronting the sources of stress. In addition, and amongst many other effects, it exerts a very beneficial anti-inflammatory effect, avoiding a blocking of the immune system and therefore an over-production of toxic substances (free radicals) the accumulation of which is harmful to the organism.

It is important to emphasise that the mechanisms of the 'stress response' are the same whatever the nature of the causative stress. Psychological anxiety or physical aggression – there is no difference: the body reacts each time with a secretion of cortisol and adrenaline. This 'stress response' presents us with clear evidence of a close relationship between the body and the mind. Unhappily, it is also the means by which our negative thoughts and emotions contribute to the development of numerous illnesses.

In fact, as Hans Selye indicated, the 'stress response' is designed to produce a speedy adaptation of the organism to threats in its environment. Alerted by emotions such as fear or anger, the body mobilises its energy, protects itself by fleeing or defends itself by attacking, and thus ensures its integrity. Once the danger is set aside, the sympathetic system calms down, and the activity of the hypothalamic-pituitary-adrenal axis slows down. The 'red alert' is no longer needed. Unfortunately, human beings often invent reasons to become stressed without there being any real life-threatening danger. Man's imagination is a wonderful tool for adaptation and evolution, but can also become an immense handicap. Because the persistence of bad or negative thoughts and emotions continues to put the body under tension, the continuation of the resulting augmentation of adrenaline and cortisol ends by producing very harmful effects on health.

To begin with adrenaline: raised levels increase blood pressure, the blood flow intensifies; turbulence in its flow damage the internal lining of the arteries; blood cholesterol – raised in a situation of stress – infiltrates the damaged linings; an inflammatory reaction involves the creation of calcium deposits; atheromatous plaques are formed; the calibre of the arteries is reduced and small vessels become blocked. Over time, arterial narrowing disturbs the blood supply to the heart, and any additional physical effort or mental stress will be enough to create a dearth of oxygen, so that the cardiac muscle suffers and there is a risk of the development of a heart attack or myocardial infarction.

Then the cortisol: in the long term its anti-inflammatory action provokes atrophy of the lymphoid organs; the immune system becomes profoundly disorganised and susceptibility to infection increases. Sometimes the immune cells become habituated to raised levels of cortisol; in other cases the hypothalamic-pituitary-adrenal cascade is exhausted and the level of cortisol drops dramatically; each time there follow chaotic immune reactions, inflammation intensifies and toxic substances – the free radicals – damage the organism's tissues. Persistent psychological stress therefore appears to be more or less an aggravating factor in or cause of a range of illnesses called 'auto-immune'.[28] Sometimes the damage may be such that some entire organs cease to function, provoking diabetes, hypothyroidism or an insufficiency of the adrenal glands. In other cases, what has by then become an autodestructive inflammation reaches the liver, the intestines or the joints, causing, for example, auto-immune hepatitis, Crohn's disease, haemorrhagic ulcerative rectocolitis or severely handicapping rheumatic diseases.[29] All these pathologies progress by attacks.[30] The stress, by increasing the prevalence of bacteria or viruses can accentuate the severity of the problem, for example in multiple sclerosis or stomach ulcers.[31]

However, the damage caused by the increased levels of cortisol does not stop there: insulin function is less effective, the level of sugar in the blood rises and there is a risk of diabetes; appetite is increased and fats accumulate in the abdomen.[32] The muscles atrophy because their proteins are used to increase the production of glucose in order to supply the energy required for the 'stress response'; the bony mass diminishes; the skin develops wrinkles and wounds heal less well; water retention contributes to raised arterial pressure; an attack on the neurones of the cerebral hippocampus is followed by memory loss;[33] and a series of effects on the cerebral cortex provoke fatigue, irritability, depression of mood, loss of libido, insomnia, agitation, anxiety, tears or a feeling of despair.[34]

Finally, apart from the augmentation of cortisol, stress entails a whole series of other hormonal changes intended to mobilise energy for fight or flight: the pancreas liberates glucagon which, together with the suppression of insulin, raises sugar levels in the blood; the thyroid hormones stimulate the metabolism. Faced with danger, in a condition of stress, there is no need to mate, reproduce or grow. At one stroke, CRH produced by the hypothalamus and the prolactin secreted by the pituitary gland also inhibit several hormones involved with libido and sexuality; ovulation is disrupted, even stopped; growth hormone production slows. The hormonal disruption is complete; the programming at the basis of the finest adjustments of the organism and the whole chemistry of the body are profoundly disturbed. In the long run, the consequences of such a disorganisation often end by being disastrous for health.

3
DISTURBING: THE DANGERS OF STRESS

THE ILLNESS UNDERLYING DISEASES

Stress – everywhere and all the time

According to a report by the American Stress Institute,[1] 75 to 90% of medical consultations are motivated by problems related to stress. In other words, numerous diseases result, at least in part, from prolonged psychological tension. This figure is sometimes considered to be an exaggeration. Nonetheless, recent development in understanding the subtle mechanisms of mind–body unity has brought some evolution in medical thinking. Slowly, but surely.

Not long ago, the idea that psychological stress could favour the development of a condition as banal as the common cold was considered bizarre. I remember a surgeon, a colleague of mine, who in 1993 mocked one of his patients because she was convinced that she had developed a cold as a result of the stress she experienced at the prospect of undergoing surgery. 'A cold is a matter of a virus. Your mental state has nothing to do with it!' he had said, raising his eyes to heaven. As I was present at this scene, I remarked to my colleague that a century earlier, Louis Pasteur had said: 'Germs are nothing, the ground is everything.' 'That may be,' he replied, 'but no one has been able to show that psychological stresses influence the "ground" on which the cold virus sets off the disease.' Wrong! In 1991, Sheldon Cohen, professor at the Carnegie Mellon University in Pittsburgh, published – in the highly respected *New England Journal of Medicine* – a trial in which he noted that, having introduced cold virus into the nostrils of several hundred volunteers, the sensitivity to the virus of the subjects tested was directly related to their experienced psychological stress.[2] In addition, Cohen found that the higher the level of stress, the more pronounced were the symptoms of cold. This was most marked in the production of mucus in the respiratory tracts.[3] An important observation was that *acute* stress did not appear to have any influence on susceptibility to the virus, while, contrariwise, *chronic* stress clearly augmented the risk of infection.[4]

This difference needs to be emphasised, since stress as such is not always negative but is sometimes actually necessary. 'No stress, no life, no progress. No tension, no creation, no evolution' I was told by a shaman in the region of Uxmal in Yucatan. We are compelled to admit that difficulties met in life prompt and stimulate us to learn new strategies to adapt and evolve. The endocrinologist Hans Selye coined two meanings for the word 'stress'. He underlined that events that are quickly resolved are *eustress* (positive), in contrast to chronic states which he defined as '*distress*' (negative), because they challenge or test our resistance and end by exhausting our resources until we fall ill.[5] Unfortunately, in modern societies, despite material progress, comfort and security, chronic stress never ceases to increase. One finds it in every area of everyday life. The reasons for this are no longer as much physical as psychological.

Why? Our obsession with progress and growth justifies all sacrifices. Imperatives to perform, obligations to compete, restriction of time and overloads of work form a fundamental rhythm of life that is effectively infernal. And this from a very early age. For example, at school, excessive programmes, an imbalance between intellectual and physical activities, as well as an elitist system of evaluation bring about a nearly permanent state of stress amongst the pupils. Abdominal cramps, eczema, otitis and recurrent colds are unlikely to be strangers to such a mode of life, since, like all chronic tensions, school-based stress disturbs the immune system. In evidence, a study carried out at the military college of Westpoint in the USA showed that amongst 200 students having had contact with the virus of mononucleosis, only 48 developed clinical signs of this condition. Detailed analysis revealed that those who succumbed to the disease were differentiated from those who remained well by one particular feature: all of them had a father who was very demanding – and therefore a source of stress – who expected brilliant success from his son.[6] Another enquiry, in a school of nursing, showed a close correlation between herpes eruptions and the period of school examinations.[7] Further, a study carried out with medical students showed that at the time of the end of year examinations they had more infectious problems associated with a diminution of the number of NK cells in the blood and a reduction of immunoglobulins IgA in the saliva.[8]

The same kind of findings have since been observed in people who have lost employment.[9] The stress created by certain severe difficulties of daily survival weakens the individual psychologically and physically. Feelings of isolation, of abandonment, doubts and uncertainties, fear of not surviving alone, are all sources of tensions deleterious to health.[10] Even in the cradle, the new-born separated from his mother begins to cry, activates his right cortical hemisphere and risks disturbing his immune defences.[11] Numerous studies indicate, incidentally, that infantile eczema can be a consequence of stress.[12] Later in life, the loss of a loved one triggers a weakening of the immune system, which perhaps explains the incidence of disease or death following shortly after bereavement or separation. A pioneering study in Australia, published in 1977 in *The Lancet*, showed that the loss of a spouse provokes a significant reduction of the activity of lymphocytes T and B.[13] Ten years later, a further study carried out on widows showed evidence of an increase in cortisol and a diminution of NK cells.[14]

Numerous studies prove that our health is conditioned by the quality of our emotional relationships. For example, Janice Kiecolt-Glaser at Ohio State University found that women whose marital relationship was satisfactory had a greater immunity than those whose relationship with their spouse was less good.[15] Furthermore, in an experiment in which married couples were asked to discuss a controversial subject, it appeared that at the time that they adopted a negative or hostile manner their immunity deteriorated significantly.[16] Sometimes, despite a harmonious relationship, the fear of losing love, the sorrow of seeing the loved one in difficulties, or having to care for him or her, can also create a chronic stress. Thus some people who are responsible for a spouse with Alzheimer's may have a raised level of cortisol and a diminished immune response on receiving influenza vaccination.[17] Similarly, men responsible for a wife suffering from dementia have levels of interleukin-6 – an inflammatory leucocyte that is raised in numerous diseases – four times higher than in a control group composed of men whose wives were in good health.[18] As we saw earlier (p. 37), the intensification and prolongation of inflammatory reactions involve serious damage to the organism. Finally, in a study of an unusual kind, Janice Kiecolt-Glaser showed that wounds made voluntarily on the skin heal more slowly in people responsible for a spouse with Alzheimer's than in others not faced with this problem.[19] It is for this reason that I never hesitate to communicate these observations to those who commit themselves to caring for a parent or a sick friend. If one is responsible for the care of another, one must not underestimate one's own fragility. It is precisely in such circumstances that it is imperative to take care of oneself.

Inflammation and depression

Taking care of yourself: Yvette had never thought of that. The eldest of six children, she had always been occupied with the care of her brothers and sisters. Then, widowed at the age of 30, she had devoted her life to the care and education of her three children. Her devotion and courage demanded admiration, but behind an apparent serenity was hidden profound psychological distress and intense physical suffering. But she never allowed that to be seen. However, since adolescence she had suffered from stomach ulcers and, not long after the death of her husband she had developed a polyarthritis which regularly confined her to bed, crippled with pain. At the time that I met her, Yvette was 58 years of age. Five months earlier her younger son had been killed in a road accident. Following her habitual pattern as 'an exemplary woman' she had gone through this ordeal without expressing any emotion. 'I must be in control. If I am not, everything will collapse,' she explained to me, her hands resting on her abdomen to show me the site of her pain. Several weeks after the death of her son, she had once again experienced abdominal cramps accompanied by violent diarrhoea. The gastro-enterologist who had been monitoring her gastric ulcers rapidly arrived at a diagnosis: Crohn's disease, an auto-immune inflammation of the intestine.

The fact seemed evident to me: that which Yvette forbade herself to express in words, the stress which she had contained for so many years, had disturbed her immune defences to the point of launching self-destructive inflammatory reactions. (This mechanism is described in Chapter 2, pp. 37–38.) In addition, despite her apparent strength of character, I suspected an underlying depressive state since chronic stress often leads to psychological depression. According to recent studies, it is this depression that leads to involvement of the auto-immune system.[20] In effect, feeling unable to face up to his problems, the individual loses courage, loses hope and sinks into despair; the absence of any positive thoughts prevents the formulation of new solutions, and, trapped in a vicious circle of negative thoughts, he sinks into a state of depression; the right cortical hemisphere is active and the hypothalamic-pituitary-adrenal axis runs at its maximum; finally, exhaustion of the supply of cortisol allows the destructive blaze of inflammation.

Yvette was troubled. The fact that I established a link between her various inflammatory problems – ulcerative gastr*itis*, rheumatoid polyarthr*itis*, and Crohn's ile*itis* – and her stresses and depression appeared strange to her. She believed she was being well taken care of by her rheumatologist and her gastro-enterologist; she had followed their treatments to the letter. If I were right, why had they not spoken of the necessity of changing her ways of being and thinking, and to consider why she was always preoccupied with her sorrows, her frustrations and her anguish? 'Simply because there is no proof that this would make any change in your physical problems,' they replied. I was obliged to contradict them.

In fact, there exists sufficient evidence incriminating psychological factors in the appearance and evolution of inflammatory diseases to justify the integration of measures designed to reduce the stress and depression suffered by these patients in their overall treatment. Thus, as early as 1965, two researchers at the University of Stanford showed a correlation between stress and the development of inflammatory symptoms within articulations. At that time, in the absence of a theoretical framework to explain these observations, the medical community regarded them with distrust and hastened to forget them.[21] Nonetheless, over 45 years later, numerous studies have confirmed the existence of a link between stress, an inflammatory disturbance and articulatory lesions. Thus it has been shown that certain cases of rheumatoid arthritis develop after a period of chronic stress or following recurrent multiple minor stresses. Further, in a good number of patients, a major life event preceded the triggering of a crisis.[22]

In the same way, it has now been shown that the appearance and evolution of inflammatory processes in the intestine – haemorrhagic recto-colitis, or Crohn's ileitis – depend on the psychological state of the patient. For example, numerous cases of ulcerative colitis appeared amongst the Bedouins following the psychological stresses resulting from changing from a nomadic life to a sedentary one.[23] Several Canadian researchers have also shown that stress triggers a relapse of recto-colitis in rats.[24]

Inflammation appears, therefore, to be an essential component of illnesses influenced by stress and by depression. Consequently, certain researchers do not hesitate to consider the presence of inflammation to be the connecting link between the body and the mind. For my part, I believe that as soon as one finds oneself about to prescribe an antiinflammatory treatment for a patient, one needs to have an automatic response of investigating his mental state, and counselling him to seek out help to relax, mentally and physically. Emotional calming and physical relaxation stimulate the reparatory processes of the parasympathetic system (the characteristics of which are described in Chapter 2, p. 35). As we shall see in the following chapters, it is probably in this way that alternative and complementary medicine probably have their major role to play.

A multifactorial process

If we wish to understand how stress and depression influence the health of the body, we need to envision illness as the result of a disequilibrium, where physical and psychological aspects are closely linked, each stimulating or influencing the other in a series of cause and effect reactions which form true vicious circles. The processes are complex and it is not easy to identify the factors which trigger them.

Taking the case of stomach ulcer (more correctly called peptic ulcer or peptic ulcer disease), this pathology has been considered for a long time to be an example of an illness linked to stress. For example, animals separated from their mother or subjected to electric shocks develop erosions of the gastric mucosa, and in humans a clear increase in the incidence of perforated ulcers is observed after a bombardment or earthquake.[25] However, in the 1980s, the discovery of a bacterium – *Helicobacter pylori* – within the ulcerative lesions brought to the fore an explanation based on infection as the origin of the disease. Antibiotic treatment was therefore advocated and showed itself effective in preventing the development of the ulcers. However, it was also observed that only 20% of those carrying this bacterium developed the pathology. The presence alone, therefore, of *H. pylori* did not offer a full explanation.[26] It was then necessary to consider a broader-based explanation. Susan Levenstein, a gastro-enterologist specialising in psychosomatic medicine, proposed that peptic ulcer disease should be considered as the physiological and behavioural result of stress. On the physiological front, the chronic stress reaction diminishes the immune defences, reduces the blood flow to the digestive mucosa, enhances the motility of the stomach, but decreases that of the duodenum, and increases secretion of acid. On the behavioural front, psychological tension provokes poor alimentary behaviour, disturbs sleep and increases the consumption of alcohol and tobacco. The total of these various changes entails a diminution of the defences of the digestive mucosa: *H. pylori* multiplies largely; an ulcer forms and, in some cases can even degenerate into cancer.[27]

A similar kind of multifactorial process is the basis of coronary illness which leads to myocardial infarction. Here too, stress engenders changes in eating habits, and consumption of alcohol and tobacco increases which, combined with hyperactivity of the sympathetic system, favours the development of inflammation of the coronary arteries and the formation of atheromatous plaques in the wall of the coronary arteries (this mechanism is described in Chapter 2, p. 37). Two psychological factors seem to be especially implicated in this process: hostility and depression. People in a state of hostility live under permanent tension, they become angry for no reason, the least opposition releases a reaction of stress and their organism is dominated by the effects of adrenaline and cortisol. As Gregory Miller, who studied the influence of hostility and depression at Washington University of St Louis in Missouri, has stated: a 'hostile' individual directs his anger at others; when he becomes depressed, he turns his resentment against himself. Depression appears, therefore, as self-directed hostility.[28] Now, we have seen that depression exacerbates inflammation; that in turn accelerates the formation of atheromatous plaques in the arterial walls, involves the rupture of existing plaques and so potentiates the phenomenon of coagulation of blood implicated in the formation of clots and thromboses. It is clear that a depressed psychological state can precipitate the occurrence of heart attacks.[29]

Several years ago I presented these theories to a small group of medical students, when one of them asked: 'If we accept that the larger part of illnesses result from a multifactorial process, that inflammation is present in most pathologies, and that psychological processes enhance the close links with the inflammatory state, cannot we conclude that the greater part of illnesses are caused or at least influenced by psychological factors?' The suggestion is audacious, but in the light of all we shall explore together is not without sense.

THE DEBATE ON CANCER

Some suspicions

At the age of 38, Christina, brilliant professor of oncology, found that she had a breast cancer. The seriousness of this diagnosis appeared to her to be relative when compared with the drama she had lived through. Six months earlier, Christina had lived through horror: nothing worse could happen to her. She had discovered her son had hung himself in the cellar of her house. She told me: 'I knew it: since the death of my son I felt that something was happening in my body. In similar circumstances, some women lose their hair. Others see their periods stop suddenly following the hormonal disturbances provoked by stress and depression. I created a cancer. I understood that simply by looking at my eyes in the mirror.'

Like Christina, many people recognise a connection to a precise event occurring not long before the illness. A study in Australia showed that 40% of women suffering from breast cancer were convinced that their disease arose from a stress:[30] the loss of a dear one, a disappointment or an unexpressed rage. Every time, the emotional shock and the psychological tension were clearly identified. Yet, although a few rare studies seemed to confirm this connection,[31] most publications concluded that, from a rigorous scientific viewpoint, there is no proof of a link between a particular stress and the appearance of a cancer. At the University of Leeds, for example, David Protheroe could find no argument in favour of a connection between breast cancer and a stressful experience during the five years preceding the appearance of the disease.[32] At the University of Harvard, a study carried out on a substantial number of nurses showed no relationship between the development of a cancer of the breast and the experience of professional stress.[33]

In addition, patients are frequently convinced that they had 'fabricated' their cancer by 'gnawing inside themselves'. Some mention having experienced recurrent depressive episodes for many years. Others speak of 'a lack of desire to live' in the course of several months before the diagnosis of cancer. This idea is not new. In the second century AD, Galen stated that melancholic women developed tumours in the breast.[34] Nevertheless, apart from a study carried out by researchers at the University of Illinois at Chicago,[35] no serious epidemiological study could confirm a direct connection between depression and cancer.[36] On the other hand, depressive symptoms appearing shortly before the discovery of the disease could be due to immune and inflammatory processes arising from the tumour; in that case, depression would not be a cause, but above all a consequence, of the cancer.

There is an inconsistency between the subjective impression of the patients and the results of epidemiological studies. Must we conclude that the connection between stress and depression on the one hand and cancer on the other results from a too fertile imagination? Does the belief in the existence of a psychological cause for cancer respond to a specific need of the human to make sense of experience? Such arguments are not to be neglected. In fact, the discovery of a cancer often provokes an acute awareness of the value of life and its finite nature. Some patients attempt to put their existence in order, and they hope to find solutions to some of the problems which interfere with living a full life. One might then think that these patients, looking back, attribute their disease to past psychological pain but that this is, in fact, mistaken.

A hypothesis

'The fact that no study has established a direct connection between stress, depression and cancer proves nothing,' Christina said to me. 'Inasmuch as I am an oncologist, I know that cancer is a multifactorial disease. It arises from numerous causes: some genetic predispositions; behaviours such as smoking tobacco and drinking alcohol; toxic substances contained in food; pollutants in the environment; and even bacteria and viruses. Why not, therefore, stress and depression as well?'

This hypothesis warrants the trouble of examination. We know that the cancerisation of one cell is produced by the effect of carcinogenic agents damaging the DNA of the cell's chromosomes. Normally, specialised enzymes make the necessary repairs. However, in the case of these failing, the build-up of lesions leads to the transformation of the cell, which begins to multiply anarchically. Fortunately, in a good number of instances, nature has provided autoprotective mechanisms: the NK cells of the immune system destroy the now cancerous cell before it has had time to multiply. The organism, therefore, possesses at least two means of preventing the development of a cancer: one is preventative – the repair of DNA – and the other is curative – the elimination of affected cells. It appears that stress and depression can interfere at both these levels.

First, at the level of prevention, several studies have shown that stress and depression compromise repair of chromosomes.[37] One such, published in 2004 in the prestigious American review *Proceedings of the National Academy of Sciences*, indicates that chronic stress provokes the shortening of the telomeres – a sort of hood protecting the ends of chromosomes – and in consequence provokes a premature ageing of the cells. The most highly stressed subjects in this study showed telomeres comparable with those of people more than ten years older.[38] These results are disturbing, since shortening of the telomeres is associated with several serious diseases, including certain cancers.[39]

Next, at the curative level, we know that negative emotions reduce the activity of the immune system's NK cells. At the University of California in San Diego, Waymond Jung and Michael Irwin showed that the diminution of the activity of the NK cells in depressive subjects was more marked in those who were smokers. Those subjects who were free of depression, *whether smokers or not*, retained normal NK functions. It is, therefore, the conjunction of smoking *and* depression that had an especially negative effect on immunity.[40] These results corroborated those of a huge epidemiological study published in 1990 which showed that depressed smokers were four times more at risk of cancer than non-depressed smokers, so that it appears that depression in the absence of smoking does not significantly increase the risk of cancer.[41]

In theory, Christina's hypothesis seems plausible: a chronic state of stress *could* involve an accumulation of errors at the level of the human genome; cells prematurely aged become more sensitive to carcinogenic factors; a cancer may appear, and in the context of weakening of the immune system because of stress or depression, the malignancy can proliferate out of control.[42]

Certainties

There is a similar scenario that may lie at the origin of certain cases where the cancer appears to declare itself especially suddenly following an emotional shock and proliferates with extreme rapidity. I remember the case of Sylvane, aged 52, in whom ultrasound examination showed a malign tumour 8cm in diameter on the right ovary. Six months earlier the same ovarian examination was completely normal. During the interval, a violent dispute with her son had shaken her severely and, progressively, a dull pain appeared in her right side.

Many researchers doubt that a cancer can form as quickly as this. Nevertheless one can imagine that the cells not as yet cancerous but already threatened by various toxic agents or a chronic stress can become malignant very suddenly through the effect of biological disturbances due to an intense stress. To be sure, this is no more than a hypothesis, but in the face of the current rise in the incidence of a number of cancers, it merits serious exploration.

In the meantime, numerous studies carried out on animals have clearly demonstrated the negative influence of stress on the evolution of cells already affected by cancer. Thus rats already carrying cancer and subjected to electric shocks that they could not escape showed a reduction in their immunity and an explosive development of the disease.[43] Similarly, in mice onto whom malign cells had been transplanted before stressing them by rotating their cage, a close correlation between the number of turns of the cage and the growth of their tumour was observed.[44]

In order to evaluate the part played by psychological causes in the process of cancerisation, it would be necessary to arrange prospective studies conducted on a large number of subjects over several decades, covering various biological factors and a precise evaluation of the degree of stress and/or depression. It would also be necessary to distinguish between the direct and indirect effects of stress and depression on the cancer, since, as we have seen in the development of peptic ulcer disease and myocardial infarctions, eating habits, alcohol intake or tobacco consumption, commonly following from psychological problems, can in themselves favour the appearance of malignancy. The problem is therefore especially complex, as Christina specified (she has since been cured): 'In practice, such prospective studies are extremely difficult, perhaps even impossible, to carry out. Certainties about the role of stress in cancer will therefore take longer.'

REFUSING INEVITABILITY

Conditioned to fight

Time: we need it to note facts, sharpen our curiosity, ask questions, find answers and make progress. The story of Meyer Friedman and Ray Rosenman is a perfect example. During the 1950s these two cardiologists shared a practice in San Francisco. At that time, the incidence of cardiac problems was growing in the population. In common with many of their colleagues they sought reasons for this 'epidemic'. One detail, apparently innocuous, brought them an answer. They had noticed that the chairs in their waiting room were unusually worn, not on the seats as such but on the front edges of the seats and the ends of the armrests. Surprised by this curious observation, they decided to observe how the patients sat, and to their considerable surprise they noted that the patients never relaxed. On the contrary: they remained constantly alert, ready to get up, impatient to see their turn come, regularly asking the secretary how much longer they had to wait. Friedman and Rosenman identified this kind of behaviour as one of the factors favouring the development of cardiac problems. Aggressive and impatient, the personalities at risk they called 'Type A', in contrast to the characteristics of 'Type B' – much less stressed.[45] When this theory was publicised, it met with great scepticism in the medical world. Ray Rosenman mused: 'Perhaps it is because many physicians, especially many cardiologists themselves, have a very marked "Type A" profile....'[46] Who knows? In any case, we have seen this confirmed, and today there is no doubt: the hostility of 'Type A' is damaging, not only for their coronaries, but their whole organism.

'I can easily recognise the dangers; it is not easy to escape "bad reflexes",' said a patient who had just survived his third myocardial infarction. 'It is as though I have been habituated to react aggressively, that the brain is programmed to do so.' It is very difficult for a hostile personality to avoid falling into the trap of his hyper-reactivity because the slightest annoyance triggers an exaggerated 'stress response': adrenaline is secreted in enormous quantities and the hypothalamic-pituitary-adrenal axis produces an excessive amount of cortisol. Animal studies show that sometimes the origins of this hypersensitivity to stress develop before birth.[47] At the University of Lille, France, Stefania Maccari demonstrated that rats born to mothers who had been stressed during pregnancy had a distinctly raised level of anxiety. At the slightest stress, their cortisol level rose very rapidly and remained abnormally high for a long time.[48] It seems that mothering lavished by the mother after parturition does reduce the damage caused by the antenatal stress.[49] Nonetheless, once arrived at adult age, certain rats continued to manifest abnormal anxiety, memory defects, broken sleep, a propensity to consume drugs, changes in their feeding behaviour and exaggerated weight gain.[50]

It is very probable that the same phenomenon of pre-natal imprinting occurs in humans. Numerous recent studies also indicate that certain emotional and behavioural problems in children reflect the emotional state of the mother during pregnancy.[51] Similarly at the university of Utrecht in Holland, Jan Buitelaar and Anja Huizink showed that the stress experienced by the mother during her pregnancy had compromised the psychological and motor development of the infant when examined at the age of eight months.[52] Further, at the University of California at Irvine, Elysia Poggi Davis noted that antenatal stress negatively influenced the adaptation of unweaned babies to novelty or change.[53] Finally, according to a team of researchers at the University of Aarhus, in Denmark, there is reason to think that antenatal stress plays a part in attention-deficit hyperactivity disorders, conditions that are now increasingly found in children.[54]

'Studies of this kind seem to wish to lay the responsibility for behavioural problems in children at the doors of their mothers,' said one young woman, as she was struggling with the immoderate agressivity of her two children. I doubt that this was the intention of the researchers. However, we cannot but suspect that the conditions of stress in which numerous women live during pregnancy may not be ideal for the future of their children. One must therefore hope that the current studies will help to raise awareness of the consequences of the conditions of life that we impose on ourselves. This will, perhaps, induce us to find other ways of living: gentler and less stressful.

Perhaps it is not too late

'It is probably impossible to change a "Type A" personality completely but is it always possible to learn, with benefit, the behavioural patterns of "Type B",' said Meyer Friedman, and frequently added to his patients: 'Sweetness is not weakness.' He himself, a perfect example of a 'Type A' character, had a first cardiac alert at the age of 45, and two myocardial infarctions at 55. He then decided to follow the advice he gave to others: he stopped criticising his wife and avoided lecturing his children, interesting himself in what he called 'the three Ps' (pets, plants, people) and in order to learn to calm his own impatience, read in three sessions the seven volumes of Proust's novel, *À la recherche du temps perdu*. Subsequently, he lived in perfect health to the age of 90.

So we can hope. Imbalance leading to illness is not always irreversible, even if sometimes its origin lies before birth. Thus, in 2004, researchers at the University of Toronto, Canada, published a study in which they showed that the reduction in the numbers of root cells in the brain caused by antenatal stress in hamsters is reversible after birth, if the young received attentive care from the mother.[55] The phenomenon of 'neuroplasticity' was unknown only a few years ago. When I was a medical student, we learned that the brain was a 'frozen organ' incapable of regeneration or reorganisation. Today we know that the opposite is true. A hundred billion neurones, ten thousand connections per neurone carrying electrical messages at a vertiginous speed of 300 km an hour: the immense brain network is the seat of constant restructuring. New cells appear; certain little-used connections tend to disappear; while others, more used, are reinforced; neuronal circuits are activated or de-activated according to need.

This huge plasticity of the brain is the basis of conditioning, memory and learning.[56] We therefore understand that, if one experience leaves an engram in the nervous system, we are not condemned to remain in that furrow. Our behaviour can be re-educated and our brain re-modelled. Some pitfalls in our past can be cancelled – to the greatest benefit of our health.

4
REASSURING: THE POWER OF THE MIND

WHEN PSYCHOLOGY BECOMES POSITIVE

Martin Seligman was born a pessimist. That may well be why he passed his life in defending the virtue of optimism.[1] Professor of Psychology at the University of Pennsylvania, this man, with his face rounded by good humour, became head of a new line of thought in psychology. For him, 'to be a psychologist is more than treating mental illnesses: it is also, and perhaps first of all, to help people to bring out the best in themselves'.

Throughout a long period, psychology interested itself solely in negative emotions. Depressions and psychoses were highlighted, but we knew nearly nothing about happiness. However, recent discoveries in psycho-neuro-immunology have clearly demonstrated the beneficial effects of positive emotions on health. Therapists have become increasingly convinced that an optimistic attitude to living is the most powerful and the cheapest medicine that humanity has ever had at its disposal.

What 'positive psychology' is currently discovering is something that Buddhism had known for ages past. This philosophy, in developing a true 'internal science',[2] advocated the transformation of five emotional poisons into five wisdoms essential to the achievement of happiness. Regular exercises enable the transformation of pride into humility, greed into detachment, jealousy into joy at what has happened to others, anger into patience and tolerance, ignorance into knowledge of the true nature of mind.

'There is nothing good or bad but thinking make it so,' wrote Shakespeare. In themselves, events are neutral. It is we who attribute feeling to them, and whatever we may think, we always have the choice between 'a glass half-full', and 'a glass half-empty'. Our interpretation of reality influences what we feel, and what we feel shapes our reality.

These essential principles make up the secret of the capacity for extraordinary resilience shown by some humans. Confronted by the worst situations, overwhelmed by the most terrible suffering, they survive. Better still, they *live*. Richard Davidson showed how women who had succeeded in surmounting traumatic experiences are capable of moderating their negative emotions when their painful memories are evoked. It seems as though the part of the cerebral cortex linked to positive emotions is capable of inhibiting the amygdala of the limbic system. At once, fear and distress are calmed, the hypothalamus does not initiate its hormonal chain reaction, and the blood level of cortisol remains normal.[3] All this happens as though these women had trained their brains to produce positive reactions. The pessimistic thoughts are swept away by optimistic ideas; they choose hope rather than discouragement. Inevitably, this attitude influences every cell in their bodies. The dominant activity of their left cerebral hemisphere arouses the best immune defences, and, protected from depressive mood, they escape the procession of inflammatory disturbances that are toxic to the organism.

Educating the brain to 'positivity' seems to be a priority. Research on neuroplasticity shows this is possible (see Chapter 3, p. 51).

The choice of happiness

Every ten years the American Psychological Association sets a theme that reflects the interests of their researchers. The decade 1990 to 2000 was devoted to the brain, while that of 2000 to 2010 concerns behaviour and positive psychology. This choice could suggest a somewhat utopian ideology aiming at research into happiness at any price. I see in it a necessary reaction to the growing importance of health problems arising from stress, all the more since numerous researchers agree in saying that the ravages caused by negative emotions are still under-estimated.

'Positive psychology' invites us to consider the fact that we have more power over our lives than we think. Its target is to help in the transformation of problems into a source of creativity and health. In working as a therapist, it is necessary to learn to identify the conditioning, the beliefs and the ideas that impede thinking in a positive way. This approach is not always simple because inherited ways of thinking are deeply imprinted on our minds. A great deal of humility and persistence are necessary to efface these negative habits.

The background discussed thus far suggests one piece of evidence: negativity hides fear, and the fear prevents us from actualising our deepest desires. In my consultations, I hear people say that they will never realise their dreams, that there is no solution to this or that difficulty, that in every way no one is interested in them. They are full of the fear of not meeting the standards of others, of not living fully, of not deserving the love of others. Through the power of the pessimistic voice within them, their predictions come to fulfilment: they live this side of their potentialities, they do not have what they desire, and they feel themselves to be alone. Thus the negative thoughts that assail us greatly increase the risk of sinking into depression. Pessimism is a dangerous poison.

Another pioneer of positive psychology, the American psychologist Mihaly Csikszentmihalyi thinks that pessimism is an attitude that prepares one to defend oneself more effectively: envisaging the worst allows the exploitation of unexplored resources. At the same time, one must avoid responding to pessimism with pessimism because the negative expectation sets up a stress which gets in the way of inventing effective solutions to the growing problems ahead. Now, pessimism is contagious. This is the reason that Cardinal Mazarin, in the 17th century, asked anyone who sought to enter his service if he considered he had real chance in the world. Positive emotions stimulate creativity. As a sensible statesman, Mazarin knew that to surround oneself with optimists created the enthusiasm needed for success.

Mihaly Csikszentmihalyi describes very well why it is a good thing to choose a precise objective to motivate one's actions. The tide of our experience leads us then towards a realisation of this aim and gives us a sense of well-being which leads us then towards success.[4] All the same, we must not forget an important detail: the secret of happiness depends upon our choosing reasonable targets. We must, therefore, recognise our limitations; not want too much too quickly; take account of the constraints of the environment and to choose priorities that respect our essential needs. To chase the unattainable creates too much stress. Frustration brings discouragement and the loss of hope will plunge us into depression.

A good way of escaping from this descent into hell is to learn to cultivate positive thoughts. This was shown by a study carried out by Barbara Fredrickson. Some students were questioned about their attitude to life. Those who had positive thoughts at the time of the first interview showed them even more strongly at the following session. Their willingness to develop, their wish to meet others, and their desire to create new projects were asserted more strongly at each interview.[5] To think positively starts a real ascending spiral of achievement, satisfaction and happiness. Solutions to problems emerge more quickly, self-confidence is established more deeply, it is easier to be open with others, and they, in return, make one's life easier. The positive attracts the positive. We all know this even if we do not always find the means of creating this ideal reality.

Martin Seligman insists that we should inculcate these principles in children from the youngest age onwards. Even if we cannot necessarily control events, the way we choose to react influences the conditions of our existence. Everything depends upon the meaning we give to facts. For example, the way in which others behave towards us is not very important: it is the way in which we react in the light of their attitude which counts. What we feel *is* under our control, and at every moment in life we can escape becoming a victim of stress. This is greatly comforting. Even so, we have to learn to balance our two cerebral hemispheres emotionally.

Laughter

A legend of the Apache tribe relates how, having equipped the human being with a whole series of qualities, the Creator frowned, sat down on a rock and put his head in his hands. His creation could talk, run, see, hear... and yet it lacked an essential quality. The human being must be able to laugh! Immediately, both men and women began to fall about laughing. They laughed from the bottom of their hearts for a long moment. Then the Creator smiled: he was satisfied. He got up and saluted the men and women who were wiping away the tears of joy. 'Now you are ready to live,' he said as he left.

As children we laugh more than 400 times a day for sheer pleasure, without reason. Once adult, we laugh no more than perhaps 20 times in the course of a day. This is a shame, because in arousing positive feelings, laughter exerts a very helpful influence on health. Even more, a sense of humour makes us more attractive in the eyes of others. Standing back and detaching ourselves makes us less aggressive. Hence we are more easily integrated into the community, and this also helps to maintain good health.

Laughter entered the medical scene in 1976 when the very serious *New England Journal of Medicine* published a statement by Norman Cousins, a journalist, who claimed that he had been cured of a serious rheumatic disorder (ankylosing spondylitis) without the help of conventional medicine.[6] Paralysed and condemned by his doctors to finish his days on a hospital bed, Cousins decided to cure himself by ingesting strong doses of Vitamin C and watching comic films. Six months later he recovered the use of his limbs and could take up his profession again full-time. Subsequently, Cousins devoted himself to the study of the connections between the psyche and immunity and he taught in the faculty of medicine at the University of California, Los Angeles.

At the Center of Neuro-Immunology at Loma Linda University in California, Lee Berk and David Felten, the man who had demonstrated the sympathetic innervation of the organs of the immune system (see Chapter 2, p. 25), ran a series of studies on the effects of laughter. These were carried out first on subjects in good health: watching a humorous film resulted in an increase of IgA in the saliva, an increase in the NK cells and a whole group of immune defences, the effects of which lasted at least 12 hours.[7] Then the programme was moved to cardiac patients who watched humorous films in the course of the year following a myocardial infarction. The results spoke volumes: 30 minutes of comic film twice a day significantly reduced the risk of further myocardial infarctions compared with a control group. Arterial tension remained lower, disturbances of cardiac rhythm were less frequent and need for medication was reduced.[8]

A study in the *Journal of the American Medical Association* showed that patients who were allergic to dust and to spiders developed less acute skin reactions to the allergens when they had watched an amusing film.[9]

So around much of the world, humour is beginning to be seen as an effective remedy. Troops of clowns are invited into hospitals. In Japan, for instance, this method is used to reduce the pains of patients suffering from rheumatoid arthritis.[10] In India, Dr Madan Kataria teaches 'the yoga of laughter'; since he launched this approach in 1995, more than 2,000 'laughter clubs' have been set up around the world. Thousands of people come to learn the exercises that release hilarity. Madan Kataria is convinced that the positive attitude created by laughter, as well as improving health, works towards creating harmony and peace in the world.

IN SEARCH OF MEANING

Writing

At the time that I set out on the journey which leads to self-knowledge, I set myself quite spontaneously to writing as though I had been called to it. Every day, I opened my diary to confide to it what I had experienced. Each time that I closed it again, I was satisfied. My ideas became clearer, and the meaning of the events of my life seemed changed. Convinced as I became of the benefits of such writing, I recommended this practice to the people around me. I was unaware of the fact that I was prescribing a remedy the power of which had already been tested in the laboratory.

A study carried out at the University of Texas, had shown that the students who wrote regularly about any difficult events in their lives were better humoured and fell ill less often.[11] 'Emotional writing' seems to reinforce immunity. An experiment to confirm this was carried out with a group of medical students. Over four days, certain students poured out their inner thoughts on paper; the others wrote about neutral subjects. On the fifth day, all the students were vaccinated against hepatitis B. A blood sample was then taken to measure the immune response to the vaccine. The results were conclusive in that the students who had written about their emotional experiences showed a significantly greater production of antibodies compared with the others.[12]

The same kind of study was proposed to asthmatic patients and to others suffering from chronic painful and incapacitating rheumatism. In the course of three days, they were required to spend 20 minutes to describe in writing the details of events that they found stressful. Published in 1999 in *The Journal of the American Medical Association*, the results showed a biological improvement that was statistically significant and which remained present four months later. David Spiegel, professor of psychiatry at Stanford, signed the summary of the study and concluded that if such results had been obtained through medication produced by the pharmaceutical industry, the impact from the media would have been massive and the molecule would have been prescribed on a large scale.[13] Obviously, 'emotional writing' is not a commercial proposition: the solution seems too easy. All the same, it works.

Some studies carried out on patients after a major stress (Post Traumatic Stress Disorder) showed that the memory of traumatising experiences activates those parts of the brain serving sight and emotion, while those serving language and expression seemed to be de-activated. Written expression seems to restore the connections between these different zones. Putting words to the image of a painful experience permits its reinterpretation in the present. The perspective changes, and positive meaning may be given to the disturbing feelings. Certainly this could be the function performed by myths and legends: the moral of the story rephrases the experiences of those who no longer understand the meaning of their life and who feel 'demoralised'. It is not at all surprising that since the earliest times, diviners, clairvoyants, astrologers and other 'creators of meaning' are consulted by members of all kinds of societies – priests, kings and presidents included – whether nomadic or settled, agricultural or industrial.

Keeping a diary becomes part of the steps taken towards the creation of meaning. The depth of what one may reach by this activity depends upon the honesty and regularity that one brings to it. There are patients to whom I recommend that they devote themselves to this approach who reply that they do not have the time available. This is exactly the present that I propose that they give themselves: three minutes a day, solely for themselves; a few moments of intimacy with oneself. This would certainly be worth as much as all the life assurances for which we work without taking the time to live – a few lines on paper to help our brain recycle our stress. It is the unity of our body and our mind which benefit from it.

Hoping

'To have hope is not to say that we think all will be well. It simply means that we think that things will have a meaning,' wrote Vaclav Havel. This meaning – it is we who give it to events. Positive or negative, it influences our thoughts and thus the whole of our body. This means that whatever faith within the human spirit fulfils an obvious biological function. In giving meaning to terrifying events in their environment, our ancestors were able to calm their fears and free themselves to create solutions to the difficulties of their existence. The evolutionary advantage of faith and hope then explains why we find systems of such beliefs in all cultures, and in all periods of human history.

In order to exert its calming power, faith needs to be blind: there is no room for doubt. *What* we believe is not very important as long as we truly believe it. It is this which stands out from a study conducted by Caryle Hirshberg and Mark Ian Barasch.[14] Having analysed cases of spontaneous recoveries in the medical literature, they showed the importance of a solid faith in the system of healing chosen by the patients.

Hope helps to live. In the early 1980s, two studies published in *Science* demonstrated this: rats carrying a cancerous tumour and given electric shocks did not survive unless they could avoid shocks by pressing a lever. Deprived of that possibility, the animals became discouraged, their immune defences sank and the cancer propagated itself virulently.[15] Hope is at the heart of healing. To bring it to life within oneself it is necessary to imagine a favourable outcome or a target full of meaning and, in anticipation, to feel the joy that would accompany its achievement. At the level of the brain, this perspective activates the circuits rich in dopamine implicated in motivation and reward. From that moment, mood improves. Once the sufferer begins to hope, his left cortex develops positive thoughts which inhibit the feelings of fear produced by the limbic amygdala. Immediately, the cascade of stress is interrupted and the endorphins – hormones reducing pain and favouring positive thoughts – are secreted into the blood stream. The body relaxes automatically and pain is reduced. In return, the brain is informed of this improvement, emotions again become more positive and the left cortex continues to feel hope. This reinforces the inhibition of the amygdala, the secretion of endorphins continues, pain is further reduced and the information reaching the brain remains positive. As a result, the immune defences function optimally, the reparatory processes are activated and healing begins.

On the other hand, let us imagine that the patient continues to suffer. The continuing pain signals arriving in the brain create negative thoughts. The left cerebral cortex has difficulty in maintaining its good mood. Sooner or later, the right cerebral hemisphere gains the upper hand, discouragement begins, the amygdalae are stimulated and the stress cascade begins. If this gets out of control, the sufferer plunges into depression, inflammatory reactions become excessive and his state of health deteriorates rapidly.

To explain, encourage, ease pain and emphasise the first signs of improvement of an illness are therefore highly therapeutic acts. Unfortunately, this aspect of the art of healing is often neglected; in most medical schools it is even ignored.

The rage to live

At the time I met John, he was 50 years old. Eight years earlier, a blood test had shown the unthinkable: he was HIV-positive. When he was told this, he was plunged into a profound depression. Then, little by little he had recovered his taste for living – just up to the date when his best friend was killed in a road accident. 'That was not fair,' he told me. 'I should have gone. He was so young and so talented.' Over the following month, John lost four kilos. He looked grey and his eyes were sad. I became worried. 'Everything is alright, I just want to die,' he replied in an ironical tone. The following day, dark blotches appeared on his legs. The dermatologist at the hospital confirmed my fears: it was a Kaposi's sarcoma, a cutaneous cancer which supervenes in patients whose immunity is weakened. In just a few days, John went from the sero-positive state to the full state of AIDS. Immediate medical treatment was needed.

Two weeks later, John telephoned me. His condition had deteriorated; he could not tolerate the medication prescribed and he did not want to continue with the treatment. 'What do you think, Doctor?' he asked me, his voice full of anxiety. I replied that I did not know. The medicines certainly had some value, but I could not imagine what would make him take them. It was not *I* who was the patient. It was *he* who had to feel and decide what would be right for him. Irritated, he said that he wanted advice. I repeated that I was sorry, but I could not advise him. My reply angered him.

And that was what I wanted. In my experience of therapy, I had learned that anger is a very powerful force, the same as the *élan vital*, our 'rage to survive'. Surprised by the power of the anger that shook him, John decided to use that energy to get moving. He took up sport, consulted an acupuncturist and took a massage every two days. To his own stupefaction, he even recovered his wish for a sex life: 'And this time in broad daylight!' he told me firmly.

When he was seen at the hospital, his doctor was impressed by the improvement in his general condition. John explained his recipe: no more medicines, just exercise, acupuncture and massage. The physician raised his eyes to heaven and replied that this course could produce a transitory improvement but in no case a cure. If John did not start again to take his medicines, his chances of survival were very slender, his remaining time being counted in days or at most in months.

As soon as the consultation was over, John telephoned me. He was distraught: on the one hand, he felt better, almost as well as before he fell ill, but on the other, his doctor had told him he would die. I reassured him by saying one should believe only what one sees – and for now, we had to admit that his regime worked better than the medicaments prescribed by his doctor. All the same, John was in doubt. What if the specialist in infectious diseases knew better than he himself what would be good for him? What if his apparent improvement was only an illusion? Frustrated, John decided to take his medicines again. His appetite declined, his strength left him, he stopped his sport and he could not find the energy to go to see his acupuncturist.

Ten days later I found him in deep depression. Again he asked me what I thought, and again I said that I could not put myself in his place. I told him that I thought his doctor was afraid of giving him false hope, and that he had to mistrust those who cast spells. I told him a number of stories of voodoo witch-doctors (see Chapter 1, p. 13).

John reacted instantly. 'That's right,' he said, 'I am the only one who can know. I have no wish to let myself be condemned to death by this doctor. He should bring proof for what he says. After all, it's my life. *I* shall decide.' Once again, this experience confirmed me in my belief that an essential element in healing is the anger of the patient. Not the destructive anger which takes on the whole world, nor the suppressed revolt which ends by exhausting him who cannot express it openly, but the strength to assert what one wants and to mobilise the energy to accomplish it. I therefore found John's attitude very reassuring. Because how can one imagine that a patient could mobilise all his strength to fight against that outside enemy called 'AIDS', if he allows himself to be put down by the catastrophic prophesies of a High Priest of modern medicine? How can one survive without hope?

John decided a second time to abandon the medicines and he took up sport, acupuncture and massage again. 'I enjoy this,' he said jubilantly. Today, three years later, John is still alive. He takes no medication.

I always hesitate to tell the story of John because it would be dangerous to draw hasty conclusions. In fact, every case is unique. I would never allow myself to advise a patient to stop taking medicines: that would be dangerous. On the other hand, I always try hard to hear what he is trying to tell me: that which he does not dare admit to himself – because to me it is essential to help the other to reach autonomy. To do so demands that I inform, discuss, but never impose. Who has the right to impose? What certainty do we really have? How much do we know about the pitfalls in our beliefs, be they scientific, philosophic or religious?

John clearly wanted to resume control of his life, and his illness was an opportunity for doing so. Until then he had never accepted his homosexuality: he had lived his life hidden, in shame. He had no self-love, he wanted to be someone else.

Steven Cole, researcher in the haemato-oncology department at the University of California at Los Angeles, has followed some homosexual men for five years in order to observe the development of their health. His studies showed that the subjects who hid their homosexuality developed three times as many cancers and infections as those who had fully accepted their sexual identity.[16] Accepting what we are seems therefore to be an essential element for maintaining good health. In another study, Cole showed that those homosexual patients who were infected with the HIV virus did less well if they felt shame at the fact of their sexual orientation.[17] John's development of AIDS caused him to understand his lack of self-esteem. As long as he thought of himself as a victim of the illness, he was incapable of responding to his real needs, so handed over his power to others – the human immunodeficiency virus, his doctor, fate. His immune system was thus inhibited. He felt himself to be disempowered. As soon as he grasped his essential desire to live life to the full, without shame, he dared to assert the truth about himself. Then he felt the lust to live, and automatically his morale and his physical state improved. His psyche and his immune system no longer submitted to *de*pression. He had decided on the *ex*pression of his self-determination.

Some time later, I had a visit from Lawrence, a friend of John's, also infected with HIV. Lawrence wished to experience the same 'miracle' as John. He wished to stop his medical treatment but his doctor had quoted some disturbing statistics, and he asked my advice. Instead of replying I questioned Lawrence about what he felt. 'Fear,' he replied, biting his lips. I assured him that I would equally feel afraid in his place – but I was not in his place. I then mentioned a third study published by Steven Cole.[18] It showed that patients infected with HIV and treated with a tritherapy continued less well if they lived under stress. The results were significant in that blood samples from those patients who were able to free themselves from stress were four times less infected by the virus. The study concluded that the tritherapy was more effective in people who were unstressed. As soon as I had finished commenting on these studies, Lawrence got up and gave me his hand. 'Thank you,' he said, his eyes bright with emotion. 'I have understood: the target is to live without strain, without shame, without anguish, without fear. I am not ready to give up my medicines – I am too frightened. I will continue the treatment but now I will think of them as a positive help – it might make them easier to bear. And then I will try to stop being eaten up with my fears. I will seek pleasure above all. It must be the best way to help myself.'

John, Lawrence and other patients whom I have had the privilege to know have taught me a wonderful thing: there are no two identical human beings. Each one has to be treated uniquely. We must take account of the beliefs, conscious and unconscious, of each one. Therefore we must stop thinking of people as parameters in a statistical equation. On the contrary: we must listen to their desires and hopes.

A psychotherapy?

In 1989, David Spiegel published the results of a study carried out in the Department of Psychiatry at the University of Stanford, in *The Lancet*. In the course of one year, some women with breast cancer that had metastasised had taken part in weekly discussion groups, as well as receiving sessions of hypnosis for reducing pain. In a quite spectacular way these women had survived 18 months longer than those who had not had psychological help.[19] Several years later, at the University of California at Los Angeles, the psychiatrist Fawzy Fawzy obtained similar results. The purpose of his study was to measure the effects of setting up psychological help as soon as possible after a diagnosis of cancer of the skin (malignant melanoma). For six weeks, the patients followed a programme of health education: they learned to relax, and they were given psychological and social help. Compared with a control group, the patients given psychological help had more, and more active, NK cells. Six years later, the relapse rate was lower and they had survived in greater numbers.[20]

The possibility that a psychological process could improve the survival of patients with cancer shook the medical community. It stimulated other clinicians to attempt the same kind of experiment, but often with less success. Finally, in 2000, Pamela Goodwin, oncologist at the University of Toronto, repeated the study carried out by Spiegel in women with metastasised breast cancer. Here the results showed no prolongation of survival following group therapy. All the same, the women who had taken part reported an overall improvement in their morale, and, compared with a control group, complained less of pain.[21]

The question of an eventual benefit from psychological intervention on the survival of cancer patients is not yet answered. Further work must be attempted to answer it. Meanwhile, as we saw in Chapter 3, there are good reasons to believe that being given psychological care can exert a helpful effect on the development of certain cancers or other diseases. In addition, it is possible that the reduction of psychological tensions increases the efficacy of certain treatments. Further, it has been shown that in mice the action of anti-tumour drugs is reduced if the animal is stressed by rotation of its cage.[22]

Amongst the secondary effects of chemotherapy, an excessive diminution of white blood cells sometimes requires the interruption of treatment. In some cases it is even necessary to have recourse to mitogenic substances that can stimulate the proliferation of the deficient cells. Thus Barbara Andersen, professor of psychology at Ohio State University, showed that among stressed patients the proliferation of white blood cells in response to these mitogenic substances was less good.[23] In a study published in 2004, she attempted to examine the influence of psychological care on the response to mitogenes in 200 women who had been operated on for breast cancer. Half the patients, selected by drawing lots, received psychological support in small groups once a week over four months. Compared with the women who did not receive this support, the patients spoke of an overall reduction of anxiety, an improvement in their personal relationships and their eating habits, as well as a reduction in their use of tobacco. When blood tests looking at the response to the mitogenes were carried out, the production of white blood cells showed itself as stable or raised in the patients receiving support, while it was reduced in the others.[24] These results demonstrated that by reducing stress, psychological support could help to prevent too great a drop in the white blood cells during chemotherapy.

Barbara Andersen's study also confirmed the benefits of psychotherapy for the quality of life of these patients. The diagnosis of a serious illness is always a source of stress and anxiety. This is enough to justify provision of psychotherapy. Further, those patients who received psychological support often accepted the constraints of the treatments more readily and used a better general hygiene. These factors themselves could exert a favourable influence on the course of the disease.[25]

One may ask what kind of psychotherapy to choose. There seem to be more than 400 different kinds of psychotherapy. Many studies have been carried out to try to decide if any one or other of these approaches is better in any way. The results are negative: any one therapy seems as good as any other.[26] An experiment carried out with psychologically disturbed students indicated that it is the relationship between the therapist and the patient that determines the efficacy of the sessions. Some students were given the care of experienced therapists while others were seen by teachers with charisma and empathy. A third group left to themselves, served as a control. After 25 hours of sessions, the students in the two groups who had been listened to felt much better than those in the control group. Meanwhile there was little difference between the students who had been seen by a psychotherapist and those who had met a teacher.[27]

Hans Strupp, former professor of psychology at Vanderbilt University and the author of the study we have just considered, states that every psychotherapeutic approach rests on a theoretical model – working within an interpersonal context characterised by empathic listening allowing an understanding of the meaning of emotions, desires and fantasies – and reaches a reformulation and reinterpretation of this meaning.

In fact, all psychotherapies set up a relationship of help, a well-defined healing framework, and follow a particular ritual.[28] Here we are not far removed from the systems of shamans and sorcerers. As Claude Lévi-Strauss remarked, in those two situations the experience of the patient is interpreted through symbols full of meaning. In psychotherapy, the patient constructs a mythology from elements of his past. In shamanistic practices the myth comes from outside in accordance with the culture of the patient.[29] Psychotherapy and shamanism are therefore 'medicines of meaning'. Attributing meaning permits the recovery of morale in a demoralised patient. The transformation that follows sets off a whole series of therapeutic results linked to the emergence of positive emotions. Psychotherapy and shamanism base themselves on the placebo effect. That is probably why it is so difficult to study them 'scientifically'.

CALMING THE BRAIN TO RELAX THE BODY

The reflex of tranquillity

Find a peaceful place, make yourself comfortable, close your eyes and relax your muscles one by one, from your feet to your head. Breathe through your nose and with each out-breath repeat in your head an expression or a word that feels positive to you. Concentrate, so that you do not fall asleep. Stay in a passive posture, without reacting to the emotions that invade your body, without allowing room to the thoughts that arise in your mind. Breathe through your nose and breathe out while repeating the positive phrase or word. Over a few minutes your body will relax progressively, the rhythm of your breathing eases, the consumption of oxygen lessens, the heartbeat slows, blood pressure reduces, muscular tension diminishes, and the brain, set between waking and sleeping, develops the alpha rhythm. Relaxation is deep. The feeling of well-being deepens.

In an article published in *The Lancet* in 1975, Herbert Benson suggests that this exercise should be practised for ten to 20 minutes twice a day, every day. The intention is to activate the autonomic parasympathetic nervous system and thereby promote the development of a whole series of reparatory processes. With a little practice, this 'relaxation response', as Benson called it, becomes progressively easier to obtain and its effects become more and more lasting. A true 'reflex of tranquillity' is established. When stress invades our thoughts and tenses our body, this reflex is sufficient to relax us.[30]

In fact, Herbert Benson did not invent this. He has simply validated scientifically a practice thousands of years old which all the spiritual traditions of humanity knew to be beneficial for the peace of the body, the soul – which we could also call the emotions – and the mind. In developing this approach in the course of his research into hypertension at the University of Harvard, Benson demonstrated the beneficial influence of relaxation in numerous physical ailments, from the pains of the premenstrual syndrome, to the ischaemia of the cardiac muscle, passing through migraine, infertility and anxiety.[31] And, as we could have expected, numerous studies have established that in stimulating the parasympathetic system, relaxation stimulates the immune system.[32]

A state of mind

The 'relaxation response' advocated by Benson is the opposite to the stress reaction 'flight or fight' described by Hans Selye or Walter Cannon, much as peace is the opposite of war – peace for which tools must be made. One of the most effective tools for this is meditation.

There are many ways of meditating; every spiritual approach recommends its own. Nevertheless, whether practised in the silence of a monastery, or more simply in the course of the ordinary activities of everyday life, all techniques share the development of vigilance without reaction. One can then meditate 'with full attention' in concentrating first of all on breathing, then on bodily sensations, emotions and thoughts. This practice of mindfulness, already taught 2,500 years ago in *Theravada* Buddhism, is arousing increasing interest, paralleling the rapid growth of Buddhist teaching in the West.

One may also meditate 'with concentration' by choosing to focus one's thoughts exclusively on an object, a mental image, a mantra – a word or sacred syllable to which is attributed a spiritual power in Hinduism and Buddhism – or a physical sensation. Transcendental Meditation, named so by the Maharishi Mahesh Yogi, who imported it into the United States from India at the beginning of the 1960s, is very close to the exercises proposed by Benson. It is also recommended to be practised for 20 minutes twice a day. Today more than 6 million people practise transcendental meditation around the globe. A network of registered teachers has been organised and one finds adepts of the technique of every age within every religion.

Meditation is a state of mind. It consists in creating an altered state of consciousness, a kind of autoregulation of attention. As in the 'relaxation response' obtained by Benson, it is designed to ensure that the meditator does not *react* to whatever may arise in his mind while remaining fully alert and concentrated. This attitude or state fosters the development of full self-awareness, of one's full presence in the present moment, in-breath after out-breath, moment after moment. Relaxation and physical fluidity accompany a change in the brain's electrical activity, which adopts the alpha rhythm characteristic of intermediate states between waking and sleeping. This change in the activity of the brain promotes a more favourable setting for creativity, and a kind of trance state follows in which re-interpretation and reprogramming are easier to achieve.

Numerous schools of meditation recommend the use of a mantra to shield the mind from disturbance. A study published in the *British Medical Journal* in 2001 by Italian, English and Portuguese cardiologists described how the rhythms of the yoga mantra 'om-mani-padme-om' and those of the rosary 'Ave Maria' recited in Latin, are very similar, and produce the same beneficial effects on arterial pressure and the blood flow in the brain. Reciting mantras is therefore shown to be as much a health-promoting activity as a religious one, and it was probably not by chance that this kind of practice has endured through thousands of years.[33] Even Benson, in his endeavours to medicalise this practice, has kept the repetition of a phrase, a word or a positive sound, at the time of relaxation exercises.

A growing number of benefits from meditation have by now been documented: reduction of stress, facilitation of reinterpretation of stressful events, improvement of mood. Amongst depressed patients, meditation has been shown to be as effective, or even more so, than antidepressants.[34] Once established, the effects last a long time and reduce the number of relapses.[35]

A study carried out with people suffering from hypertension who had used meditation over six months, demonstrated a reduction of the thickness of the carotid artery walls, suggesting a regression of the atherosclerosis secondary to the reduction of stress stimulated by the practice of meditation.[36] Reduction of hypertension, improvement in the level of blood cholesterol, reduction of obesity, better recovery after a myocardial infarction; at a time when the costs of the health services have rocketed, the education of the public in meditation could have a considerable impact on the development of public health.

At the Medical College of Georgia, in Augusta, the effects of transcendental meditation were analysed in 50 obese and hypertensive adolescents. Over four months, 15 minutes twice a day, these adolescents had meditated to the sound of a calming mantra. Published in 2004, the results showed an overall diminution of arterial pressure in comparison with a control group who had not practised meditation. When one realises the importance of the risk to these adolescents of developing a cardiovascular disease, we can see the positive influence meditation could have on their future.[37]

Meditate to shape the brain

Richard Davidson at the University of Wisconsin evaluated the effects of meditation in the context of his research on cerebral hemispheres and the immune response (see Chapter 2, p. 34). He asked the employees of a business to practise meditation regularly for two months. At the end of this period, an electroencephalogram (EEG) showed a significant increase in the activity of the anterior part of the left hemisphere, associated, as we have seen, with positive emotions. A vaccination test provided evidence of an overall improvement in immunity in the subjects who had meditated. This correlated positively with the increase of activity in the left hemisphere. Davidson concluded that the positive emotions engendered by meditation created a real benefit in immunity.[38]

In a study in which the French Buddhist monk Matthieu Richard took part, Davidson compared the cortical activity in people who were little accustomed to meditation with that of monks who had spent more than 10,000 hours in meditation. Meditation involves developing a compassionate state, allowing feelings of love to enter the mind without other thoughts interfering. Recording the electrical activity of the brain showed a difference between the novices and the monks. The monks showed a major increase of gamma waves: related to intense mental activity. Further, this increase was correlated with the time spent in meditation: some young monks who had spent 40,000 hours in meditation showed more gamma activity than some of the older monks who had spent no more than 10,000 hours in the practice. It therefore seems that a mental training allows one to reach a higher level of consciousness.[39] On the other hand, the images obtained by functional Magnetic Resonance Imaging showed an overall increase of left frontal activity in connection with positive emotions among the experienced monks. When photographs of suffering were shown to them, the cerebral areas governing purposeful movement were immediately activated. Thus we can say that, while the practice of meditation by monks involves developing compassion, it prepares them to take up action to give help to those who need it.[40] 'Spending time in meditation, far from the world, prepares one to be more just when one acts in the world,' Matthieu Ricard told me in commenting on these results.

These observations tend to prove that the phenomenon of neuroplasticity can be induced by the influence of purely mental signals. Certain changes appear in several minutes or hours. Others, more profound, take more time. Discipline and practice, essential elements of all spiritual progress, do not affect only thought. They provoke a veritable reshaping of the arrangements of the cerebral cells. Inevitably this eventually rebounds on the functioning of the body.

FROM VISUALISATION TO AUTOSUGGESTION

Some images that impress on the body

The influence of thought constitutes a considerable evolutionary advantage. And with reason: constructive ideas stimulate positive emotions and so exert a protective action on the body. Obviously, like all advantages, this influence can become an inconvenience. The damage caused by negative emotions proves the point. The imagination is therefore a two-edged sword. However, the human race would never have been able to survive without its influence. Imagination allows one to visualise an ideal, to hope for a favourable future, to mobilise positive emotions, to stimulate the immune system, to release the repair mechanisms in the body, to invent new strategies, and to deploy the energy with which human beings have been able to construct the pyramids of Giza, the Great Wall of China or even the Apollo lunar module.

The shamans of traditional societies, deprived of sophisticated technologies, employed the power of the imagination as a true medicine. Images are information. Now as we saw in Chapter 2 (p. 27), information is expressed in the forms of matter and energy. During the 1970s, the oncologist Carl Simonton proposed exploiting this energy for therapeutic purposes. Like a shaman of modern times, he led his patients into an imagined world in which the white blood cells attacked the cancerous cells, where robots captured the microbes, or where favourable liquids penetrated the sick cells to heal them.[41]

In 2002 a study published by Antony Bakke of the Oregon Health and Science University at Portland showed that this kind of guided visualisation improved the feeling of well-being in patients treated for breast cancer and, an altogether surprising observation, significantly increased the number of the immune system's NK cells.[42] These results obviously do not prove that guided visualisation can heal a cancer. On the other hand, it seems altogether reasonable to consider that positive emotions stimulated through this exercise stimulated the immune system and favourably influenced the course of the disease. Moreover, several studies have shown clearly that visualisation can reduce and even suppress the undesirable effects of chemotherapy.[43] In effect, having undergone chemotherapy, some people then feel real nausea at simply recalling their experience of the treatment. We may therefore suppose that an opposite suggestion may suppress or at least diminish the disagreeable experiences of the treatment.

In my practice I recommend patients to visualise the perfusions of chemotherapy as a golden liquid penetrating the cancerous cells to destroy them. And if they have to undergo radiotherapy, I suggest they visualise the source of the radiation as a sun whose energy will explode the sick cells. Once I have advised using such images, my patients mention secondary effects much less. It is very probable that the positive feelings so aroused help the immune system to eliminate the cells destroyed by the medicines or radiation.

Sometimes some of my patients look at me with suspicion. 'You think of yourself as a sorcerer?' Louis, an adolescent in treatment for leukaemia, asked me one day, before adding that I could keep my 'charlatan ideas' for others and that I could not make him swallow 'never mind what'. Instead of justifying myself I asked him to close his eyes and imagine a beautiful lemon, bright yellow, cut in two. That moment, his mouth filled with saliva. Image is information and evokes bodily reaction. This demonstration was enough to convince Louis. Revolted by the impotence into which his illness had plunged him, this adolescent found in such visualisation a way of participating actively in his treatment. This is not the least of the arguments in favour of such therapeutic support. Abandoning the status of victim to replace it by becoming an agent of healing gives meaning to the trial of suffering. The motivation accompanying this attitude helps to draw on his deepest resources to fight against discouragement and weakening.

Training

In the Rehabilitation Service of the Cleveland Clinic in Ohio, Guang Yue studied the influence of thought on functional recovery after a trauma. In one experiment, he asked subjects in good condition to imagine a contraction of the abductor muscle of their little finger or of the biceps muscle for 15 minutes a day over three weeks. The results were impressive: the strength of the biceps had increased by 13.5% and that of the abductor of the little finger by 35%, improvements that lasted once the experiment was ended. Recordings of the brain activity showed that the subjects' concentration activated the cerebral areas controlling the innervation of the muscles visualised. It is therefore possible to increase the strength of a muscle without physical training simply by the power of thought.[44]

This type of visualisation, which is commonly employed by the best sportsmen, facilitates the improvement of motor abilities.[45] The power of visualisation of a situation brings about a real conditioning and releases the bodily reactions needed to deal with that situation in reality. It is also possible to train the body mentally to develop motor capacities for actions that are especially complex to perform.[46]

During the 1950s, numerous studies showed that it is possible to modify the curves of an electrocardiogram, to develop the cerebral alpha rhythms and to become deeply relaxed simply by mental activity. These observations were used for treating headaches or chronic pain appearing after tensions or muscular spasms, to reduce stress and anxiety, to train voluntary physiological functions or involuntary ones such as arterial pressure, urinary continence or intestinal peristalsis.

Today, sophisticated equipment makes it possible to record information arising within the body, such as, for example, cardiac rhythm, skin temperature, muscular resistance, or the cortical waves which they convert to audible or visual signals. In following the variations of these signals on a screen patients discover what kind of breathing, what attitude or way of thinking improves or degrades the various parameters recorded. In this way, continually informed as to the state of the body, the mind can adapt in accordance with real biological feedback.

For sceptics, 'biofeedback' is an effective way of learning the relationship between the mind and the body. We know, for example, that the variation of cardiac rhythm is a natural process which depends upon the effort made by the organism and the movements of breathing. The greater this variability, the stronger is the heart. Asthmatic patients show a reduced cardiac variability. These observations enabled a group of researchers at the Robert Wood Johnson University at Piscataway in New Jersey, to teach asthmatic patients to control their cardiac variability with the help of abdominal breathing. The results of this treatment by biofeedback, published in 2004 in the review *Chest*, were rather encouraging, since six weeks later the doses of corticosteroids taken by the patients were reduced by a third and asthmatic crises were halved when compared with a control group who had not received biofeedback.[47]

If the variability of the cardiac rhythm seems important, the consistency of this variability is perhaps even more so. Researchers at the Institute of HeartMath, in California, showed that 'cardiac coherence' could be established by learning to regulate breathing while visualising the heart and recalling happy memories. The technique of biofeedback establishes profound breathing and mobilises the left hemisphere and its positive emotions. All at once, the parasympathetic system is activated and the neurological balance which commands cardiac activity is re-established. Automatically, the heart is freed from chaotic irregularities, caused by sympathetic accelerations and parasympathetic slowing. This is followed by coherence of the cardiac rhythm, a feeling of emotional well-being favouring relaxation of the body and the optimal operation of all the biological functions of the body.[48] Harmonious breathing, emotional balance and cardiac coherence seem therefore to be inter-related elements and guarantees of a good bodily fluidity. With the help of cerebral plasticity, this state of profound well-being is established more and more quickly; it becomes a real 'reflex of fluidity'.

WHEN SUGGESTION BECOMES HYPNOSIS

Mistrust and reticence

Sitting in front of a computer screen for some 12 minutes, Michael watches the curve of his cardiac variability scrolling in front of his eyes. A sensor attached to his index finger sends his heartbeat to the machine. He breathes in calmly and deeply, then breathes out, taking time to empty his lungs completely. A slight smile is on his lips. He is thinking of his wife and his children. He feels his love for them and, unconsciously, he raises one hand to his heart. On the screen, the curve is nicely regular and a percentage shows in one corner. Michael can check the result of his concentration: he now manages to maintain a good cardiac coherence. He is relaxed, totally absorbed by the curve on the screen. Things happening around him do not reach his awareness now: he is effectively hypnotised.

This kind of hypnotic state is altogether natural. All of us experience this more or less consciously, when we focus our attention on something about which we are fully alert while at the same time being possessed by a numbness close to sleep. In this somewhat special state of consciousness, we seem to be especially open to suggestion and we become able to initiate changes that are comparable to actual psychological re-programming. Hypnosis and suggestion are therefore closely linked. It is in this way that television exercises a noticeable influence on the behaviour of those watching it, absorbed as they are by the programmes they watch. In the same way, a loved one can preoccupy us to the point that we separate ourselves from reality. Do we not say that love is blind?

'Hypnosis is like being absorbed in a good book while the world turns around us. Obviously we have to want to read the book,' said Elvira Lang, professor at the University of Harvard. One day when she was preparing to change an intestinal catheter under radiological guidance, her patient suddenly panicked. Not knowing how to manage this situation, Elvira accepted the help of the technician in charge of the X-ray equipment who claimed to be able to calm the patient in a few minutes. Elvira was sceptical. All the same, the simple fact of breathing deeply and listening to the technician who encouraged the patient to imagine a more pleasant setting than the hospital was enough to calm the patient, to the point where changing the catheter was easier than it had ever been. Convinced by the efficacy of hypnotic suggestion, Elvira decided to resort to this technique systematically. From then on, the staff of the radiology service at the Beth Israel Medical Center at Boston were all trained in the use of this technique.

In a study published in *The Lancet* Elvira Lang showed that the use of hypnosis in radiological interventions allowed an overall reduction in the dosage of analgesics or tranquillisers, kept arterial pressure more stable throughout the time of the operation, shortened the time taken, and involved costs half those of a standard procedure.[49]

'Such results argue in favour of more general use of hypnosis in medicine,' a psychiatrist colleague of mine who was in treatment in Professor Lang's department, told me with enthusiasm. It is true. Nonetheless, a climate of suspicion opposes this. Firmly anchored in our thinking, this suspicion began in the 18th century when Franz Anton Mesmer tried to explain the phenomenon of hypnosis by postulating the existence of a magnetic fluid. This theory, which is today described as pseudo-scientific, was quickly demolished and placed in the category of unfounded beliefs (see Chapter 11, p. 178). This is certainly unjust, since trance states close to 'mesmerism' were used in certain traditional societies, especially for operating on patients without incurring perceived pain. Early in the 19th century, James Esdaile, an English medical officer who had assisted at this kind of practice in India, induced hypnosis in his patients before operating. In a quite extraordinary way, the postoperative mortality rate, normally around 40%, dropped to 5%. These results would probably have been enough to rehabilitate hypnosis if William Morton and John Collins Warren had not invented anaesthesia by means of a cloth soaked in ether in 1846, at Harvard. A century later, finally, hypnosis regained a little of its credit thanks to the reports of surgeons who used it successfully for anaesthetising the wounded on the battlefields of the Second World War.

In itself an example of medicine working on the body and the mind, hypnosis inspired many therapists. Initially, Sigmund Freud used it at the beginning of his career before abandoning it because of its intrusive character, which he saw as in conflict with his concern for an objective analysis of the human psyche. Then there is the American psychiatrist Milton Erickson who completely reconsidered this approach. Handicapped by many attacks of poliomyelitis, Erickson attempted his own rehabilitation by putting himself in a trance state which allowed him to recover his childhood memories. At once he recovered the physical sensations that brought about movement before his paralysis. And, quite unexpectedly, he recovered part of his mobility. The autohypnotic state described by Erickson allowed him to overcome his pain. He then began to teach his patients how to use their natural suggestibility to allow the emergence of their own solutions from the 'reservoir of the resources' of their unconscious. Respectful of each individual, Ericksonian hypnosis became a way of mobilising the therapeutic creativity of the patients.

In the early 1930s, inspired by the work of Emile Coué, the German neuropsychiatrist Johannes Schultz sketched an approach combining autosuggestion and relaxation. The scientific character of the name he gave to his technique – autogenic training – helped its acceptance by the medical community. Numerous clinical studies were published, and a recent analysis carried out of around 60 research reports confirmed his interest in taking on problems as varied as pain, hypertension, stress, anxiety, insomnia, asthma or eczema.[50]

Finally, in 1958 the American Medical Association decided to integrate hypnosis in the therapeutic arsenal. On the other side of the Atlantic a paper published in an issue of the *British Medical Journal* in 1963 described the possibility of suppressing the appearance of a skin reaction in response to a test of immunisation against tuberculosis, simply through hypnotic suggestion.[51] Because these results did not fit into the medical knowledge of the time, they were largely ignored. Thirty years later, as we have seen, developments in psycho-neuro-immunology provided at last a theoretical framework to explain these phenomena.

Since then, hypnosis has been used successfully in the treatment of pathologies such as asthma, various allergies, skin diseases, functional problems such as a spastic or irritable colon, and psychological difficulties such as phobias. The same kind of suggestion has been prescribed to help weight loss, stopping smoking or improving sports performance. And since 1996, the American National Institutes of Health has recommended hypnosis to manage pain in cases of cancer and chronic illnesses.

Thus, little by little, hypnosis is losing its scandalous image. The time of cabaret performances where hypnotised people end up by undressing under the stare of a magician with bulging eyes is long gone. Modern hypnosis is a scientific discipline and if, perhaps ten years ago, the specialist journals refused to publish articles about the subject, today the most prestigious universities raise funds for the exploration of this still ill-exploited human capacity.

Apollo or Dionysus?

David Spiegel, psychiatrist at Stanford, identifies three components in the hypnotic trance: first, *absorption*, which, like a magnifying glass, emphasises the awareness of details and reduces awareness of peripheral matters; second, *suggestibility*, the result of a highly concentrated attention which blocks the critical sense from exercising its judgement; third, *dissociation*, comparable to the waking sleep of a motorist on the motorway. This last phenomenon brings about an altered state of consciousness during which rational thought in the cerebral cortex is short-circuited to the limbic system where information is treated automatically without the intervention of reflection. This happens particularly at the time of trauma or psychological shocks, perhaps to allow speedy mobilisation of reparative mechanisms. Some people are capable of putting themselves into this state very easily: they 'disconnect' or 'float away' very willingly.[52]

It is obviously impossible to hypnotise someone against their will. Further, not everyone reacts in the same way to hypnotic suggestion. In Elvira Lang's experience, the most anxious preoperative patients were the most adept at self-hypnosis. It seems as though the capacity to imagine a negative scenario (the origin of the anxiety) can be used to create positive autosuggestion.[53]

Herbert Spiegel, professor of psychiatry at the University of Columbia, and his son David, professor at Stanford, identified different types of personality in terms of their natural predisposition to trance. The least susceptible to hypnosis – termed 'Apollonians' in reference to the Greek god of reason – had a rational intelligence which gave little room to feeling. In contrast, the 'Dionysians', named after the Greek god of wine, Dionysus, were much more sensitive to the details of their environment. Their marked capacity for concentration and their propensity to dissociation made them very open to influence. In marked stress, such personalities are more frequently susceptible to post-traumatic stress disorder of which we spoke earlier in this chapter (p. 57). Between these two groups we find the 'Odysseans' – referring to the voyage of Odysseus – who are the most numerous. They move from one tendency to the other, reacting sometimes with their heart, sometimes with their reason, and seek a balance between their internal world and the influences of their environment.[54]

A questionnaire prepared by the Spiegels allows a clearer understanding of how a patient functions in relation to the outside world, and that helps to choose a treatment adapted to the personality of the patient. This idea seems essential to me and should be taught to all who wish to work in healing. One does not approach an Apollonian as one would approach a Dionysian. Barbara Ann Brennan, an American healer with whom I have often worked, frequently told me: 'One must enter into relationship with another by the door that is open.' Thus in my consultations, if I meet someone with highly developed intellectual abilities, I take the time to describe his treatment very rationally, without hesitating to explain numerous scientific details. On the other hand, if I find myself faced with someone more intuitive, I avoid long descriptions and explain the treatment with the use of metaphors, and suggest that we begin work straightaway, starting with the realities of his body.

Certain very Dionysian people have an impressive capacity for suggestion – I would even say to the point of danger. Quite often they meet a stream of doctors, therapists and healers and allow themselves to be convinced by sometimes very contradictory discussions. My task is to help them define who they are in order to develop their critical sense. This is essential because the eagerness of certain Dionysians to respond without judgement to all stimuli, plunges them into stress and agitation which can be damaging to their healing. Happily, every disadvantage can become an advantage, since when these people become calmer (under the influence of relaxation or hypnosis for example), they can easily enter into contact with their capacity for self-healing.

The opposite phenomenon is to be found in the Apollonians. In effect, since they are less easily affected by exterior stimuli, they manage to protect themselves from negative influences. Unhappily, they deprive themselves at the same time of some suggestions or circumstances favourable to the maintenance or recovery of good health. As the Buddha taught: the road to follow is in the middle. That is the way taken by the Odysseans: while protected by their critical sense, they keep enough flexibility of mind to integrate helpful influences, even if they are hypnotic.

Pain – differently

At the University of Montreal in Quebec, Pierre Rainville asked some subjects to put their hands into water at 47°C, a temperature at the limit of tolerance. He had previously suggested under hypnosis to some subjects that the water was boiling and to others that it was very cold. A questionnaire completed by the subjects after the experience showed that those who believed they touched boiling water had felt pain markedly more intense than those who believed their hands went into cold water. The expectation of pain therefore increases its perceived intensity. The interest of this study by Rainville is that he observed, with radiological examination, the reactions of the brain after the hypnotic suggestion. In this way he was able to demonstrate a stronger activation of the brain pain circuits in those convinced that the water was very hot. Depending on the words used, the suggestion clearly exercised its influence on the cortical zones associated with the affective or the pain-sensitive constituent.[55] Such results show to what degree the pain experience can be affected by the attitude of those that manage it. Close attention, reassuring answers and some well-designed suggestions certainly permit the reduction of excessive doses of analgesics prescribed to the ill.

Marie-Elisabeth Faymonville, an anaesthetist at the University of Liège in Belgium, understood this well. For ten truly pioneering years she had helped more than 4,300 people as they underwent surgery. Whether the operation involved the excision of a skin tumour, an insertion of mammary prostheses, a face lift, the removal of the uterus, or an ablation of the thyroid gland, every patient was invited to recall pleasant memories to the sound of gentle music in the muffled ambience of the operating theatre. Moment by moment, Marie-Elisabeth talked to them and enquired after their comfort. A light sedation and local anaesthesia were used in the most painful cases to supplement hypnosis. The doses used were one fifth of those for a classical anaesthesia and therefore postoperative nausea and vomiting due to the anaesthetics employed were markedly reduced. Only 18 times was it necessary to apply general anaesthesia. When hypnosis could be used the patients were less tired, their pain was reduced and they recovered more quickly. For example, the patients undergoing thyroid surgery under hypnosis resumed their normal activities 13 days earlier than those who had undergone the same operation under general anaesthesia.[56]

'Hypnosis is a gift of nature like art or music,' was the summing up of Marie-Elisabeth Faymonville. 'Everyone has some vestige of this capacity, some are beginners, others virtuosos.' According to Helen Crawford, psychologist at the Virginia State University, this natural capacity to respond to suggestion is linked to the anatomical layout of the brain, especially at the level of the corpus callosum, a structure which connects the two hemispheres and which, in its anterior section, is specifically involved in the process of attention.[57]

Functional Magnetic Resonance Imaging can refine our understanding of this phenomenon. At Liège, for example, Marie-Elisabeth Faymonville showed that a state of hypnosis involved an increase of activity in cortical and sub-cortical zones affecting the sensory, cognitive and behavioural components of pain.[58] In Quebec, Pierre Rainville demonstrated an increase of activity in the anterior cingulate cortex, intervening in the process of attention and in motor control. Various areas of the brain are therefore called upon, especially the thalamus, implicated as it is in sensory and emotional perception, and the brain stem, linked to the spinal cord by which sensory information is passed. In addition, it seems to decrease the activity of the parietal lobes of the brain which are involved in the perception of the boundaries between the body and the environment, and at the same time, a stimulation of the visual cortex which favours the production of mental images.[59] Therefore the hypnotic state seems to be the result of a combination of specific activation and inhibition of neuronal circuits involved in the control of consciousness.

All evidence points to the fact that hypnosis is far from the superstition denounced by its detractors. On the contrary: it is a neurological phenomenon which is becoming better and better understood. Some researchers are even beginning to study it in 'real time'. For example, in the Major Burns Department of the University of Washington in Seattle, the psychologists Hunter Hoffman and David Patterson, with the help of Paul Allen, co-founder of Microsoft, have produced a helmet which projects three-dimensional images that can induce hypnotic suggestion. When this device was used during the changing of bandages on burns patients, it reduced pain by 25 to 30%. Some patients can even avoid all analgesia. Functional Magnetic Resonance Imaging (fMRI) carried out concomitantly showed an overall diminution of activity in the cortical areas mediating pain.[60] The proof is irrefutable: hypnosis works on the activity of the brain in a specific and effective way.

Differently from a classical video film, virtual animation allows complete absorption in the reality pictured. This, as we have seen, is precisely the kind of absorption that leads to hypnosis. Lying on the table of the fMRI scanner, heads in the virtual reality helmet, the patients of Hoffman and Patterson had the impression of flying over a snow-covered canyon. The illusion was perfect: they were not disturbed by the immobilisation of their heads or by the infernal noise of the machine. In the opinion of these researchers, this experimental method opens a new era in research in the neurosciences because, in addition to the hypnotic phenomenon, it allows observation of cortical activity in real time during a series of virtual experiences, exactly as if one were in a real situation.[61]

No one can now doubt that the progress in medical imagery clarifies many obscure areas of the mind–body unity. At the same time, the enthusiasm aroused by these recent developments in brain science must not lead us to forget that the human being is not composed just of a mass of neurones. One part of the answers to the questions we pose ourselves is hidden under the skin, in the bones, the muscles, the ligaments, the membranes and the organs of the body. This is, therefore, the direction that we must take to pursue our enquiries.

PART TWO
A MEDICINE OF THE BODY TO HEAL THE MIND

5
OBSERVING THE BODY THAT SUFFERS

IT'S ALL THERE IN FRONT OF OUR EYES

Three in one

I remember my amazement when, as a student in the second year of medicine, I understood how, starting with a single cell, the increasing complexity of evolution culminated in a body capable of developing consciousness of itself. An unbelievable epic which extends over billions of years summarised in 40 weeks of pregnancy. The study of embryology seemed to me to carry a poetic dimension which was lacking in the somewhat arid lessons of physics and chemistry. All at once the Meccano pieces come together and, as though by magic, the living matter acquires meaning.

The story begins at the moment when, winner of a competition between 500 million of his like, a tiny spermatozoon forces itself through the thick membrane of a large ovum. From this meeting arises a cell containing all our potentials. This multiplies and, three days later, has formed a mass of eight cells. Then 16, then 32, then 64. With the cell division, the size of the embryo grows at a prodigious rate. After two weeks one can already detect a shape: it has a top and a bottom, a front and a back. Ever more numerous, the cells align themselves in three layers – the endoderm, the mesoderm and the exoderm – three structures that give birth to all the tissues and the organs.

The plan of this construction has a remarkable precision. At the fourth week of life, the endoderm finally forms a tube from which develop the lungs and the digestive organs – intestines, stomach, liver and pancreas. At the same time, one part of the ectoderm turns in on itself to form another tube, this time neural, which gives birth to the nervous system – brain, spinal cord, nerves and sense organs – while the rest becomes the skin. Finally, between these two, the mesoderm creates the bones, the muscles, the blood vessels, the heart, the spleen, the bone marrow and the blood which is made there, the kidneys and the testicles or ovaries, the lymphatic vessels and the connective tissues which fill the space around the muscles and organs and extends itself between the cells and finally forms the fibrous skeleton at the core of the cells, where the codes of hereditary transmission are stored.

Each of these embryonic layers specialises therefore, in very specific functions. Arising from the endoderm, respiratory and digestive organs ensure the acquisition and absorption of matter and energy. Developing from the ectoderm, the skin and the nervous system have a function of perception, analysis and motor control. Finally, the mesodermal structures play a role of support and of linking the organs and other parts of the body.

Some strange correlations

In this way, embryology allows us to understand the logic of the body, as long as one possesses a sufficiently developed right cerebral hemisphere to mark the analogies, identify the relationships and acquire a vision of the whole, where the left hemisphere can see only the details without seeing their interconnection. The American physician and psychologist William Sheldon had this kind of ability. During the 1930s, having met Sigmund Freud and especially Carl Gustav Jung – the latter's classification of psychological types especially fascinating him – he set himself an apparently ridiculous question: is there a connection between morphology and psychology?

Analysis of several thousand photographs taken from the front, the back and in profile led him to identify three major types of morphology. By detailed examination of each anatomical form, Sheldon concluded that these developed preferentially from one of the three embryonic layers – endoderm, ectoderm and mesoderm. Thus the *endomorphs* show a round and pear-shaped body. Organised around the abdomen and the digestive system, their body has a tendency to enlarge very easily. On the other hand, the *ectomorphs* can eat without gaining one gramme. It is the nervous system which predominates in them. They have a large cranium, their silhouette is thin and slender. Quite different again, the *mesomorphs* have a skeleton that is well-constructed and covered with a strong musculature which gives them the look of a natural athlete.

In the course of his research and discussions, Sheldon ended by identifying the temperament associated with each of these morphological types.[1] The endomorphs appeared to be the most relaxed, convivial, sociable and affectionate. Careful of their physical comfort, they appreciate the pleasures of the table. In a group, they mix easily with others, they are tolerant, and if in difficulty, they seek company. Their intestines are very developed, lengthening the time required for digestion; they sleep easily and deeply; their metabolism, rhythm of breathing, heartbeat and style of movement are all characterised by their slowness. In fact, one might say that their voluminous digestive apparatus betrays a need for assimilation both relational and alimentary. Sheldon described them as socially extrovert and biologically introvert.

Ectomorphs have a very different personality profile. Equipped with an overdeveloped nervous system they spend their time protecting themselves from excess stimulation. Like a giant aerial their body needs time to integrate the mass of information that they perceive. Very sensitive to pain, ectomorphs have a tendency to isolate themselves and take shelter in solitude. Endowed with a great power of imagination, they live inside themselves, seek intellectual stimulation and are very creative. In company, they remain largely silent, watch the others and seek out individual contact. When in difficulties, they appreciate intimacy. The stomach is not highly developed and is quickly satiated; they are frequently hungry, lack energy and eat frequently. Their sleep is light. Biologically extrovert, they are socially introverted so that these sensitive and original people seem at first glance to give an impression of mediocrity. It takes time to get to know them.

Time is exactly what the mesomorphs lack. Their powerful musculature involves them in action. They cannot bear to be enclosed in small spaces. Rarely tired, they eat quickly, they are careless about meal times and sleep little. They are daring and strive to dominate. In groups, they take charge of others, they love power and seek competition. Pragmatic and authoritarian, they are easily angered. Their character recalls the 'Type A' personalities which we discussed in Chapter 3 apropos of their risk of myocardial infarctions (see pp. 48–49).

These descriptions are obviously somewhat nuanced, and in reality shade one into another. Sheldon himself considered his classification as a basic tool, most individuals presenting a combination of at least two morphological types. In addition, Sheldon demonstrated some differences linked to gender: women's bodies showed less mesodermic features (muscles) and more endodermic (fat) than men. This explains why when women gain weight, this is most commonly in the thighs and buttocks, so that their body develops the shape of a pear, whereas men, who accumulate fat at the level of the belly, keep slender legs and have an apple-shaped body.

At the University of California in San Francisco, Elissa Epel studied the relationship between morphology and the mode of reaction to stress. Set various intellectual exercises, pear-shaped women were less stressed and showed a less marked increase in blood cortisol than those with an apple-shaped body. Abdominal accumulation of fat is therefore correlated with a greater sensitivity to stress and thus creates a greater risk of cardiovascular illnesses.[2] The observations made by Elissa Epel confirm Sheldon's morphological observations: an endodermic morphology (pear-shaped) is paired with a calm and relaxed temperament, whereas people with a mesodermic profile (apple-shaped) are much more stressed and inclined to hostility, and as such are more subject to cardiovascular risk. This should console women who are distressed at gaining weight in the buttocks: it is thus that they avoid troublesome cardiac problems.

The intuition of the ancients

Sheldon's conclusions also corroborated various observations made in India several thousand years before our era, starting with the oral traditions and later written in the books of the *ayurvedic* medicine.

An assembly of practices designed to heal the individual in his totality, *ayurveda* – 'science of life' – was built on an intuitive appreciation of the great organising principles of the living creature. Before the use of microscopes made the identification of the three layers of the embryo possible, it was an acute sense of observation that brought the wise men of the *ayurvedic* tradition to explain the laws of life in terms of energy – *energeia* in Greek: force in action, the capacity of a system to produce work. They considered each human being as a unique combination of *kapha*, *vata* and *pitta*, the three fundamental energies – or *doshas* – that animate living beings. According to which of these three energies is dominant, the individual presents some specific morphological, physiological and psychological characteristics. Good health depends upon the harmony between the *doshas*. The aim of *ayurvedic* medicine is then to prevent or to correct imbalances between the three fundamental energies.[3]

The predominantly *kapha* individuals are large and well-built. They have a tendency to obesity and contain a good deal of vigour which they express very little. Calm and affectionate, they avoid confrontation. They sleep well and do not like to get up in the morning. They learn slowly and forget equally slowly. Some of these characteristics are very endomorphic.

The *vata* individuals are slender and light. Almost too thin, they have little strength, but use great efforts. Easily frightened, their mood is changeable. Their sleep is light and often broken with periods of wakefulness. They learn quickly and forget easily. One can recognise their ectomorphic characteristics.

Finally, the *pittas* are of average size and weight and are well-proportioned. Their energy is variable, they seek out competition, they easily become angry, they are jealous and stressed. They have an intense appetite. They sleep well and get out of bed easily. Their profile is undeniably mesomorphic.

Sheldon's observations and the theories of *ayurveda* teach us that the basic temperamental characteristics of an individual are functions of his morphology. All the same, these theories remain very controversial. They are too subjective for some, insufficiently documented for others, and do not take account of a fundamental question: is it the morphology which determines the characteristics or rather, in contrast, the behaviour that determines the characteristics of the body? A few studies, carried out principally on twins, indicate a genetic and innate component in character. At the same time, most scientists consider that the environment and the experiences of life are the principal determinants of behaviour.[4] This does not exclude the possibility of hereditary transmission of personality traits through the influence of fears, beliefs and habits which, while not transmitted by the genes, pass from one generation to the next. We need to know whether psychological experiences can actually influence the appearance of the body.

REPRESSION OF EMOTIONS

Tensions and distortions

Early in the 1930s, Wilhelm Reich interested himself in the question of the possible influence of psychological life on morphology. A former pupil of Freud, he postulated the existence of a 'bodily unconscious'. His method attempted to identify the physical traces of psychological pain. In contrast to psychoanalysis, which, by means of free association, seeks to know *why* the child represses his feelings, Reichian analysis endeavours to understand *how* this control is exerted. Since emotion is expressed in the body, it is there that Reich studied the mechanisms of repression.

For Reich, fear, grief, anger, pain – and every emotional event – provokes movements and characteristic postures. Tensions and imbalances automatically then become established in the body.

At the slightest stress, the arousal of the nervous system provokes the contraction of certain muscles. The perception of emotions is deadened and, at the level of the brain, the awareness of the unpleasant feelings is attenuated, even suppressed. Thus this muscular tension eventually allows a real separation from the self, a kind of emotional anaesthesia.

This process is useful in the case of acute stress because too vivid an awareness of the emotions in the body could prevent the arousal of the reaction of fight or flight. All the same, if the situation is prolonged, muscular tension due to hyperactivity of the sympathetic system hinders respiration, blood and lymphatic flow are slowed, toxins accumulate and the acidity of the tissues increases. Finally, cell activity is disturbed and, instead of increasing our power, the development of intense sympathetic activity renders us more fragile.

This made Reich remark that it is necessary to be able to relax the tension quickly in order to profit from the reparatory properties of the parasympathetic system (see Chapter 2, p. 35). In the opposite situation, in trying to avoid feeling the stress of what we experience, we develop a kind of 'affective paralysis'. Body and mind become rigid. This lack of flexibility prevents us from breathing freely and we block natural movements of contraction and relaxation. Falsely protected by our physical and mental stiffness, we simply risk breakdown.

The body tells us

Wilhelm Reich identified seven concentric segments which, from the head to the feet, are the sites of contractions provoked by repression of the emotions: these segments are ocular, oral, cervical, thoracic, abdominal, diaphragmatic and pelvic. Since Reich never mentioned this, it is troubling that these seven zones correspond to the seven *chakras* of the *ayurvedic* tradition. Once again, the ancient insights seem to have identified both a psychological and a physiological reality. (We shall examine the theory of the *chakras* in Chapter 10, pp. 157–161.) Examination of the muscular contractions and rigidities allows the identification of the veritable 'characterological armour' which holds the unexpressed emotion.

In his 'Analysis of Characters' published in 1933, Reich came to the conclusion that there are five personality types which are the result of traumatic experiences in life, and in particular in the development of the child and the adolescent.[5] Bodily contractions and tensions arising from these emotional wounds can become chronic. Reich postulated the establishment of actual conditioned reflexes which come to a head in profound bodily changes. Each psychological type then determines the morphological characteristics which reveal the wounds and the underlying conflicts.

In the light of the concepts of neuroplasticity we can now understand better how reflex contractions can impress themselves deeply on the postures and shape of the body. The framework of reading the body, proposed by Reich, then becomes a code allowing the deciphering of the intimate history of the individual.*

Thus some intense emotions felt in the course of pregnancy, or in the first six months of life, can favour the emergence of a profound

---

* A detailed analysis of the fears, the defences and the morphological types described by Wilhelm Reich is discussed in my book *Le travail d'une vie*, Paris, Robert Laffont, 2001.

existential fear, as if the hostility of the environment challenged the right of the individual to live peacefully and in full security. Inevitably this fear gives rise to a defence characterised by a flight into imagination, a loss of contact with reality and difficulties in forming deep relationships with others. Reich identified this behaviour as *schizoid*. Rather tall and slender, with fragile limbs, the body of the person concerned seems to float several centimetres above the ground. Large expressionless eyes emphasise the impression of absence. Twisted, fragmented, disarticulated, badly co-ordinated in its movements, the body lacks harmony. Angular and tense, it moves like a robot. Sometimes a scoliosis distorts the spine and a lopsided posture makes the silhouette almost ghostly, as though evanescent.

The inevitable frustrations of the first months of life lead the baby to fear being abandoned. Vulnerable and dependent, he prefers to deny his needs in order to avoid the occasion of being let down or else he complains in an exaggerated way in the hope of being heard. This demanding behaviour – qualified by Reich as 'oral' – hides feelings of despair and awareness of impotence. Muscular tone is weak, the shoulders drop, the torso is hollowed and the pelvis is strained forward. Even after development, the body remains immature and the eyes express the need to be cared for.

Sometimes the infant, frustrated in his desire for omnipotence, tests those around him to evaluate the limits of his power. He discovers that manipulation is an effective way of getting what he wants. Described as *psychopathic* and *narcissistic* by Reich, such manipulative behaviour is widespread in our contemporary societies. It is now aggressive, now seductive. The body builds itself in the service of dominance. The limbs are thin and the pelvis is narrow. The over-developed chest impresses the adversary. Piercing eyes exercise constant control over the environment.

In other circumstances, humiliated by the frustration of his desires, he prefers to bury his feelings and hide his rage behind a mask of gentleness. Meanwhile, he expresses himself plaintively and reproachfully. The body of the *masochist*, as Reich named this, controls the energy of his anger. The locking of the head and the torso leads to a clenching of the teeth and creates a shortening and thickening of the neck. The back becomes rounded as though to 'receive blows'. A further blocking between the torso and the legs favours the development of stoutness around the pelvis. Small and deep in their sockets, the eyes express a feeling of defeat and suffering.

Finally, some children choose to conform to the perfect image they believe is demanded by the parents. To do this, they refuse spontaneity. Their feelings are suppressed to the centre of a tense body, well-muscled, athletic and well-proportioned. The back is arched and the pelvis retracted as though the sexual area, thought shameful, must be hidden. A lack of suppleness in the ocular muscles makes for a cold expression, empty of emotion. The bodies of such *rigid personalities* seem without soul.

Obviously, like the classification of Sheldon or those of *ayurveda*, in reality the categories of Reich are not always clearly defined, and with good reason: in his development, an individual goes through all the stages and all the frustrations that the Reichian analysis describes. For example, when examining my own body, I found the stigmata of the schizoid infant hidden under the rigid carapace that I had fabricated to protect myself in order to survive, a shell that did not prevent me, according to the circumstances, from lowering my shoulders and hollowing my torso when facing an oral fear of being abandoned, nor, contrariwise, inflating my chest and exercising a psychopathic control by means of my piercing looks. Sometimes I surprise myself eating secretly, like the masochistic baby who fears being humiliated or restrained. Then, much to the annoyance of the perfectionist in me, my rigid shell is enveloped by a layer of protective fat, which damages the idealised image I have forged for myself.

The art of observation

Having experimented with Reichian analysis in consultations over about ten years, I remain astonished at the information which it allows me to access. Certainly, no classification can pretend to cover completely the subtle complexity proper to every individual. We must remain careful, all the more so because the force of wishing to validate a theory can make one deceive oneself by selecting only those elements that confirm the original hypothesis.

All the same, the frameworks of Reich, Sheldon or *ayurveda* for reading the body have the merit of sharpening one's observation and focusing attention on the body of the client. Then we understand that the body shelters a sensitive being who has a painful history, from which he continues to suffer. As we decode the defences inscribed in postures and bodily shapes, the subject of our interest quickly appears different. We no longer see him as one of those who are 'haughty and difficult to reach', 'who blow the air', 'whiners constantly demanding', 'seducers, aggressors or manipulators', 'too obsequious to be honest', 'cold, rigid and without heart' – but as hurt children who fear rejection, abandonment, betrayal, humiliation or imperfection.

In a consultation, for example, the capacity to see behind the appearances allows one to adopt an attitude adapted to the fears of the other. One can then put questions in such a way as to have a meaning related to the story which the patient's body tells.

The first time I met a practitioner 'initiated' into Reichian decoding, I asked myself what kind of sorcerer I was dealing with. In a few minutes, he had penetrated to my most intimate secrets. The precision of his analysis was almost surgical. And in a disturbing way his questions made me become aware of suffering once hidden in the shades of my unconscious. I asked him if he saw himself as a clairvoyant. 'No,' he replied, 'I am simply a psychotherapist aware that well before words, the body is a vector for language'.

6
INTERROGATING THE BODY THAT REMEMBERS

PSYCHOCORPORAL THERAPIES

Freeing energy

On 13 March 1895, Sigmund Freud wrote to his friend Wilhelm Fliess: 'Today, Mrs K. has again presented with pain in the chest [...]. In her case I have invented a bizarre treatment: I search for a sensitive zone, press on it and arouse trembling, which gives relief.'[1] Without knowing it, the father of psychoanalysis had just opened the door by which those who disagreed with him would rush in to go straight to the heart of the body–mind mystery. The first amongst them was certainly Wilhelm Reich. The 15 years between 1933 and 1948 which Reich devoted to the development of his 'vegetotherapy' became the occasion of a revolution in psychology, the importance of which we have hardly begun to grasp.

For Reich, who had demonstrated the muscular armouring caused by emotional stress, healing came via the release of tension. It is therefore necessary to treat the areas of resistance. Movement, pressure, massage and breathing exercises can trigger intense emotional discharges: convulsions and tremors overcome the body, the energy contained within the contractures is released and a profound feeling of well-being accompanies the subsequent relaxation. Reich compared the pleasure then experienced as akin to that of orgasm.[2]

As its name suggests, vegetotherapy works on the autonomic nervous system (also termed 'vegetative') since it corrects the imbalances due to sympathetic hyperactivity. Now, to restore the sympathetic/parasympathetic balance is to allow neurological, hormonal and immune system information to circulate in a fluid way throughout the organism.

During the 1950s, Alexander Lowen and John Pierrakos, two physicians and former patients and pupils of Reich, translated the concept of bodily tensions into terms of blockages of energy, and analysed their psychological and physiological repercussions. Psychologically, negative emotions paralyse the individual, his desires vanish, and, in time, his mood becomes depressive. Physically, action is inhibited, although the organism is in a state of arousal, and if that continues too long, the immune defences are weakened. When relaxation appears, the physical energy discharges itself in movement and the psychic energy is expressed in the form of positive emotions and new desires, of which Goethe wrote that they were the presentiments of our potentials. Negativity therefore gives way to creativity. (For the influence of positive emotions on creativity, see Chapter 2, p. 31.)

Lowen and Pierrakos called their approach 'bioenergetic analysis'.[3] This consists of a Reichian reading of the body, the examination of the life of the patient and a series of exercises adapted to each case. Thus, for example, lying on a big ball, the belly stretched, the patients discharge old tensions. Then, raising the level of energy by breathing and movement, suddenly, just as a dam gives way under too great a pressure, they let out a shout, tears and anger – a rage of which they had had absolutely no awareness, buried for years and which they often had turned on themselves, in judging themselves negatively or in preventing themselves from expressing their needs. Behind all anger is hidden a fear, a frustration and a need.* The therapist invites the patient to discharge his rage in striking a mattress or some cushions with a racket or a baseball bat.

All the evidence points to the fact that feeling anger is more important than talking about it. As was already said by the English physician and philosopher William James (brother of the writer Henry James) in the 19th century: 'What experience of fear would remain if one could not feel the accelerated beat of the heart, shortness of breath, trembling lips, weak limbs, stomach pain? I find it impossible to imagine: can we imagine anger without ferment in the belly, reddening of the face, widening of the nostrils, or clenching of the jaws, and in their stead flaccid muscles, quiet respiration and a calm face?'[4] Thus the physical experience of an emotion gives it body. The energy that it contains becomes a tangible reality, a potential available to us. Again, it is necessary to us to learn to express it, not in aggressivity towards others or towards ourselves, but, as was well shown by the psychologist Marshall Rosenberg, in the affirmation of one's boundaries and needs.[5]

My first contact with bioenergetic therapy was a deeply moving experience. It took place in a workshop conducted by the American psychiatrist Elisabeth Kübler-Ross whose life was dedicated to accompanying the dying. Completely cut off from my usual emotional feelings, I watched the other participants from behind a sort of mask of serenity, a detachment of which I was unaware at the time, and which was a way of protecting myself. Suddenly, Linda, a woman with cancer

---

* These ideas are explored in my book *Vivre en paix*, Paris, Robert Laffont, 2003.

of the colon began to express the rage that lay buried in her body. A profound unease arose in me, and without the slightest empathy, I declared this to be 'a theatrical performance, ridiculous and useless'. In fact, I found it terrifying. Thinking and judging seemed to me to be much more comfortable than feeling. I could not then imagine that the energy of rage could be used in the service of healing. (This aspect of healing is discussed in Chapter 4, pp. 59–62.) And, equally certainly, I was unaware that, not much later, I would be hitting the cushions in my turn, and, even less expected, that one day I would be helping some patients to do the same.

Words or sicknesses?

Picture a therapy group: Liza, Michael, Frank, Valerie, Nicole... Around 15 participants sitting in a circle, each with his own load of conscious and unconscious suffering, all firmly determined to relieve their troubles. Michael describes the difficulty he experiences when he tries to express the anger he feels towards his father. At that moment my attention is drawn to Frank. The pale face, the jaws clenched, the fists tight, the man is patently annoyed. I ask him immediately what he is feeling. 'Nothing,' he replies. A murmur runs around the group. Nicole rises and says she had noticed the tenseness of Frank's face. 'I would say that he is annoyed. Perhaps he is angry,' she says, a little embarrassed. I encourage Frank to tell us what he feels in his body. Mutely he puts his hand on his stomach. I ask him to breathe to relax himself. Suddenly he says: 'I have a weight on my stomach, a lump in my throat... my back hurts too.' I ask him if he feels angry. 'I don't know,' he replies, frowning. Aware of his difficulty in putting words to what he feels, I ask him if the fact that he had heard Michael speak of his problems with his father had made him uneasy. 'No,' he replied dryly. I suggest that he expresses what he feels in his body by gestures. Slowly and progressively, his limbs stretch, his torso straightens, his fists unclench. The whole of his body begins to move as though he were warming up to run the 100 metres and suddenly he begins to bang his fists and stamp his feet. One hand on his shoulder, I encourage him to let sounds come out of his throat. He must breathe in and out deeply to draw out the force that is roiling in his belly. Tears rise in his eyes, his legs begin to tremble, he stamps harder and harder with his feet and suddenly he shouts. Around us, the other participants all have their fists clenched as they re-live their own angers. Frank continues to shout, like a wild beast. This is the experience that is waking inside him: his emotional brain is letting go of his anger. At that precise moment I ask him to let words out without thinking, in a spontaneous surge. In a few seconds the shouts give way to abuse. We understand that he feels something terrible towards someone. Rage pours out of him like lava from a volcano. Amongst the shouting and tears, the name of his father appears at last.

After a few minutes, Frank becomes calm. He relaxes deeply. His muscles and eyes are relaxed and his gaze expresses joy. 'I would never have believed I would feel so much life in myself,' he tells us. 'It is like electricity from my hands to my feet.'

Frank then explains to us that he had undertaken group therapy because a year earlier he had had an operation for a gastric cancer, 'a hell that opened for me six months after my father died'. Then, breathing deeply he declared: 'By contacting my anger so suddenly, I realised that this illness is a lump in my stomach, something I cannot digest.' As if his memory had just been freed, Frank described the suffering that he had endured as a child when his father had beaten him. He also told us of the disarray that he had experienced when his father died. At last he understood why, every time he was in the presence of his father, his jaws and hands clenched and his heart speeded up. 'I could have killed him, my anger was great enough.'

Alexithymy

Like Frank, certain people experience enormous difficulty in decoding their own emotions. They feel it all in their body, but they remain incapable of expressing them in the form of feelings. One person in seven suffers from this impossibility of identifying and communicating their emotional life. This is the case more commonly amongst men. Really cut off from themselves, they do not understand the meaning of their malaise and they have great difficulty in making others understand.

Modern medicine has put a name to this isolation: alexithymy (from the Greek *a*: lack of, *lexis*: word, *thymos*: emotion), that is to say the inability to put words to the emotions. It is likely that this difficulty becomes established in early childhood because the parents are unable to name the feelings experienced by the child and do not help him to identify or express what he feels. Imagine, for example, an infant who is hungry. The discomfort provoked by that sensation leads to tears and bad mood. If the parents make the connection between the discontent and the sensation of hunger, they are helping the infant to decode what he feels. If not, the experience leads to a kind of emotional illiteracy.

A study by means of functional Magnetic Resonance Imaging carried out on alexithymic men by the French psychologist Sylvie Berthoz, showed disturbances at the level of the anterior cingulate gyrus, a cerebral area that connects the limbic emotional system to the cortex.[6] Alexithymy appears to be an actual deficiency in the cognitive appreciation of emotion.

It seems that participation in sessions of group therapy can be very helpful to alexithymic people. Progressively, in listening to other people express their feelings, each participant can learn the words which are appropriate to his own feelings. He discovers that other people have experiences in common with him and that the emotions are messages which are important to listen to, to express and to communicate to others.

To work on the body seems, in this context, especially effective because one meets the defences of the individual head-on. The words and the images of the mind can re-awake memories, as can the postures and movements of the body. The patient is then very vulnerable and the therapist must employ a precision that is almost surgical to expose the connection between discomfort and emotions, to establish links between the pains and words and to build a bridge between the body and the mind. In increasing the energetic charge with the help of breathing and movement, the physical sensations are emphasised. It is probable that at the cerebral level, once a certain threshold has been reached, the lock on the cingulate gyrus opens and suddenly the cortical functions are mobilised. All at once, meaning can be associated with sensation and, sometimes, memories become re-attached.

The first time that I put this kind of phenomenon to the test was an altogether unexpected experience. Several hours earlier, I had taken part in a group therapy session. In the course of that session, several participants had 'let the body talk', accepting the discharge of their suffering through gestures and words in order, in the end, to experience a profound muscular relaxation and a real calming of the mind. Faced with their pain, my own discomfort was revealed: I felt burning in my stomach, I felt oppressed and found it difficult to go home while in this state. The therapist for the group encouraged me then to breathe deeply 'to free the tensions'. That is what I did in the following two hours. Somewhat relieved, I was about to leave, when suddenly I began to sob. A childhood memory surged into my consciousness. Pictures that were extremely vivid rushed in front of my eyes, accompanied by sounds and smells, and I understood the origin of the physical suffering I had experienced. This memory released a series of insights, whole sections of my life became clear, so much so that this experience is still one of the determinants of my life.

Listening to the body

In contrast to the verbal therapies, where thoughts and memories inform the body of their content with the help of the associated positive and negative emotions, in the psychocorporal therapies it is the effects within the body which, translated into feelings, end up releasing the memory. Insights which arise in the course of psychocorporal sessions are in direct contact with the emotion and the trauma of the patient – intellectual discourse having no hand in the process. In comparison with approaches based on words, the risk of 'cheating' is thus reduced. Moreover, one learns very quickly to distinguish from the tone of voice between those patients who remain within their intellectual defences and those who truly feel what they verbalise. That undoubtedly explains why, in contrast to certain interminable analyses, the therapies involving the body produce quick and profound results.

Psychoanalysis thinks about the body. The psychocorporal therapies aim at experiencing it. They permit the development of a self-awareness there and then, as much physical (the postures and the tensions of the body) as psychological (the memories and beliefs underlying these postures and tensions). To be fully present to oneself helps to escape from the conditioning of the past in order to choose new behaviours. To leave the vicious circle of the defences then becomes the way that leads to true freedom. Take the case of Frank: every time he meets someone who reminds him of his father he feels himself invaded by an intense anger. The tension in his body is such that he forgets to breathe. Having made this process of cause and effect conscious, he has learned to choose to relax. A few deep in-breaths then help him to free himself from his conditioning.

In other circumstances, attentive listening to the body allows one to recognise the signs which appear when the tolerance of the individual is surpassed. Personally, since the time that I developed consciousness of my body, it has become impossible for me to ignore the symptoms of stress. I see them as real warning messages. Because of this I now respect my essential needs better, which, as we have seen, is an excellent way of preserving physical and psychological health.

Additionally, much like the example of numerous patients, I have noticed that an increased sensitivity to bodily messages gives rise to the development of intuition. As was shown by Joseph LeDoux, emotional reactions often show themselves in the body even before we have been able to analyse consciously the situation that has aroused them (see Chapter 2, p. 30). Learning to recognise the signals given by the body helps us to recognise whether our experiences are favourable or not for maintaining our integrity. Once we have become aware, through the body, our instinct for survival becomes an intuitive sense much more powerful than most of our convoluted reasoning.

Despite this, numerous therapists neglect the bodily expression of emotion. For myself, this attitude was dictated by the difficulty of governing my own emotions and my own suffering, a difficulty experienced by many people, and which spares neither physicians nor psychiatrists, psychologists nor other therapists – and with good reason: their academic training explores the emotional dimension from an intellectual point of view. This is an approach which is antinomic or self-contradictory at the very least, since without bodily experience it is impossible to understand the nature of emotion. It is through feeling in the body the wounds of the past that one learns not to fear them any more. Taming these discomforts allows us to use the powerful energy contained in our defences. This aspect of therapeutic practice is vital because the meeting of sufferer and therapist always brings together two hurt children, each trapped in his own defences. Failing to hold this in mind prevents the establishment of true healing. In effect, it is difficult to point to the road which leads to future freedom if one oneself remains prisoner of the shackles of the past.

Meanwhile, we must remain aware that the emotional discharge which sometimes occurs during a body–mind therapy is not in itself the end. Moreover, this catharsis does not always have to be spectacular. On the contrary, in the opinion of numerous body–mind therapists, the therapeutic work can be carried out calmly. Thus simply drawing the attention of a patient to a muscular contraction is sometimes sufficient to plunge him into emotional reaction which permits him to become conscious of a repression, a fear, or an unhappy memory, and this may trigger off a series of associated thoughts, which, in the classical psychoanalytic sense, bring meaning to his experience. That is already a good beginning. Subsequently the body can be questioned in depth through movement and relaxation of tensions.

With hindsight, having experimented with both kinds of approach – verbal and psychocorporal – for myself and for my patients – I am convinced of the importance of addressing the body–mind unity of the individual throughout his therapy, whether this is on the grounds of a psychological problem or a physical disease. Sometimes the body–mind approach presents too powerful a threat to the defences of a patient. Nothing need stop one offering him verbal therapy while recommending in parallel that he develop his awareness of his own body by, for example, having massage, following a course in dancing or singing, practising yoga or *tai-chi*, or learning the methods of Alexander or Feldenkrais (see Chapters 8, 9 and 10). Made supple, conscious and sensitised, the body becomes a precious tool for psychological work.

The finger on the wound

Jeannine is a rheumatologist in a well-known Paris hospital. For four days she had suffered from intense pain in the left shoulder. The pain had appeared suddenly while she was eating breakfast. Her partner, an orthopaedic surgeon, palpated a muscular contraction around the scapula. However, no abnormalities were shown on radiological examination. Since the pain did not respond to anti-inflammatory medication, Jeannine decided to make an appointment with Frédéric, a friend who was a physiotherapist.

The latter immediately proposed using Rolfing, a technique invented in the 1960s by Ida Rolf, a biochemist, when she attempted to heal the result of a fall from horseback. Inspired by the practice of yoga, the work of Reich and the innumerable research programmes carried out at the Esalen Institute (see Chapter 7, p. 115), Rolf's approach focused on the connective tissues of the body: ligaments at the level of the articulations, tendons at the extremities of muscles, and the fascias around the muscles and organs.[7] With the help of hard palpation, pressure and vigorous manipulation, the practitioner draws out and loosens the tissues made rigid by tension and contractures.

Lying on the massage table, Jeannine let it happen. The sensation was not comfortable. At certain points it was even painful. Suddenly she felt a surge of emotion arise. Accustomed not to show anything, she attempted to suppress her desire to weep, she choked, her jaws clenched. It was a lost effort: a flood of tears spurted and she began to sob like a child. Incapable of arresting her tears, Jeannine let them flow. She felt the muscles of her back relax. The pain diminished. And suddenly images of her childhood passed before her eyes: she relived the explosion of a lorry in front of the door of her house: the light of flames, the smell of smoke, the shouts of her father who caught her violently by the shoulder. At the end of the session, Jeannine, severely distressed, apologised to her 'Rolfer' friend, who comforted her, reassuring her that this kind of manifestation commonly arises 'when the body remembers'.

The childhood memory which Jeannine had just recovered was an experience which, at the time, had profoundly traumatised her. She had talked lengthily about that event in the course of the psychoanalysis she had undertaken during her medical studies. She thought that she had freed herself, but this was clearly not so. Astounded, Jeannine suddenly realised that the pain in her shoulder had appeared on 12 September 2001, several hours after she had watched the television re-transmission of the collapse of the Twin Towers of the World Trade Center. It was as if that catastrophe had reawakened an unconscious memory in her body at the same point at which her father had seized her to save her.[8]

This kind of memory recovery is not the purpose of Rolfing (see Chapter 8, p. 122), nor is it necessary to obtain the relaxation, looseness and realignments sought by this technique. It simply shows that somatic states are intimately linked with a traumatic memory.

THE BODY REMEMBERS

The strata of memory

From the 1960s onward, the American psychologist Arthur Janov explored the nature of memories stored in the body in the course of psychotherapy, mingling individual sessions with group sessions. These are distributed over a period of three weeks during which the patient is isolated from the outside world, compelled to write a diary and asked to remain in contact with objects or photographs of his own past. This therapy, termed 'primal', sensitises the patient to a high degree and eventually activates the painful memories which Janov locates precisely in terms of the function of the cerebral layer in which the trauma has been remembered. (The different layers of the brain are described in Chapter 2, p. 28.)

Janov defines suffering at three levels – first, second and third – according to whether the trauma occurred at an instinctual, an emotional or a cognitive level. Thus, contrary to some commonly accepted beliefs, memory does not need language in order to encrypt. Thus preverbal events, experienced in the earliest days of life, at the time of delivery or even during pregnancy, can show themselves in physical problems – such as colitis or palpitations – which, later in life, regularly re-emerge at times of anxiety, though the original cause has been long forgotten. According to Janov, no tears and no words can express these ancient memories: only physical symptoms can do so, because the first level (earliest) memory is prior to both emotional and intellectual processes.

During a session, the primal therapist can follow quite directly the re-awakening of the traumatising memory by observing physical phenomena such as body temperature and arterial pressure. Janov relates the case of a patient who was delayed by a traffic jam on the road leading to the Primal Center in Venice, California.[9] Late for the session of group therapy, in a nervous state, the man explained his difficulty. As he spoke about his anxiety, his pulse speeded up, his body temperature increased from 37 to 40°C, and his blood pressure rose from 125/90 to 200/100. These reactions are produced every time that a painful memory rises into consciousness because the body is preparing itself to confront aggression. Within a moment, the man felt again the emotion arising from a time in the past – when his parents stopped him from acting as he wished. Overwhelmed with anger he began to beat on the wall while howling. He saw again a scene from his childhood when his mother had forbidden him to play football after school. At that exact moment, his blood pressure and temperature fell, and, like a small boy, he wept for half an hour. Then, quite suddenly, he fell into the foetal posture. These signs tell the therapist that the patient is reliving the experiences recorded at the time of birth. The physiological parameters rose brusquely once again, but briefly because at the moment that the patient feels again the sensation of being stuck, he can no longer breathe, he feels at the point of death, his blood pressure falls to 95/55, and his temperature to 35°C. Prostrate on the ground, he does not speak, and simply groans without weeping. Like a foetus stuck in the vaginal canal he struggles and pushes with his head for 40 minutes until, eventually he becomes calm. Once he is lucid, and profoundly relaxed, insights rise to consciousness. Now he understands the link between his adult behaviour and the trauma he has just re-lived.

In Janov's view, repression is *the* fundamental biological defence against pain. When his inner processing is disturbed, the individual is forced to become agitated, to talk a lot, to masturbate compulsively, to over-eat, to drink alcohol, to smoke, even to take drugs. If the traumata are emotional or instinctual, intellectual understanding is not sufficient to free the individual from them. Only work synchronised with the chronology of the engrams allows one to go back, layer by layer, as far as the origin of the suffering. Janov therefore distrusts certain therapies using breathing strategies, such as rebirthing, where hyperventilation favours the brutal reappearance of primary layer memories embedded long before the cerebral cortex became active and which are therefore impossible to verbalise. According to him, the danger lies in the patient protecting himself from pain by escaping into his imagination, to the point of sinking into hallucinatory delusions, which, depending on the culture of the patient and the beliefs of the therapist, may refer to previous lives or other symbolic metaphors.[10]

Having myself observed at numerous such sessions, I must admit that the spectacular aspects of primal therapy can be off-putting. To heal by reviving suffering is not necessarily the most appealing route, especially in our hedonistic societies, accustomed as they are to various forms of anaesthesia. Precise and intrusive, primal therapy must be managed by an expert. That is its principal limitation since qualified therapists are rare. Nevertheless, the results seem to justify the means. Patients have reported that blood pressure diminishes, chronic pain disappears, drug use stops, digestive problems improve, and the repetitive cycle of a whole series of neurotic behaviours is interrupted. Arthur Janov also reported an increase in growth hormone resulting from the process of post-traumatic recovery, and an overall improvement of the immune defences relating to the re-establishment of balance in the autonomic nervous system.

Inherited suffering

There is no proof that memories reawakened in a session of bioenergetic analysis or of primal therapy are real. Some researchers think that such recall might involve reconstructed memories designed to give meaning to the emotional experience. At the very least, the evocation of a trauma triggers off a whole series of sensory perceptions, physiological disturbances, biological changes and motor reactions. Whether reconstructed or no, these memories express real suffering. Arthur Janov also noted the appearance of bruises on the skin of certain patients when they revived the memory of violence that had been inflicted on them in childhood.[12]

This may seem unbelievable. Nevertheless, because of the principle of brain plasticity, we know that every experience leaves a print in the network of the cerebral neurones (see Chapter 3, p. 51). According to Antonio Damasio, in his 'Theory of somatic markers', every such trace is associated with the condition of the body at the moment when the experience had been committed to memory.[13] The calling up of a memory then re-arouses the associated physical manifestations, and at the same time a particular physical experience can trigger off the recovery of the memory of a specific experience. Thus Frank had clenched his fists in anger every time he met his father, simply because in his childhood he had clenched his fists when his father beat him. It is therefore not surprising that hearing Michael talk about his relationship with his own father was enough to trigger off a bodily reaction in Frank. Nevertheless, he had not been able at the beginning of the group therapy session to make the connection between the emotions he was expressing in his body and the wounds of his childhood (see above, pp. 92–93), simply because he was avoiding the feelings associated with his memory. We know that an alexithymic experience prevents the physical sensations provoked by emotions from entering the mind, and so becoming conscious and verbalised. Now it seems that alexithymy is more common in patients suffering from what we call 'psychosomatic' pathologies. It is as though being incapable of putting words to feelings stimulates the somatisation of those feelings into organic disturbances and bodily symptoms.

Ghislain Devroed, professor of surgery at the University of Sherbrooke in Quebec, described very clearly this process amongst women who had been sexually abused in childhood. At the moment of defecation, some of these women have poor co-ordination between the contractions of the rectum and those of the anus as though one part of themselves wished to expel the faeces while another, unconscious, prevented all opening of the perineum. Listening to the bodies of these women, Devroed often avoided operating uselessly. Through 30 years, his experience as surgeon-psychotherapist was punctuated by surprising cases. Thus one constipated woman was cured instantaneously on the day her father died. Or another patient, who had presented repeatedly with constipation and urinary retention, when asked if she had been abused in childhood felt an intense rage, and suddenly remembered that her abusing father had ordered her to 'shut it'. By expressing her anger through an intense catharsis, she was permanently cured.[14]

Sometimes messages appear to be imprinted on the body before they can be understood by the intellect of the child. Ghislain Devroed tells the story of Charles, a child with constipation since birth, in whose case no other abnormality could be found. A troubling fact was that his mother had had a difficult pregnancy during which she had repeated non-stop: 'Come on, baby, we are holding back.' In time, he had eventually learned to relax through biofeedback (see Chapter 4, p. 70). But after his parents had divorced, every time that he went to see his mother he became constipated again. It was then that his mother told him that she too suffered from constipation. Curiously, he became angry towards her for having put him into the world. One day, this anger was expressed towards a holiday supervisor, when he threw an axe at the man's head. Frightened, his mother decided to tell him her 'secret'. In Charles' childhood she had been the victim of a rape attempt, and her father had insisted she keep it secret. Comforted, she entered psychotherapy. Soon Charles was cured. He was never again constipated.

'Some children express their parents' sufferings through their own body, as if they were trying to protect them and relieve their pain,' Ghislain Devroed commented. This is not limited to functional problems: there are children who go as far as developing intestinal inflammation, like Sacha, a little boy who had anal bleeding due to Crohn's disease, an illness that his mother had developed during her pregnancy with him, and which had gone when the child developed the condition in his turn. Devroed added: 'There are many cases like this; it is enough to open one's eyes and ask questions.'

I have had the same experience. I remember, for instance, Patricia, a young woman of 19, whose liver had been completely destroyed by an auto-immune hepatitis. Her disease had appeared a few months after the death of her father, who died of alcoholic cirrhosis – another form of destruction of the liver. Fortunately, Patricia had received a liver transplant in a major hospital in the United States. Nonetheless, it seemed to me that I could read sorrow in her eyes. 'I am not sad,' she told me, 'I am angry. How could I not be? I passed the whole of my childhood trying to satisfy my parents by acting the model little girl. All that time my father was destroying his liver with alcohol and my mother never stopped lecturing him and me. I put up with all that and never said a word. All that – for nothing!' (The relation between stress, depression and the auto-immune diseases is discussed in Chapter 2, p. 37 and in Chapter 3, pp. 41–43.)

I remember also the case of Leah, a three-month-old baby who refused to take food. After a long conversation, her mother at last revealed to me that she herself had become anorexic during her childhood because she had herself had trouble in tolerating being separated from her own mother when she was sent to a boarding school. I then asked her to speak to her little girl to tell her that she need not bear the sadness of her mother, and that, even if she herself had wanted to die, her baby had the right to live. She was sceptical but did what I had asked. The same day Leah began to suck at her bottle: the message had been well transmitted.

As noted by the French psychoanalyst Françoise Dolto, this kind of transmission of information to a child raises questions. How does an infant whose cerebral cortex is not yet capable of understanding words and syntax understand the meaning of speech?

The question of preverbal communication is among the most complex enigmas which science has yet to solve. How can one understand the fact that little Sacha had decided to 'relieve' her mother of the Crohn's disease she had suffered during pregnancy? Was Charles' constipation the consequence of a message heard *in utero*, or simply an accident? How can one explain, as was noted by the psychotherapist Anne Ancelin Schützenberger, that a little girl drew a picture of herself in the belly of her mother with a large dagger pointed at herself, at the time when an amniocentesis was carried out during the pregnancy, knowing that the disclosure of this episode, the occurrence of which she had been unaware, had produced a definite improvement of her symptoms?[15] We know that the foetus dreams synchronously with its mother and can recognise his mother's voice.[16] Can the unconscious images of the mother be transmitted to the child? This seems difficult to conceive in the present state of our knowledge, because, until we get proof to the contrary, we believe that the nervous system of the foetus is capable of feeling but not representation. Do we need to imagine the existence of a mode of transmission and perception of information as yet unknown? Who knows? We need to remain humble and to remember that it is not long ago that we believed that the foetus was completely isolated from the outside world. Nowadays no one disputes the fact that the womb is a sensory bath in which the child receives experiences that determine the maturation of his nervous system. We saw in Chapter 3 (pp. 49–50), that more and more studies show that stress in the mother during pregnancy influences the behaviour of the baby after its birth.

From one generation to another

Here is another great enigma to resolve: the phenomenon of transgenerational memory. In 1975, Anne Ancelin Schützenberger was prompted by the case of a young woman who developed cancer at the same age at which her mother had died of an identical pathology, to search systematically in the family histories of her patients for repetitions, and unconscious identifications with a loved one.[17] She then observed that, in certain families, a birth, a marriage, a false pregnancy, an illness or a death could occur at the date or the anniversary age of a major event that had occurred three, four, or even eight generations earlier. These observations corroborated those of Josephine Hilgard who had spoken in 1957 of the 'anniversary syndrome' to describe the statistically significant repetitions of accidents and psychiatric admissions in adult hospitalised patients in the United States admitted at the same age as a forebear had had an accident or had been admitted to hospital in the past.[18] After lengthy enquiries, the Hungarian psychoanalysts Ivan Boszormenyi-Nagy, Nicolas Abraham and Maria Török, suggested the concepts of 'invisible loyalty', of 'crypt' and of 'phantom' to describe what appeared to be a real transmission of family secrets. Thus from unconscious to unconscious the unspoken crosses the generations. Sooner or later they end by expressing themselves in the body of a member of the family in the guise of strange symptoms or an illness.

Such cases are astonishing. Nicolas Abraham tells the story of a man truly handicapped by two obsessions: one, that, as an amateur geologist, he spent every Sunday in gathering stones to break later; the other, as a butterfly hunter, he trapped butterflies in order to kill them in a jar of cyanide. After several periods in psychotherapy and an analysis, he undertook some transgenerational research. This yielded information about a grandfather of whom no one had ever spoken. The unacknowledgeable secret the family had kept hidden was of a shameful stay by their ancestor in a penal colony. Continuing with his research, he discovered that his grandfather had spent the last years of his life breaking stones before dying in a gas chamber. The behaviour of his grandson seemed therefore to demonstrate the shameful and concealed destiny of the grandfather.[19]

The psychoanalyst Yolanda Gampel reports numerous descendants of the victims of the Holocaust whose fate seems shaped by the sufferings of their ancestors. For example, she, a forensic scientist whose life was dedicated to the dead, had discovered that her father had been sent to an extermination camp where he was forced to collect the dead and throw them in the common grave.[20]

The weight of family heritages can be very heavy. Ghislain Devroed and Anne Ancelin Schützenberger describe how a brother and sister had refused to follow in the profession of their father who had died from a cancer. Nevertheless, both of them ended by re-enacting part of the paternal drama ten years later. The son developed Crohn's disease and began to bleed 'from behind' like the lorry full of corpses which had haunted the nightmares of his father, a former combatant in the Algerian war. The daughter had a cerebral attack on the anniversary day of the same attack that had brought down her father several weeks before he died from cancer. An emergency scan showed that she had a tumour of the brain![21]

I remember Emma, a young woman who never succeeded in becoming pregnant, the undoubted result of an excess of male hormones responsible for the hypertrichosis, almost amounting to hirsutism, that she exhibited, but also because of the fact that not one of her relationships lasted more than a few months. Whenever Emma talked of men it was in a reproachful tone, her voice full of anger. I suggested to her that she should examine her beliefs and expectations of the masculine. The result was plain: 'You can't have any confidence in them! My sisters and my cousins agree: there are no more real men. And so they too remain single!' I then encouraged Emma to ask her grandmothers how they saw men. It was as well that she did so, because her maternal grandmother revealed a secret that she had never told anyone: six generations earlier a forebear had been murdered by her homosexual husband. The belief that was then passed down the generations was that men are women and traitors and one cannot rely on them. All the women in this family had adopted very masculine behaviour in order to survive. This masculinity was so deeply embedded that it manifested itself in a hairy body impregnated with testosterone and which, whenever it gave life, brought only girls into the world!

Conditioning, autosuggestion, psycho-neuro-endocrino-immunological reactions, genetic selection and mutation: the mechanisms invoked to explain transgenerational phenomena are numerous, and for the moment hypothetical. Some researchers speak of an 'internal familial clock' which is responsible for stories at the outer limit of the believable, like that of the actor Brandon Lee killed while filming by a bullet forgotten in a revolver supposedly loaded with blanks, an accident that happened 20 years after the death of his father, the actor Bruce Lee, killed by a cerebral haemorrhage while filming a scene in which he was playing the role of a man killed accidentally by a revolver that should have been loaded with blanks.

Thus a new discipline appeared: psychogenealogy. Examining the cases concerned yields evidence that is difficult to verify in a rigorously scientific way. To prove the somatic expression of unspoken ancestral secrets requires the identification of such a family secret and observation of its impact on the descendants of the holders of the secret. But a known secret is no longer a secret. It is therefore difficult to imagine prospective studies or how to establish the statistics usual to research. Because of this, psychogenealogy is condemned to rely on individual cases, which may appear only anecdotal; nonetheless in view of the consistency of the mechanisms that emerge from their analyses one cannot be content with simply attributing them to chance.

It is probably not by chance that the pioneers of psychogenealogy originated in central and eastern Europe, countries profoundly scarred by the results of the Second World War. A study directed by the psychologist Nathalie Zajde amongst the descendants of Holocaust victims showed that they were frequently haunted by nightmares linked to the Nazi persecution. The precision of their nocturnal dreams is remarkable, and a good number of the subjects questioned said that they had suffered from such problems from a young age, even before their parents had mentioned their traumatising memories.[22] The re-emergence of the wounds of the past in the present perhaps offers them the opportunity of making them conscious and so healing them. The materialisation of an unspoken ill as an ill-ness then seems like an attempt to heal the individual, the family and even the society in which it evolves. That is, I am sure, why the trees of psychogenealogy grow in the field of post-war suffering. At a time when the ancestral memories are occluded by the rational pragmatism of Western science, it seems appropriate to help with this spontaneous impulse towards the forgotten past. Personally, I see in it a wider expression of a society which knows that no tree can grow without strengthening its roots.*

SHOW ME WHERE IT HURTS, AND I WILL TELL YOU WHY

The body's symbolism

Early in his career, Freud made several allusions to the role played by ancestors in the appearance of physical symptoms. However, he neglected to explore this transgenerational phenomenon in order to concentrate on the demonstration of the sexual origin of the neuroses.

---

* I develop these ideas in the chapter entitled 'Faire la paix avec les morts – La psychogénéalogie au secours des vivants', in J.P. de Tonnac and F. Lenoir (eds) *La Mort et l'immortalité. Encyclopédie des savoirs et des croyances*, Paris, Bayard, 2004, pp. 1655–1668.

Perhaps an unconscious reason prevented him from stirring up a memory that was too painful. Is it not troubling to learn that, haunted by the memory of a young brother who died of a gastric illness, Freud himself suffered violent stomach pains every time he visited his mother for a meal?[23]

The correlation seems obvious. The body sometimes expresses the conflicts that trouble the mind so clearly that the symbolism of these manifestations cannot be missed. Remember Frank who had been operated on for a gastric cancer and talked about the violence inflicted on him by his father as 'an undigested weight in the stomach' (see above, pp. 93–95).

Or Patricia who had received a liver transplant following an auto-immune hepatitis (see p. 101). Compelled to respond to the expectations of her parents, this young woman no longer knew what she wanted to be; she had no self-confidence; she admitted no dream. 'In fact, I have made myself into shit,' she wrote in her diary. 'Life made me into shit, everybody made me into shit.' At the same time she began to suffer from terrible diarrhoea. As if her body spoke for her, a new auto-immune illness – ulcerative colitis – was diagnosed. I also remember Pascale, a young woman of 35, recently operated on for breast cancer, who told me: 'I have always said that I would prefer to have a cancer than to be left by my husband.' Having discovered that her man had been unfaithful, she fulfilled her expectations…

Unfortunate coincidences? Mental set? Interpretations without objectivity dictated by the need to make sense of experiences? These questions need to be asked, though answering them is not simple. As we saw in Chapter 1, with the placebo effect a human being is conditioned by both biology and culture. Everything is expressed in language: innate, transmitted or acquired. His reflexes are subject to conditioning; his physiology is influenced by his beliefs; suggestion is at the centre of all his relationships; his survival is intimately dependent on his imaginative capacities.

Currently, there is no framework allowing us to understand clearly how memorised information or fantasies are able to work on our physiology and to use the body as a means of symbolic expression. Some researchers are therefore tempted to doubt the veracity of observed facts, to minimise the importance of the phenomena or even simply to deny their existence.

At the opposite extreme of this attitude, others do not hesitate to assert ways of reading psycho-physical symbolism, which they use to facilitate the insights, vital, according to them, for the healing of the patient. The German physician, Ryke Geerd Hamer, is the leader of a movement. In the 1980s he developed the idea of a 'New Medicine', in which an illness is thought of as the result of psychological conflicts rooted in the family or personal history of the patient. Based on a very detailed embryological rationale, precise correlations are described between each type of pathology and 'programming' and 'releasing' conflicts.[24] This theory is seductive, but has never been validated in a rigorously scientific way. If it were to be, there should additionally be evaluation of the degree to which becoming conscious of something psychological influences the healing of a bodily lesion. We have seen that there are cases, such as constipated or anorexic babies, in which verbalisation of a psychic conflict triggers off the resolution of a physical problem. Nonetheless, even when a psychological cause is believed to be the origin of an illness, we must not lose sight of the fact that some bodily processes are sometimes too advanced to be reversible. Humility is then in order, as is prudence.

Even so, following Hamer, numerous physicians and therapists recommend abandoning all treatment other than that which aims at bringing into consciousness the psychic conflicts hidden behind the physical symptoms. Rich in clinical experience, these decoders of bodily symbolism construct new theories, mixtures of 'new medicine', psycho-genealogy, and traditional inspirations. 'Total biology', 'psychosomatic analysis', 'psychobiological decoding' – such approaches are multiplying.[25] And the public is becoming increasingly interested, especially, it seems, in francophone countries. The growing success of this approach reveals an intense need for meaning which patients fail to satisfy in listening to the cold and rational explanations of scientific and technological medicine. 'The world has become disenchanted with too much materialism and reductionism', said Arnulfo, the Mexican healer we encountered in Chapter 1. A symbolic approach to the understanding of illnesses is perhaps a way of re-enchanting the human being.

The idea of a bodily symbolism is not new. It has been supported in the sacred literature of the great cultural traditions. Thus, in the same way that there is a disconcerting correspondence between the work of William Sheldon and the theories of *ayurveda* (see Chapter 5, pp. 84–85), we find similarities between the bodily symbolism in Hebrew, Indian and Chinese texts.[26] This is not surprising since all of these different approaches represent thousands of years of observations. Often they refer to the scientifically established functions of the different parts of the body and consequently their approach is stamped with logical deduction and common sense.[27]

The fact of drawing attention to the emotional meaning of bodily suffering can help certain alexithymic patients to put words to what they feel. From one association to another they can reassemble the chronology of their psychic suffering and admit problems long repressed. Even so, there is a danger in following this route because veneering a symptom with a complete explanation runs the risk of preventing bringing into consciousness a more profound suffering. In psychotherapy, even the 'bodily', questions are worth more than statements. It seems important to me to remember this; I have actually met numerous patients completely conditioned by the symbolic correlations imposed dogmatically upon them – to the point of re-inventing their personal histories in order to make them fit with the therapist's cause-and-effect diagnosis! This is a shame because a human being is much more important than a theory.

The keys for decoding bodily symbolism give the therapist a power of which he is not always conscious. And with good reason: a need to control the illness and the sufferer hides itself in the shadow of every therapist. (Fear of illness and of death, often unconscious, is discussed in Chapter 1, p. 17.) To ignore this is dangerous, the more so since patients often are ready to hand over their own power to 'one who knows'. Having myself experienced some of these approaches, I am convinced that, instead of imposing on the patient the meaning of his illness, it is better and right to help him express his own truth. Bernie Siegel, surgeon and pioneer of body–mind medicine, summarised this necessity well when he wrote: 'I have a dream, and this dream is to help patients to find their own dream.'[28] This takes time and patience – two virtues indispensable to all medicine.

Caution! Nocebo effect!

The interpretation of the symbolism of illnesses raises another problem. We saw in Chapter 1 that suggestion can influence the state of health and the appearance of symptoms. We must be on our guard lest certain theories favour the appearance of the diseases that they predict simply through a 'meaning effect' which indicates which diseases are valid for explaining a poor fit in a medical context or a specific culture.[29] 'In our society, the language of the body and of disease is the most acceptable that we have to talk about suffering', according to Anne Harrington, professor of the history of science at Harvard.[30]

The story of Sylvia and her sister Nora illustrates this very well. At the time that I saw her for a consultation, Sylvia complained of pain in her left knee. Lying down on the table with difficulty, she began to explain: 'I read in a book that it developed because of my divorce. Pathology in a knee is always connected with a difficulty about flexibility, accepting things as they are. The left side is the *yang* side, that is, the masculine: my ex. I have not accepted that my husband has left me.' When I did not reply, Sylvia continued: 'The only thing that bothers me is the left side because I saw a therapist who told me that it is the side of femininity, and that does not fit with what I had read in my book about the meanings of illnesses. About the divorce I am certain: it is the cause of the inflammation in my knee. But one of my friends lent me another book. According to that, with a *"genou"* [knee] it is always a problem of *"je-nous"* [I – us]. It's obvious: it's all about me and my relationship with my ex-husband.' Irritated by my silence, the young woman added: 'What do you think, Doctor? I know that you have an open mind for all these things. No? Not like my brother. Imagine: he dared laugh at me. And when I talked to him about the theory of *"je-nous"* he asked how I would translate that into Chinese or English!'

I answered that the stress due to her divorce had perhaps favoured the appearance of the inflammation in her knee. All the same, other causes were possible. The only thing of which she could be certain was that the end of her 'couple' represented an extremely painful trauma for her. The wound was perhaps so vivid that the least pain in her body was an occasion for her to talk about her psychological suffering. This did not necessarily mean that there was a real cause and effect connection. This reply seemed to me to be the only one that an 'open mind' (as she said) could give to her question. At the present time, no serious study has been carried out to examine the truth of the theories of the bodily symbology, and it has to be said that some of them contradict each other.

'You are too Cartesian, Doctor. I am certain: this knee is the result of my divorce. You must help me free myself of my negative emotions. If not, it will never heal!' The die was cast. Her reading and her therapist had strongly conditioned Sylvia. In the weeks that followed, she felt very guilty at the fact that she could not heal her emotional suffering more quickly. 'My knee reminds me that I must bend, Doctor. Alas, I can't, so I go on suffering in my body.' As we worked on this feeling of guilt, Sylvia's pain diminished progressively, though not without the help of several sessions of acupuncture and even, on some days, anti-inflammatory medication. 'The pain is gone, but even so I still have not digested this divorce,' she said with surprise. I remarked that she had 'bent' in another way: she had accepted her own emotions and put her beliefs completely in perspective.

Several months later, Nora, Sylvia's sister, consulted me. She too suffered from an inflammation of the left knee. When I suggested treatment by acupuncture, she explained that that would be useless. 'I understand it all,' she told me. 'This pain is caused by my boyfriend. I can't stand that he goes away at weekends with his friends. I am jealous. It's a problem of "*je-nous*". I cannot accept the relationship in which we actually live.'

Nora seemed to somatise her psychological stress in the same area as her sister had claimed that her emotional setbacks had shown in her own body. It was as though the knee had become a shared means of expression between the two sisters. I therefore explained to Nora that the interpretation of the origin of the problem belonged to the culture that produced them. Some African sorcerer would perhaps have advised her to protect herself against an evil spell cast by an enemy. Another, perhaps an Amerindian healer, might have expelled the spirit of an angry ancestor. For now, I suggested that she should relax by seeing a Vietnamese masseuse who lived a few doors away from herself…

7
TOUCHING THE BODY THAT RELAXES

A FUNDAMENTAL NEED

Breaking a taboo

Wilhelm Reich probably never considered himself to be a rebel when he decided to include the body in his analytic practice. On the contrary, the reunion of the mental and the physical seemed to him to be at the centre of Freud's vision. The problem was that, in order to succeed, Reich did not hesitate to upset several established dogmas. Touching a patient and putting oneself face to face with him in order to create contact – that method was judged to be heretical. Adding Reich's communistic ideas put him beyond the pale of the psychoanalytic movement.

All the same, Freud himself explained the importance he gave to the body in his earliest cures, when he kneaded and applied pressure to the legs of his patients, massaged and stroked their painful abdomens or pressed their heads between his hands in order to assist the revival of their old memories.[1] One may well ask about the reasons which, very soon, led to the banning of bodily contact in psychoanalytic practice.

Part of the answer lies in the beliefs and prohibitions dominant at the end of the 19th century. Think about the time when Luther Emmett Holt, eminent professor of psychiatry at Cornell University, advocated – in a book which was a best-seller even as late as the 1930s – that an infant should never be comforted, but left to cry for as long as necessary for him to become quiet. In the same period, John Watson, a founding father of behavioural psychology, wrote: 'There is only one rational way of treating children: never take them in your arms, do not embrace them, never take them on your knee. If necessary, give them a kiss on the forehead when they go to bed and a handshake in the morning.'[2]

Such statements remind us that medical science is not protected from intellectual blindness. It is tragic to see entire generations following the advice of specialists who are convinced by such extremely doubtful truths.

'When the gods die and value systems collapse, only the body remains for the human race in its search for landmarks,' was said to me by a yogi whom I met at Thanjavur in the south of India. We cannot wonder that the Occident, having lost itself in the shadows of ideological battles, now strives to recover the wisdom of the body. The skin, the muscles and the bones are not abstract concepts. On the contrary, they are tangible objects which express an objective reality. Suddenly, a whole series of therapies, physical and psychological, arose, centred again on the body – and, a sign of the times, more and more people with illnesses turned to them.

Nonetheless, the prohibitions of the 19th century are still powerful in the background. There reigns in the West a terrible confusion between love, sex, feelings and touching. And let us not deceive ourselves: the fear that hides behind avoiding physical contact is that of sexual arousal and abuse. With this background, it is not surprising that many people, physicians and therapists included, avoid touching the body of their patient.

This must surely be regretted, since touching is a very powerful form of communication. Numerous studies have shown that the simple fact of being touched when meeting someone profoundly influences our attitude. In a restaurant, for example, customers who have been touched by the waiters leave a bigger tip, even if they do not consider that the food or the service were of particularly good quality, than the clients who had not had any physical contact.[3] In another study, students who had been touched by a librarian when they borrowed a book, had more positive feelings towards the library even if the bodily contact lasted only half a second and even though half of them did not remember the contact.[4]

Learning to touch and to let oneself be touched in complete security: this aspect of human relationships must be taught to all and particularly to health professionals, in order that they may integrate touch in their practice without ambiguity and within the boundaries defined by their therapeutic framework.

The resistances and inhibitions shown, especially in certain workshops which I arranged for health professionals, are especially important. I remember a fellow surgeon of about 40 who considered it 'absolutely ridiculous' to have to form a circle in which each participant massaged the back of another. It had been his assistant who had encouraged him to join this 'masquerade'. He certainly never shook hands with patients and some of them complained of having to go into the scanner without his having laid a finger on their abdomens, because 'technology is sufficient to diagnose tumours' he had explained with full conviction. Evidently, this brilliant technician never took account of the fact that ill people expect and merit more than a simple diagnostic procedure on the part of their therapist. 'If they come to talk and be touched, they need only consult a "psy",' he retorted, a little irritated.

A psychotherapist, formerly practising as a psychoanalyst, who also participated in the workshop, explained that many therapists and, *a fortiori*, some psychoanalysts, were as unable as some physicians to touch a patient. 'Really! As though they had gone to see a masseur!' replied the surgeon, more and more irritated. I allowed myself to remark to him that that did not prevent his patients from feeling a need to be reassured by his touch – because, whatever specialist with whom they have business, patients are not made up of separate pieces. To touch someone is to recognise them in their totality. My colleague shrugged his shoulders. I therefore put a kindly hand on his back.

At the end of the day, when we came back into the circle as in the morning, I saw a childlike smile illuminate the face of the surgeon. He clearly had a great sense of well-being from having touched and been touched by the other members of the group. In leaving the workshop he suddenly began to sob. Several days later, I received a letter from him describing his sorrow at having waited so long to experience this quality of contact. He felt the sorrow of never having been touched by his parents in his childhood. The letter ended: 'Obviously, this is not very scientific!' Wrong.

The first of the senses

The skin, originating from the ectoderm, is the largest organ of the body: about 600,000 tactile receptors connected to the spinal cord and to the brain by more than half a million nerves. An immense sensory receptor turned towards the outside world: 'the skin is no more separated from the brain than the surface of a lake is from its depths…. they are two points on a continuum… it is a single functional unit from the cortex to the fingertips. To touch the surface is to shake the depths,'[5] wrote Deane Juhan, former professor at the Esalen Institute in California. Some consider the skin as the exterior surface of the brain, and that the brain constitutes the deepest layer of the skin.

Eight weeks after conception, at a time when the embryo measures no more than two centimetres, the skin is already well-developed. The first of the senses to appear in the course of evolution (unicellular organisms have a sensitivity to contact) touch is therefore the first of the senses developed in the foetus.

The need for being touched and touching is essential and universal. It is found in every species and every culture. Baby mice die if they are not suckled and baby monkeys huddle in a corner of their cage if they are deprived of contact. Without being touched, growth and development are impossible. This is, naturally, why traditional societies encourage contact between mother and child. Amongst the San hunter-gatherers in the Kalahari, for instance, it has been calculated that mothers carry their baby more than 90% of the time. In the United States, this is reduced to two or three hours a day during the first three months of life, and even less later.[6]

The reduction of tactile stimulation in our societies worries the specialists. Already in the 1950s the work of Harry Harlow showed that baby monkeys preferred a mother-substitute stuffed with soft material to one made with wire wool, even if the latter provided nourishment.[7] Subsequently, an experiment on baby monkeys placed behind a barrier of Plexiglass through which they could smell, see and hear their mother showed that, amongst all possible sensations, it was that of touch which was indispensable for their harmonious development and the maintenance of good immunity.[8]

The psychiatrist René Spitz compared the development of nursing babies raised by their mother in the prison in which the latter had been confined, with those of babies separated from their mothers and placed in a crèche where they received the best medical, dietetic and hygienic care possible from an overworked staff. Contrary to what might be imagined, the babies raised in the comfort of the crèche developed much less well than those that stayed in prison. Separated from their mothers, the former lacked an essential: the staff looking after the babies did not have the time to take them in their arms and communicate a little affection.[9]

Lack of tactile stimulation results in a reduction in the production of growth hormone, sleep difficulties and a stress that damages the immune system. Infants deprived of contact with their mother show more constipation, diarrhoea and respiratory infections.[10] It also seems that eczema and allergies are similarly more frequent in children who have been insufficiently touched.[11] The famous anthropologist Ashley Montagu tells the story of two young asthmatic women. Twins, their mother had died at their birth, and they had been cruelly deprived of touching contact during their childhood. Montagu had advised one of these young women to have a massage regularly. Her asthmatic attacks ended not long afterwards. Several years later the health of her sister improved following her marriage. Unfortunately, after she became divorced, she died of a renewed respiratory crisis.[12]

Numerous reports provide evidence of a connection between lack of being touched and aggression in children. Cultural differences may be involved in this phenomenon. Thus a study carried out by the American psychologist, Tiffany Field, in two McDonald's restaurants, one in Paris, the other in Miami, showed that the French mothers touched their children more often than the American. There was a related observation: in the fast-food play area, the young French children showed themselves to be less aggressive toward other children than the young Americans.[13]

Another study carried out in the same restaurants showed that French adolescents touch each other more than the Americans. However, the young Americans touched themselves more often – and were more aggressive than their French opposite numbers.[14]

Our non-touching civilisation does not take account of the damage it produces. In the face of the growth of violence and behaviour problems such as attention-deficit hyperactivity disorders, it is certainly important to encourage more tactile contact,[15] especially in the crèches and infant schools where the young children pass the greater part of their time.

THE OLDEST OF MEDICINES

The hand of the heart

Touch is probably the oldest means of healing. More than 2,000 years before our era, Egyptian bas-reliefs display rubbing of the hands and feet. In both India and China no system of medicine was without deep and scrupulously codified massage. In Greece, Hippocrates insisted that every physician must be trained in 'the art of friction', and the *kheirourgos* – the ancestors of our surgeons – treated their patients above all with the palms of their hands and the tips of their fingers on the skin. In Rome, the famous physician Galen followed the example of the god Aesculapius, son of Apollo, who healed by touching.

Subsequently the religious prohibitions of the Church in the Middle Ages and the dawn of treatment by medication progressively deleted massage from the Western therapeutic arsenal. That is, until in the 18th century, inspired by a knowledge of anatomy and physiology as well as certain traditional concepts of the nordic peoples, the Swedish physician, Henrik Ling developed a technique of massage which migrated to the United States in the luggage of Scandinavian emigrants.

However, the real rehabilitation of massage in Western culture took place much later at the Esalen Institute in California. At this institute, founded by Michael Murphy and Richard Price, philosophers, anthropologists, psychologists, artists and theologians met to examine what Aldous Huxley had called 'The Human Potential'. Sessions of meditation, prayer meetings, group therapies and body-work: there were many and varied pathways of exploration. Naturally, the benefits of touching found a special place there.

With its effleurage (light touching or brushing), kneading, percussion, tapping and rubbing, massage helps those who receive it to recover awareness of their own bodies. Boundaries are made conscious, separated parts are brought together and reintegrated into a coherent whole, and the individual is confirmed in his identity throughout the globality of his body.[16] Massaging someone signals to him that he is accepted in his entirety.

The message is strong. A deep relaxation comes about. One may think this to be quite ordinary in that the fact of being massaged by another person raises positive sensations which stimulate the left cerebral cortex and the parasympathetic system that governs muscular relaxation. This psychological mechanism, however, is not the whole story. Massaging the skin leads to a direct neural arousal which, at the cerebral level, stimulates the posterior part of the hypothalamus without passing through the cortex and, from there, stimulates generalised parasympathetic muscular relaxation.[17] For this reason, the massage does not need to be complete to achieve these effects. Massaging the feet or the calves is enough to trigger the relaxation of the whole body, hence the usefulness of massaging oneself regularly to rid oneself of the tensions accumulated in the course of the day.

As a young surgeon, I worked several months in an Intensive Care Unit. Convinced of the benefits of massage, I encouraged the medical team to massage the feet of the patients three times a day. Unmistakeably, the parasympathetic stimulation aroused by the massage reduced arterial pressure and slowed the heart rate of the patients, even if they were in coma. Therefore it is not necessary to be conscious to benefit from touch. Moreover, with children in distress born without a cerebral cortex but with an intact limbic system, stroking produces muscular relaxation and stops crying.[18] Thus every time that one touches someone one acts directly on his emotional brain. The warmth of the skin needs no words to communicate. To paraphrase Aristotle one could say: 'the heart is the organ of touching'.

It is then not surprising that one can communicate with the baby *in utero*, as was shown by Frans Veldman, inventor of haptonomy (from the Greek *haptein*: touch and *nomos*: rule).[19] It is equally unsurprising to see patients with Alzheimer's disease come out of their torpor, their faces lighting up, when they receive a caress. If the intention is positive, touch stimulates positive feelings and all the physiological concomitants that follow.

A study carried out on disturbed children in a paediatric service demonstrated the superiority of physical touch when compared with verbal contact. Divided into two groups children were consoled either by words or picked up, cradled and caressed. In the course of 40 sessions of spoken comfort only seven children appeared to feel an effective calming, while tactile comforting worked in 53 cases out of 60.[20]

Another study carried out in a delivery suite showed that a comforting touch helps anxious women to relax and to feel less pain, while words brought no help.[21]

When I worked in a hospital, every evening I went to say 'good night' to the patients before going home. I sat for a few minutes on each bed, put a hand on their leg or stroked their hand and waited for their eyes to shine again. This ritual dispersed the pains of the day and prepared the patient for a night of recovery. At first, anxious to get home, I tended to cut these visits short. However, my 'evening round' soon became virtually a drug because, as well as feeling the pleasure of helping to produce the change that appeared in the patients, I took away with me a deep relaxation and feeling of well-being. In fact, touching is a gift that one gives another *and* oneself. Thus the elderly people whom the psychologist Tiffany Field asked to massage young children, or alternatively allow themselves to be massaged by someone else, indicated major changes in their habitual ways: more social contacts, a lower consumption of coffee, better sleep, better morale and fewer visits to the doctor. Contrary to what one might expect, the effects were more pronounced in those who *gave* the massage than in those who *received* it.[22]

A SCIENTIFIC BASIS

As is the case for so many scientists, it was personal significance that led Tiffany Field to choose her area of research. Herself the mother of a premature child, she noticed that babies born before term gained more weight, had better scores on neurological tests and were discharged earlier if they had been massaged during their period in an incubator.[23] Many researchers before her had tried to help the babies by touching them, but their massage seems to have been too light. A good massage acts in depth, stimulates the activity of the organs, increases the digestive secretions, liquifies the respiratory mucous, stimulates the sebaceous glands, induces sweating and promotes the excretion of toxins. By augmenting parasympathetic activity, it leads to a reduction of stress, a lowering of the blood level of cortisol and improved immune function. Increased quantities of growth hormone are produced as well as oxytocin, a hormone that promotes attachment and the building of relationships.[24]

Convinced of the positive effects of touching, Tiffany Field founded the Touch Research Institute in 1992 at the University of Miami in Florida. Some researchers at several Universities – Harvard, Duke and Maryland – joined this venture and the Institute supported work at three other centres, in Los Angeles, Paris, and the Philippines. The project was ambitious and the results fruitful, since at last the practice of massage began to be taken seriously by the scientific community.

To begin with a psychological viewpoint, Tiffany Field showed that a back massage of around half an hour during five consecutive days considerably improved the morale of adolescents hospitalised because of depression. These patients became less anxious, much more co-operative, had better sleep and showed a reduced level of cortisol.[25] Another study, carried out with anorexic women, showed that regular massage was followed by a reduction in symptoms of stress and anxiety, as well as a lowering of the level of cortisol. These patients developed a better body-image and had fewer difficulties over eating.[26] Recording cortical activity during a massage showed that depressed adolescents had selective activity in the hemispheres, in that the activity of the right hemisphere – relating to negative emotions – was reduced, to the benefit of the left hemisphere – on which depends good or positive mood.[27] Further, in the same way that antidepressant medication acts, massage increases the levels of dopamine and serotonin.

We know intuitively that massage relieves pain, and this is confirmed by observation. In the case of sufferers from migraine, for instance, being massaged for 30 minutes twice a week over five weeks reduces anxiety, improves sleep, raises the level of serotonin and significantly reduces the frequency of migraines, when compared with a group of patients who had benefitted from a programme of relaxation which did not involve touching.[28] The positive effects of massage have been studied and demonstrated in patients suffering from fibromyalgia, severe burns, various inflammatory disorders, metastases, or postoperative pain.[29] However, the mechanisms involved have not been completely elucidated. We know that the stimulation of mechanoreceptors in the skin activates the high speed nerve fibres capable of inhibiting the pain signals to the brain which travel via the low speed fibres. Thus when you bang your knee, energetic rubbing reduces the pain you feel. We know also that the increase in serotonin arising from massage inhibits the passage of pain signals to the brain. Finally, an energetic massage involves the cortical production of endorphins which, like morphine, inhibit the perception of pain and produce a sensation of well-being.[30]

Massage equally exerts an influence on the immune defences. Thus patients who are seropositive to AIDS have benefitted from a daily massage over a month. Less anxious and less depressed, they showed a reduction in cortisol and a significant increase in the NK cells of the immune system.[31] Another study amongst adolescents infected with HIV showed that massage was more effective than simple relaxation to obtain these psychological effects and the NK cell increase.[32] John, the patient whose experience we heard in Chapter 4 (pp. 59–61), was therefore wise in choosing to be massaged, even if his doctor thought it served no purpose.

In the same way, a study carried out on women with breast cancer showed that a massage of 30 minutes three times a week for five weeks reduced anxiety, depression and anger. These improvements were correlated with a raised level of serotonin and dopamine as well as an increase of lymphocytes and NK cells capable of destroying cancerous cells.[33]

Finally, the effects of massage have been evaluated in asthmatic children. Those children who had a 20 minute massage every evening for a month before going to bed showed an overall improvement in their symptoms and the respiratory passages when compared with other children receiving daily sessions of relaxation.[34] The same protocol used with diabetic children demonstrated that blood sugar level returned to normal, and the level of stress hormones diminished.[35]

There is therefore no dearth of studies showing the benefits of massage. Efficacy and cost-effectiveness compel us to pay attention. Medical practice is also beginning to take an interest in the benefits of this oldest of medicines. A recent study in one company tested the effect of a massage carried out in a sitting position for 20 minutes twice a week over two months on a hundred employees. Compared with others who only had 20 minutes of rest in a quiet setting, the massaged subjects had a better morale, managed their emotions more easily, slept more deeply, were more satisfied with their work and showed a significant improvement in blood pressure.[37]

One might think that this kind of massage 'softened' the employees. On the contrary: the parasympathetic stimulation and the positive emotions which are associated with that, improved intellectual performance and increased vigilance (see Chapter 2, p. 31). Thus a study comparing brain activity between subjects resting and others receiving massage showed brain waves characteristic of relaxation states, but in the massage group there appeared some waves indicating a relaxed but alert state close to that of meditation. In fact, the massaged subjects, when given a series of mathematical calculations to carry out, completed their tasks more quickly and more accurately than the others.[38]

A gesture as natural as that which consists of touching the surface of the body influences the mind in a significant way. What happens if one acts more deeply, at the level of the skeleton, the connective tissue, the blood vessels, the nerves and the organs? To understand that, we must explore the fascinating architecture of the human body.

8
ALIGNING THE BODY THAT BALANCES ITSELF

THE ARCHITECTURE OF LIFE

Life and the force of gravity

Fortunate indeed are those who have had the chance of admiring the works of the American sculptor Kenneth Snelson. Without their knowing it, their eyes have scanned the complicated architecture which, from a virus to a human being, is that from which life is constructed. At Washington, for example, in the garden of sculptures of the Hirshhorn Museum, an elegant 'Needle Tower' rises to 20 metres in height. Composed of an astonishing interweaving of metallic rods linked together by suspended wires, it seems to be extremely fragile. However, if you push it, it goes back to its original form – and when the wind blows, it bends but does not break.

In fact, this fragile structure is a system in 'tensegrity' (a contraction of *tensional integrity*), a word invented by the brilliant designer of geodesic domes, the architect Richard Buckminster Fuller, to describe the ability of a structure to remain stable through the interplay of forces of tension and compression distributed between the different elements of which it is composed.

A system in tensegrity is therefore self-stabilising. An increase of tension in one of the elements is transmitted to all the others, however far removed. In Snelson's sculptures, the wires distribute the tension and the rods carry the pressure. At any given moment, some forces push and others pull. The whole is dynamic, flexible and robust.

Faced with the force of gravity exercised upon the whole of the material, tensegrity offers the most economical solution in terms of lightness and strength. It is therefore not surprising to see these principles applied at all evolutionary stages of living creatures. At the microscopic level, the double helix of DNA and the configuration of proteins are stabilised by tensegrity. At the macroscopic level, the 206 bones of the human skeleton are compressed by the force of gravity and stabilised in a vertical position thanks to the traction exercised by the muscles, tendons and ligaments. At the least impact, the mechanical energy is distributed throughout the whole structure in such a way that, if one part of the body is subjected to tension, the whole is affected. In a configuration that is vital, the different ligaments form a structure capable of supporting the weight of the body without compressing the spinal column.

The bones, muscles, ligaments and tendons can therefore be regarded as a system in tensegrity. Because of this, the least shortening or the weakest stiffening reduces the capacity of the body to absorb pressure or deformation.[1] On the other hand, as in a kind of 'anatomic unity', an injury at one point favours the appearance of other lesions remote from the site of injury.[2] The opposite is equally true: improvement of flexibility in one area influences the restoration and healing of the whole.

In the case of a slight physical trauma, the various elements recover their normal position. The body again finds its best adaptation to gravity; the nervous system transmits information in an optimal way, the circulation flows smoothly, lymphatic drainage works easily and the organs function at their best. On the other hand, if the trauma is more serious, or combines with lesions that have not been completed healed, distortions of some structures and limitations of movement become permanently established.[3] The compensatory changes which follow provoke stretching in the neural elements, blockages in the circulatory system and alterations in the lymphatic circulation. Certain underused muscles become atrophied; others subject to more demand become hypertrophied. The distribution of load between the different parts of the body changes. This involves a reshaping of the bony structure and the body undergoes real deformation.

As we saw in Chapter 5 with Wilhelm Reich (pp. 85–87), muscular contractions due to chronic emotional stress also provoke important morphological changes. Once chronically shortened, muscular fibres lose the capacity to relax. The ease of movement with which the body evolved in the context of gravity is then reduced. Some structures wear out prematurely, some organs suffer and a whole series of pathologies are set up. The word 'disease' – better: 'dis-ease' – translates this process very well.

At the beginning of the 20th century, Joel Goldthwait, orthopaedist at Harvard noticed that numerous pathologies were consequences of poor alignment of the body.[4] For example, in the case of a person who has a tendency to push the head forward, the deviation of the spinal column provokes a curvature of the vertebral arteries which reduces their calibre, the blood flow slows and disturbances of cerebral metabolism follows. These may unbalance the sympathetic/parasympathetic equilibrium from which follow digestive or cardiac problems, as well as emotional disturbances. All this is accompanied by a speeding up of wear in the cartilages of the cervix, which in the long term produces a painful and handicapping degenerative arthritis.

These chains of consequences and effects have been confirmed by other researchers. They are aggravated by age because, in time, the tissues lose their flexibility and the reparatory processes become less effective.[5] It is an essential means for the maintenance of health to maintain an optimal alignment of the body in relation to the gravitational force of the Earth. This is exactly what is suggested by the technique of 'Structural Integration' – or Rolfing – designed by Ida Rolf (see Chapter 6, pp. 96–97). The palpation and pressure of the 'Rolfer' act directly on the connective tissues of the organism, especially the ligaments, tendons and fascias around the muscles, organs, nerves, blood and lymphatic vessels, and thus on every cell of the body.

These 'connective' tissues, as is suggested by their name, are then the links between the different structures of the body. Without them there is neither shape nor tensegrity. The collagen fibres of which they are made are bathed in an amorphous substance (a colloidal gel) with semi-liquid properties. A contraction of the tissues leads to their dehydration; on the other hand, stretching and relaxation stimulate hydration.[6] The pressures applied in Rolfing can modify the viscosity of the colloidal gel. This is why it is important to rehydrate oneself after such a session. Ligaments, tendons and fascias become more supple, the body realigns itself, and, as Ida Rolf said: 'Gravity becomes the therapist.'[7] At the microscopic level, the increased porosity of the colloidal gel permits a better diffusion of oxygen, nutriments, enzymes and the substances produced by the cellular metabolism. Evacuation of waste material and toxins is eased because deep massage stimulates the blood and lymphatic circulation. The regeneration of the tissues and their cells is immediate.

The living matrix

For a long time, biologists represented the cell as a sac made up of a membrane containing a viscous gel similar to that of the extracellular connective tissues, in which the molecules float in solution. This now appears a little simplistic. In reality, the cell is occupied by a network of microfilaments and microtubules which constitute a veritable intracellular skeleton. This 'cytoskeleton' is connected to the conjunctive tissues via transmembranous proteins, and, an important detail, it extends as far as the chromosomes of the cell nucleus.[8] Thus from the skin to the DNA, a network of fibres, tubules and filaments form a continuum, a 'living matrix' the role of which is beginning to become clear.

During the 1970s, Donald Ingber, a young student of cellular biology at Yale had a happy intuition: while contemplating a sculpture by Snelson, he realised that the cytoskeleton behaves like a tensegrity system.[9]

For Ingber, who has since become a professor at Harvard, the properties of the intracellular network define the changes of the shape of the cell. In addition, because of the linkages established by the microtubules and the microfilaments between the nucleus and the cellular surface, the least pull on a receptor on the membrane – for example if a molecule becomes attached – affects the whole of the cell, including the chromosomes. Now we know that the majority of the molecules, especially the enzymes that we believe float in solution in the cell, are in fact attached to the microtubules and microfilaments of the cytoskeleton. The biochemical reactions that follow are therefore not by chance: they are guided by the intracellular structure. Consequently, every mechanical change of the cytoskeleton influences its cellular chemistry, the activation of the genes, and the manufacture of proteins coded by the DNA.

There is therefore a relationship between the structure and cellular functioning. In an article published in *Science*, Ingber's team showed that the shape of the cells controls certain genetic programmes through the 'living matrix'. Distributed in small numbers over a surface, the cells can flatten and their cytoskeleton, drawn out, begins the genetic programme of cellular division. On the other hand, if there are many cells, the lack of space compels them to reduce their volume, and the cytoskeleton, then contracted, begins the programme of cellular death. The shape of cells therefore controls their proliferation. Thus, if injured, the cells, being very flattened, 'feel' through their cytoskeleton the necessity of large-scale multiplication to heal the wound.[10] This confirms what we said in the previous chapter: touch and kinaesthesia (perception of position and movement) are the earliest sensations, the oldest senses already present at the unicellular stage and common to all living organisms.

In fact, the 'living matrix', both extra- and intra-cellular, constitutes a system of communication at once mechanical and biochemical, having developed long before the nervous, vascular, hormonal or immune systems, when an organism was made up of a small number of cells. It is then not surprising that this matrix exerts a dominant influence on the reparatory processes of the organism. From this point of view, the work of Ingber opens totally new perspectives on medical research. It also constitutes a scientific basis for understanding various treatment methods, even as far as those purely empirical treatments which, lacking a satisfying scientific explanation, were often played down or even rejected by scientific medicine.

Thus balancing posture and harmonising movement do not act solely on aligning nerves, vessels and organs in their optimal functional positions. In accordance with the principles of tensegrity, the least of these repositionings acts on the skin, the bones, the muscles, the tendons, the ligaments and all the fascias which surround even the smallest structures in the body. Inevitably, the connective tissues which unite the cells between themselves are also mobilised and, by extension, the cytoskeleton controls the biochemical and genetic changes that lie at the heart of every cell of the organism.[11]

THE FLUIDITY OF MOVEMENT

The good use of self

Frederick Matthias Alexander did not know anything of these fascinating discoveries, and for good reason: he lived at the end of the 18th century. His name would never have become part of the world of alternative and complementary medicines had he not suffered from recurrent laryngitis that put his career as an actor in jeopardy. Having consulted numerous specialists without finding help, Alexander decided to seek for the solution to his problem himself, hence the originality of his approach. From being passive, he became proactive. In looking at himself in a mirror, he noticed a slight shortening of his body every time he began to speak, as though an unconscious fear prevented himself from holding himself straight. He deduced that this bodily 'habit' caused a laryngeal malfunction which predisposed him to the hoarseness of which he suffered. He therefore decided to correct his posture by making it more upright. However, his tension reinforced the contraction of his larynx: the solution was not to be found in bodily control. On the contrary. In developing an acute awareness of his body, Alexander came to understand that his attempts to correct his posture interfered with a balanced posture and harmoniously co-ordinated movements. He concluded by deciding that there is no correct posture: the important point is the relationship between posture and movement, the target being to find bodily ease. From that moment his voice never let him down.[12]

Having devoted a decade to experimenting along these lines, Alexander developed a technique designed to unlearn bad habits. Awareness of oneself, maintained intention and a sense of responsibility were the essential pillars of his thought. This did not involve learning particular exercises or positions; it was, above all, a question of a 'good use of self' – the word 'self' being preferred to 'body', to underline the necessity of regarding the individual in his entirety.[13]

Alexander really knew nothing about anatomy or physiology. His capacity for observation and his good sense were enough. He did not consider himself a therapist before his patients, but really as an 'educator' addressing his 'pupils'. His approach had considerable success in the artistic and theatrical world, as well as amongst numerous scientists, amongst them Nikolaas Tinbergen, who praised the merits of Alexander's work in the speech he gave when receiving the Nobel Prize in medicine in 1973.[14]

Learning to feel the pressure, the weight, the position and the tone of the body upright, seated, lying down, and walking, in no matter what everyday activity, Alexander's principles echoed those of Buckminster Fuller: posture and movement must respect tensegrity. This explains the marvellous sensation of ease and lightness that one feels after a lesson devoted to his technique. In the light of Ingber's work, one can imagine how this postural re-education can influence the repair of even the most fragile zones – down to the level of cellular biology.

Nonetheless, like the majority of bodily approaches, the Alexander technique cruelly lacks basic studies to convince the sceptics of its medical interest. Those who have experimented with it feel less fatigue and tension at work, they improve their physical performance, and they are less easily damaged by repetitive movements in, for example, dancing or playing a musical instrument. They speak also of the disappearance of some chronic pains, they have a better sense of balance and fall less often. Their respiratory capacity increases, they suffer less from asthma, migraine, or symptoms such as that of irritable colon. Often they say that they gain in self-confidence, recover their self-esteem and feel less depressed.[15] This approach seems to improve both health and the quality of life. It deserves to be evaluated according to the criteria of scientific objectivity, in the manner of a study published in 2002 which showed that people suffering from Parkinson's disease who practised the Alexander technique gained a lasting improvement in both their physical capacity and their morale.[16]

In the meantime, as I was told by a patient who was very pleased that he had resorted to this technique: 'The Alexander technique has preventive virtues which should make people learn it because who, from infancy on, has not adopted bad postural habits?'

The intelligence of the body

Lynn was 45 years old. Over two years of her life, nothing had gone right: she was divorced, her children were in the middle of adolescent crises, she worked too much, she was exhausted, she had a bad back, she felt depressed. Six months before she first came to see me, a cancerous tumour on her right kidney had been removed. A sombre picture, then. When I met her I was immediately struck by her strange way of walking: the legs stiff and hesitant, her pelvis and thorax as though welded together, the neck curved forwards and her shoulders raised as though pulled by wires. She looked like a badly articulated wooden marionette. No accident and no illness explained the frozen aspect of her posture, nor the bad co-ordination of her movements. It was in her eyes that I found the answer to my questions: it was patently obvious that she was frightened, even terrified. The loss of her parents when she was four years old; a difficult school career, during which, she recalled, her teachers made her anxious; learning to read and write always put her 'under tension'; and, later, work as a secretary 'sitting all day in front of a computer' – enough to deform a body for life – without taking into account a rape when she was 14 years old, and the aunt who had brought her up and projected onto her all her own fears. Every time Lynn took an initiative, her aunt warned her to be careful, to the point when the girl no longer dared to cross the road alone.

One cannot tell at what point the fears of adults inhibit the spontaneity of children, and at the same time interfere with the acquisition of new movements. Because of fear, the child prevents the natural intelligence of the body from expressing itself. By such restrictions or limitations, the possibilities for the body's adaptation are reduced and a feeling of insecurity creates anxiety, which encourages further limitations. The individual then loses all self-confidence.

Moshe Feldenkrais described this process well.[17] Like Alexander, Feldenkrais did not belong to the medical world. An engineer with a PhD in physics, fascinated by martial arts, he founded the Judo Club of France in 1936. Like Alexander, it was seeking a solution to a problem of his own (a damaged knee) which launched him on the conscious exploration of his body. Profiting from his sporting experience, his thorough knowledge of mechanics, of psychology, anatomy and neurophysiology, he arrived at an original method designed to recover the intelligence of the body.

I advised Lynn to take lessons from a Feldenkrais Method teacher. The results were spectacular. Lying on the ground, Lynn became aware that she suffered from a virtual sensory and motor amnesia. 'It was as though there were parts of my body that were dead or missing,' she explained, surprised that she had not noticed this before. Then, by simple movements she regained the spontaneity and efficiency that she had lost a long time earlier. An anodyne posture, like taking a strong pressure on both legs, allowed her to test a confidence which she had never known. Straightening out her torso, relaxing her shoulders and throwing out her chest made her feel that she had inner resources that she had underestimated. 'In that position, it is impossible to feel depressed,' she concluded enthusiastically. And when the teacher demanded that she smile, she said spontaneously, in surprise, that this 'grimace' had created a good mood.

Thus one's psychological state influences one's physical state and in return the posture of one's body changes one's mental state. All learning is facilitated by new stimuli. By increasing certain movements one generates new information for the brain; this then reorganises its sensory and motor connections and the body is freed from its limitations.[18] The self-image is automatically modified, because, as Antonio Damasio showed, the sense of self is the result of the integration of information deriving from the body at the level of the brain.[19] Therefore it is the very identity of the individual that is redefined in the course of body-work.

This is the basis of the way in which the Feldenkrais Method is shown to be effective, as much in patients handicapped by the sequelae of accidents or neurological diseases as amongst people limited by physical pain or psychological problems. It is also claimed that it can help the elderly in preventing falls, to maintain a good self-image, and to avoid sinking into depression.

Clearly, even if this has not yet been confirmed by formal scientific research, the methods of Alexander and Feldenkrais have an action that is both physical and psychological: physically, in restoring tensegrity necessary for the optimal functioning of the body and its living matrix; mentally, in allowing a better awareness of the bodily schema at the level of the brain. Here the feeling of well-being is not due to a sporting activity augmenting the production of endorphins. There is no effort to exert, no suffering to endure. All is done gently, respecting the solutions appropriate to each individual. This is the psycho-corporal integration that produces feelings of stability, security and completeness.

Real models of somatic education, the methods of Alexander and Feldenkrais opened the way to a whole series of other approaches. A particular instance is the 'anti-gymnastic' approach, developed by the French physiotherapist Thérèse Bertherat in the 1970s, who began with the work of Wilhelm Reich on the 'armoured body' and the discoveries of Françoise Mézières on the posterior muscular chain from the neck to the big toes.[20] Another example is the Pilates Method devised in the 1920s by a German, Joseph Pilates, deriving from his experience of dance, yoga and Zen meditation, which became popular during the 1990s amongst a public frustrated by the poor bodily awareness developed in body-building, aerobic exercises or the lessons of classical gymnastics.[21]

In facilitating the development of corporal intelligence, somatic education carries two essential messages: the first emphasises the fact that we can find some solutions in ourselves, in the body's own reality;

the second reminds us that we are able to evolve and change throughout our life, especially if the transformations are inscribed within the reality of our body, and if we cannot succeed alone, there are therapists who suggest that they help us through the agency of their hands.

THE EQUILIBRIUM OF THE STRUCTURE

A controversial subject

As in the example of massage, the art of manipulating the body has been a part of every medical tradition since the dawn of time. However, since the advent of a medicine is based on clinical evidence and scientific proofs its utility is often doubted, even denied. We have moved far away from that ancient time when Galen was called the 'Prince of physicians' for having restored the use of his arms to a Roman sage in realigning his neck.

It was Daniel David Palmer, an American healer who, at the end of the 19th century launched the polemic. Convinced that he could heal a large number of pathologies by realigning the skeleton, he created a method that he called 'chiropractic' (from the Greek: *kheir*: hand, and *praxis*: action). The story relates that, in correcting a deviation in the spinal column in a man rendered deaf by an accident that had occurred 17 years earlier, Palmer had tried for the first time the power of bodily adjustment: the man recovered his hearing. True or not, this story was in any case the origin of the theory of chiropractic. Based on the fact that the nervous system controls the whole of the body, Palmer thought that the tensions in the body and the compressions and irritations of the nerves were responsible for the greater part of illnesses. He introduced the idea of 'bony subluxation' to explain the origin of the nerve damage responsible for the problem. The aim of his practice was, therefore, to 'unblock' the spinal column and other parts of the body, to treat not only muscular and skeletal disorders but also organic dysfunction.[22]

The problem is that so far there is no evidence either of the role played by subluxations in the disorders treated, or even of formal proof of their existence.[23] All the same, numerous studies have demonstrated a favourable effect on dorsal pain and the restoration of skeletal mobility. Unfortunately, in view of statistical bias and gaps in the methodology, it seems that we cannot decide the case.[24] The analysis of a few studies carried out along more rigorous lines – double blind selection of patients with a control placebo – 'sham' treatment – is no more convincing.[25] Similarly, no serious study has as yet been done to demonstrate the possibility of treating problems other than muscular and skeletal ones.[26]

In addition, in the absence of an explanation of how it works, it is proof of the effectiveness of the spinal manipulations that is lacking.[27] Patients appear to be satisfied, and despite the reticence of conventional medicine, chiropractic has been considerably developed, to the point where today it is considered to occupy third place in Western medical practices, after allopathic medicine and dentistry. I have heard numerous patients in my practice declare that they had been helped by a chiropractor. I therefore came to recommend this treatment and I even had recourse to it myself, with success. One may well wonder about the reasons for the observed benefits. Some assert that spinal manipulations are no more effective than other treatments and that it is the natural course of dorsal pain that explains the recorded results.[28] Others claim that the effects obtained are essentially a placebo phenomenon. The effectiveness of the method on animals contradicts this latter belief, but here too, the absence of studies carried out on veterinary chiropractic makes it impossible to advance the debate.[29]

It is possible that the active mechanisms of chiropractic are other than they are believed to be. It seems legitimate to doubt the possibility of manipulating the vertebrae of a horse, surrounded as they are by thick layers of muscles and ligaments.[30] If such an intervention does have an effect, it may not be due to the force applied to the skeleton. It may be that the observed effect takes place at a more subtle level and follows currently ill-understood rules. The ideas of tensegrity and the 'living matrix' could play a part.[31] In any case, it seems indispensable to encourage research in these areas.

More subtle and less clear

Several years before Palmer's work, another American, Andrew Taylor Still had also explored the possibility of treating the body by manipulation. Physician and Pastor, Still had lost three children during an epidemic of meningitis. The researches of Louis Pasteur had only just begun, antibiotics did not exist. Apart from purging, cupping and bleeding, medical resources at the end of the 19th century were poor. For all that, Still was convinced that there were other means of treatment. Trained in surgery on the battlefields of the Civil War, he had acquired a detailed knowledge of human anatomy. This enabled him to develop an extremely sensitive system of palpation, so good that in 1874 when he was called to the bedside of a child with haemorrhagic dysentery, Still had no difficulty in noting a temperature difference between the back and the abdomen of the patient, a hardening in the lumbar area and some changes in the suppleness of the spinal column. He moved his hands over the different zones, trying to harmonise the temperatures and movements and, to his great surprise, the haemorrhage stopped at once. A few days later, the child had returned to perfect health.[32]

One can imagine the suspicion aroused by this kind of miraculous story. In the light of the then current knowledge, Still suggested an explanation that could not but arouse the hostility of the scientific community. His theory, still embryonic, postulated that structure influences function and that the imbalances responsible for illness always showed at the level of the bones – hence the name 'osteopathy' which he gave to his method, a name which can be interpreted erroneously since this method is not composed simply by manipulating the skeleton. In distinction to the chiropractor, the osteopath essentially works on soft tissues. Observation and subtle palpation of the body are the core of the method – spotting 'osteopathic lesions' and 'restriction of mobility' that the osteopath has learned to recognise at the tips of his fingers. Often very gentle, his adjustments aim at restoring harmony and the fluidity not only of the fascias, the muscles and the ligaments, but also the blood vessels, nerves, glands and organs. Even if osteopathy has developed further, according to the principles dictated by Still the manipulations are always carried out to permit the body to mobilise its self-correcting mechanisms.

However, it remains for us to discover what really releases this self-healing. Again, fundamental research is lacking. As in other kinds of treatment, the placebo effect is certainly involved. To approach the individual in his totality and to draw his attention to the fact that he has his own inner resources, undoubtedly contributes the creation of meaning and the positive emotions which activate the parasympathetic nervous system as well as healing relaxation. However, this cannot be a complete explanation since numerous therapists describe observing benefits in suckling babies, and even in animals. Veterinary studies could therefore be very valuable.[33] On the physiological side, work on tensegrity and the 'living matrix' seem to provide a good path for future research to follow.[34] The mechanisms shown in studies on touch and massage may provide another avenue (see Chapter 7). But then, nothing has as yet been shown.

Serious clinical studies are equally lacking. Those that have been done principally concern muscular-skeletal problems and they are not sufficient to allow one to draw convincing conclusions.[35] This is no doubt related to the fact that osteopaths mostly work in isolation from each other, without collecting their results in line with the accepted criteria of scientific research. In addition, the variation in their practice makes it difficult to determine the real cause of the improvements noted. Some of them favour functional manipulations, others structural; others again the visceral or the cranial. At one moment they clearly touch the patient, at another they barely brush against him, and most of the time they add other techniques to the basic bodily manipulations, such as dietetic advice or psychological listening. The detractors of this technique snigger when they assert that there exist as many osteopathies as osteopaths, forgetting that, as is the case in all therapeutic approaches, osteopathy is an art. In this practice, faithful to the teaching of Still, the artist addresses his patient in his totality. Therefore the approach cannot be restrained within over-codified rules. Nonetheless, some osteopaths are uneasy about some of the derived and modified methods met in practice.[36]

Having myself referred patients for osteopathic treatment and having communicated with numerous practitioners I became curious about the diversity of their practices. Some seemed to me to be more like traditional healers than the 'scientific' technicians that their training is supposed to produce, based as it is, very solidly, on the models of classical medical studies. So far, osteopathy has not yet won its place in Western scientific medicine. To get to this point, it would be necessary to discern what really takes place in all the suggested practices. Rigorous studies are therefore indispensable. These would permit one to identify the actual content of the method and thus better select the pathologies that would benefit from it. In the absence of such an approach, osteopathy may remain an effective treatment, but purely empirical and exposed to the risk of the most dubious deviations. This would be a shame, because the principles it proposes are interesting, and an understanding of the mechanisms mobilised thereby could help to further all medicine.

Even more mysterious

During the 1930s, William Sutherland, an osteopath and a pupil of Still, asserted, contrary to current belief, that the bones of the cranium were mobile and affected by physiological movements perceptible on palpation. Baptised 'primary respiratory mechanism' (PRM), this slow and rhythmic pulsation is said to arise in the cerebrospinal liquid and is transmitted to the whole body via the dura mater around the brain and the spinal cord, as well as by the fibrous fascias around the muscles and the organs. The PRM is therefore palpable throughout the body. By their mobility, the cranial bones make up an indispensable 'shock absorber' for the cerebrospinal fluid which flows from the head to the sacrum in a closed hydraulic system. Any restriction of the mobility of the cranial bones therefore provokes a disturbance of the PRM, and from that results in problems throughout the organism. Consequently the mobilisation and relaxation of the cranial sutures could be a form of treatment for numerous pathologies.

Sutherland's theory was perhaps too original and innovative, and so provoked an outcry amongst scientists and a lively controversy amongst osteopaths.[37] However, 40 years later John Upledger, then professor of biomechanics at Michigan State University, showed by means of an electron microscope that, far from being rigidly joined, the cranial bones are separated by sutures containing vessels, nerves and fibrous tissues.[38] The movements felt by Sutherland would therefore be possible. Moreover, the studies carried out on animals, and then in humans, showed a cranial pulsation, the frequency of which was different from both the cardiac and respiratory rhythms.[39] Nevertheless, the controversy endured, and many osteopaths think that the approach is not well enough documented for them to introduce it into the teaching of their discipline.[40]

Upledger himself never entertained any doubts. Instead of focusing on the bony sutures, it seemed better to him to act on the craniosacral system of the dura mater which regulates the production, reabsorption and circulation of the cerebrospinal fluid. Using the bones of the cranium as levers enabled him to lighten the tensions in the membranes that are attached to them, so that 'craniosacral therapy' replaces the deeper manipulation of cranial osteopathy with very fine, barely perceptible, movements.

The subtlety of this approach awoke suspicion especially amongst physicians who are obviously not trained in this kind of palpation. The blind pianist, Ray Charles, 'saw with his ears'. It seemed that the craniosacral therapists 'heard with their fingers'. Having myself refined the sensitivity of my own touch, I could understand the expertise of certain practitioners. Nonetheless, I also know that autosuggestion may make us perceive sensations according to our expectations. It is therefore important for studies to be carried out comparing the reliability of sensations perceived in one palpation compared to another by a particular examiner and how these may then be reproduced by different examiners. In the case of craniosacral therapy, those studies that have been done are contradictory.[41]

A session of craniosacral therapy begins with a palpation of the whole body to test the mobility of the tissues and identify zones of restricted movement. According to Upledger, the body stores the memory of the shocks and tensions it has undergone centrally inside 'energy cysts'. These are formed following the failure of dispersion of the energy originating from the trauma. Manual freeing of these 'energy cysts' disperses the stored energy, provoking a sensation of warmth, or an emotional reaction. The body can then rebalance itself and put into action its self-healing mechanisms.

Mary Ellen Clark, a bronze medallist in diving at the Olympics in Barcelona in 1992, relates how, after experiencing terrible vertigo and being unable to find any effective help, ended by consulting John Upledger. At the first session, the latter freed numerous 'energy cysts', the results of multiple traumata stemming from dozens of daily dives from a ten metre high platform. In the second, Upledger turned his attention to her left knee. She remembered then receiving an injury to that knee during a training session on the trampoline. Upledger established that there was a compensatory torsion of the spinal column originating from the injury to her knee, and responsible for poor positioning of her head. Correction of these problems started an improvement in her symptoms. Six weeks later, Mary Ellen resumed her training and again carried off a bronze medal, at the Atlanta Olympics in 1996.[42]

The craniosacral approach thus seems still further away from conventional medical beliefs than chiropractic or osteopathy. Following the example of these two related disciplines, craniosacral therapy is based on anatomical notions the interpretation of which, original and seductive as it is, has not so far been verified within the criteria of scientific research.[43] Here too, however, the number of practitioners grows, as does the number of their patients.

An osteopath who worked with craniosacral therapy told me that he considered that the theories on which it is based are mistaken. 'All the same, they enable me to offer a way of making contact with the body of my patients,' he said. 'Later, like Upledger, I accept that intuition determines a large part of what passes between me and the patient which is quite inexplicable.' This kind of therapeutic relationship may initiate the helpful placebo effects of which we spoke at the beginning of this book. Are these practitioners modern sorcerers who, following the example of traditional healers, must have a real belief in their theories if they are to obtain a good effect? Is this effect so much more marked that, in contrast to the invisible world of the sorcerers, the body represents a tangible reality and the discourse held is similar to that of medical science? (These points are discussed in Chapter 1.) So many disturbing questions, but nonetheless unavoidable, because, 'as a tree may hide a forest',* this would not be the first time in medical history that a theory may mask mechanisms the explanation of which

---

* *Translator's note*: This metaphor may be a little obscure to anglophone readers. It may be read as 'You can't see the wood for the trees', or, more prosaically, 'Concentration on detail may distract from perception of the whole'.

turns out to be very different from those initially conceived to explain unexpected facts.

It is this phenomenon that we shall introduce when we examine how Western science explains therapeutic systems far removed from mechanistic ideas. We will pursue our enquiry in China, India and the 'New Age' setting of the Western world. It is there that the human being is regarded as a system of energy.

PART THREE
A MEDICINE OF ENERGY TO HEAL BODY AND MIND

9
BEHIND THE CHINESE THEORIES

REFINING THE CONCEPTS

Behind the tree, the forest

There is probably no better example of the tree hiding the forest than Chinese medicine. In fact, this 'medicine' consists of a collection of practices developed from shamanistic and religious ideas, the origins of which are lost in the darkness of time. Exclusively empirical, these different approaches are based on analogies observed between the macrocosm and the microcosm, between the human being and his environment. Some of them, probably the most effective, have been handed down to us, influenced in their turn by a multitude of schools of thought. So much is this so that what we call 'traditional Chinese medicine' is the result of a quite recent synthesis developed between the 1950s and 1970s in an attempt to create a uniformity which would support comparison with the Western scientific medicine that is itself so well structured and codified.

However, comparison is probably impossible, because the traditional Chinese approach remains very different from that of Western medicine. In effect, the Chinese viewpoint is concerned neither with separating into the tiniest detail, with precise measurement nor with rigorously analysing the mechanisms of physiology. Its purpose is not to describe in detail the different organs and systems of the body. What counts is the understanding of the functional relationships which unite these organs and the systems between them. In consequence, the language of traditional Chinese medicine is not scientific in the sense that we understand this in the West. It is metaphorical and analogical. Its view is never compartmentalised: it embraces the concept of globality.

Five disciplines – dietetic; pharmacological, based on plants; massage; acupuncture; energy exercises such as *qigong* and *tai-chi* – seek to preserve the harmony and equilibrium of the forces and energies responsible for good health. The approach is seductive, even rational and logical. All the same, the theories to which they refer present a substantial obstacle to their acceptance by the scientific community. The concepts of *yin* and *yang*, the theory of the five elements, and the notion of *qi* (pronounced *tshi*), are sometimes described as superstitions. This is to be regretted because a deeper analysis can often decode analogies between these traditional concepts and scientifically established facts. Sometimes a comparison of these two approaches ends up by providing evidence of formerly unsuspected physiological mechanisms. Chinese medical thought then becomes a source of inspiration and a promise of discoveries and progress.

Taking the notion of *yin* and *yang*, we have seen in Chapter 2 (p. 35) how these two forces, the one active and emitting, the other passive and receptive, translate a neurological reality embedded in the opposition of the autonomic sympathetic and parasympathetic nervous systems. The homoeostasis of the organism depends upon the balance between tension and relaxation. From the balance between these two systems come our emotions, the actual drivers of our thoughts and actions. From the point of view of Chinese medicine, an excess or a lack of *yin* or of *yang* creates chaos and sickness. In fact, Western psycho-neuro-immunology teaches us the same. A thousand-year-old observation therefore accords perfectly with physiological reality and it is easy to translate the oriental metaphor into the scientific language of Western culture.

The theory of the five elements is more difficult to define. Five *yin* organs (kidneys, liver, heart, spleen and lungs) and their corresponding *yang* (bladder, gall bladder, small intestine, stomach, colon) are related to five elements (water, wood, fire, earth and metal); to five symbolic animals; five colours; five sounds; five odours; five flavours; five emotions; five climatic seasons; and five periods of daily hours. Some cycles are established according to a natural logic where fire forms cinders and earth, earth creates metal, metal is transformed into water, water nourishes wood and wood feeds fire. This very complex theory equally postulates the existence of cycles of control, creative and destructive, always driven by the necessity of preserving the physical and psychic balance. Obviously, these multiple correspondences are difficult to verify in a scientific way, but that is no reason to reject them *en bloc* – even if prudence is counselled, because many of these concepts date from a period when entire sections of human physiology were ill-known. The heart, for example, also called the Emperor, historically played a central role in the theory of the five elements. Now, many of its attributes are displaced to the brain, the function of which was practically unknown until the development of the neurosciences.

Another source of difficulty for Western minds lies in the fact that Chinese medical theories were influenced by beliefs that today still remain unvalidated by scientific methods. It is not easy to discern the implicit part played by superstition in the process of healing. For example, a study published in 1993 in *The Lancet* showed how the astrological beliefs of Californian patients of Chinese origin influenced the progress of their health. To arrive at this conclusion, David Phillips, researcher at the University of California at San Diego, examined the age and cause of death of around 30,000 Californians of Chinese origin compared with a control group of white Californians. The results were astonishing: to a very significant level, the Californians of Chinese origin died earlier than average when they suffered from an illness which Chinese astrology and medicine associated with the year of their birth. The white Californians showed no indication of such influence. It therefore seems that the beliefs of the group of Chinese origin influenced their expectations and hopes when faced with an illness which is considered inescapable if it corresponds to the prophecies of their birth year.[1]

Suggestion, conditioning and the 'meaning effect' are certainly not strangers to a medicine in which metaphors perform the office of theories. Nevertheless, this statement should not turn us away from a vital question posed by traditional Chinese medicine: what is the true nature of the links between the macrocosm and the microcosm? Climates, seasons, the movements of the planets, a whole series of natural cycles, influence our health in a more subtle way than we think. (This point is touched on in Chapter 10, pp. 166–168.) The empirical Chinese tradition observed this and expressed its observations in words full of imagery. If occidental science were to remain open and curious, it might be able to translate these concepts into its own language. That would certainly facilitate their integration with the preventive and therapeutic aspects of modern medicine.

A question of energy

According to Taoist thought, all matter comes from the condensation of a single fundamental 'substance': *qi*. At first glance this idea appears difficult to translate into scientific language: we speak of 'energy'. Nonetheless, let us be clear: this does not refer to any of the forms of energy (electricity, electromagnetic, nuclear, calorific or mechanical) measured by Occidentals. *Qi* appears more like 'force in action' expressed by the Greek word *'energeia'*. This is an imprecise concept, following 'the breath of life' (*ankh* of the Egyptians, *pneuma* of the Greeks, *prana* of the Indians) and arising from intuitive observation at a time when man lacked the means of sophisticated analysis. *Qi* can therefore represent all the forms of energy identified by Western science, to which we must add psychic energy which, through the emotions, puts the body into motion.

The advantage of this imprecision is that it allows us to think about the human being in its entirety while avoiding all separation of mind and body. *Qi* is therefore the *link*, a kind of continuum, between matter and thought. Its manifestations are multiple, sometimes physical, sometimes psychic. And even if *qi* is invisible and intangible, its effects allow us to perceive its quantity and quality. In this sense it represents energy, since it represents the ability to perform work.

Without wishing to create a pseudo-scientific bridge with the discoveries of present times, we must note that the equation of Einstein: $E = mc^2$, together with information theory, provides a basis for reflection on the nature of *qi* (see Chapter 2, p. 27). As much matter, as much movement, force and action, as much the two at the same time. In the course of my exploration of Eastern medicines and energy therapies, I found that the word 'energy' has several meanings, according to the circumstances in which it was used: physical force (one is full of energy); emotional disposition (one feels positive or negative energy); or a particular intention (one adopts a good or a bad energy) to do something. Indeed, it is interesting to note that in our exploration we regularly refer to these different aspects of the dimension of energy in our lives. We talk readily about waves or vibrations, good or bad, positive or negative.

Whether it is energy or matter, *qi* contains information. Our actions and our words can therefore influence it. We have seen that a massage of the body or breathing exercises can re-establish the equilibrium of the nervous system, stimulate the cerebral areas responsible for positive emotions and arouse the immune defences. In the same way, a comforting word, the meaning attributed to a treatment, or simply positive thought can produce physiological effects which are equally manifestations of *qi*. Thus *qi* expresses the reality of the 'body–mind unity'. For traditional Chinese medicine, good health depends upon a fluid circulation of *qi*. In other words, the psychological and physical equilibria are indivisible. *Qi* is probably not a form of energy the existence of which has not yet been demonstrated. It is more likely that it is made up of intentions, thoughts, emotions, actions, nervous impulses, circulation of the blood, inter-cellular communication, chemical reactions between molecules, and collisions or attractions between particles. From there, one can understand better how a blockage of *qi* produces physical discomfort and psychological stress which can lead to illness.

MASTERING *Qi*

'One does not lose good health because of an illness. One is ill because of the fact that one is not in good health,' is written in the *Huang Ti Nei Ching*, the oldest of the Chinese medical texts.[2] The message is clear:

before anything else, medicine must *prevent* the imbalances responsible for weakening the body.

Amongst the tools that traditional Chinese medicine developed to harmonise the circulation of *qi*, energetic exercises constitute their foundation. Their origin is of the greatest antiquity, and they are the basis of all the martial arts. Their philosophy stands on the Taoist wisdom: 'To cede is to conquer, to bend is to stand,' wrote Lao Tseu. 'To turn is the movement of *Tao*, to submit is the way of *Tao*.' 'The principle of death is stiff and inflexible, soft and submissive is the principle of life.'[3]

Energy training

I experienced my first contact with Chinese thought affecting my body in the presence of a master of *qigong*. Slowly and patiently, this man taught me the 'work of *qi*'. Far from being a simple gymnastic, *qigong* brings together exercises of meditation, visualisation and breathing, holding postures and sequences of various movements, stretching and swaying, as well as carrying out self-massages, all done with the greatest respect for *yin* and *yang* in balance between passivity and activity. The promise made by Lao Tseu is inviting: 'To breathe in and out lets one get rid of pollutants and become fresh. Moving like a bear and stretching like a bird leads to a long life.'

Occidental medicine has been closely interested in the benefits of *qigong* for many years. An institute of research was established in Hong Kong in 1953 and numerous studies have since become available. Unfortunately, most of them are published in Chinese journals that are difficult to access in the West, and often their methodology does not conform well to scientific criteria. All the same, there is a consensus stating that the effects are real and that the researches should be continued.

Qigong puts great emphasis on breathing, some studies showing a marked reduction of the severity of symptoms in asthmatic patients. Other studies indicate a favourable effect on blood pressure, a reduction of blood cholesterol and an improvement in diabetes.[6] The preventative action of *qigong* reduced the frequency of cerebrovascular accidents and slowed the decline of cardio-respiratory function in old people.[7] As a result, numerous medical teams have decided to integrate *qigong* in their programmes of cardiac rehabilitation.

In improving suppleness, in using the muscles and developing the sense of balance, the use of *qigong* also reduces the frequency of falls in the elderly. It must be added that the gentleness of the approach means that it can be used to a very advanced age. Some studies have shown that regular practice raises the levels of testosterone and growth hormone significantly, the increase being proportionally greater in elderly than in young subjects.[8] In addition, positive effects have been noted in the elderly on the levels of activity of the thyroid and parathyroid glands as well as on the metabolism of calcium.[9] These endocrinological effects, associated with preservation of the bony mass which allows the use of *qigong* exercises, could retard ageing in a natural way without involving the consumption of alimentary or hormonal supplements. There is therefore a point of special interest in *qigong*: more than being a curative discipline, it is a preventive approach intended to preserve health.

Sometimes *qigong* helps healing. Early in the 1960s, Guo Ling, a young Chinese woman, discovered that she was condemned. At the age of 30, a gynaecological cancer left her no hope of survival. Unable to resign herself to this outlook, she decided to practise the *qigong* of her ancestors which she adapted to her own ideas. And, contrary to all expectations, she survived. The history of Guo Ling fires the imagination. The news spread and very soon, the young woman opened a training club in Shanghai. The second member of her club, a man named Wang, healed a gastric cancer which had responded neither to chemotherapy nor to radiotherapy. By the end of the 1980s, the Cancer Recovery Clubs of Guo Ling counted several tens of thousands of members. The parks and gardens across the whole of China were filled with people practising *qigong*. It became very popular.[10]

As with the majority of those experiencing 'miracles', Guo Ling probably owed her recovery to her extraordinary conviction, hope and determination to take her destiny in her own hands, which foster, as we have seen, the mobilisation of the immune defences of the organism. Her charisma, the strength of her faith and the credibility of her testimony had drawn other sufferers to the same experience. From a psychological point of view, Guo Ling's clubs compose a network of precious support in the cultural context of China which tends to marginalise sufferers from cancer. From the physiological standpoint, one can easily imagine that the reduction of cortisol,[11] and the improvement of the immune response,[12] seen in the practitioners of *qigong*, are able to relieve, even cure, certain patients.

The main distinctive character of *qigong* consists of the fact that the exercises are carried out without stress and are therefore associated with profound relaxation. A kind of meditative state is aroused by the visualisation and concentration necessary to achieve the postures and movements. The parasympathetic system is aroused. Deep breathing reinforces this phenomenon. Positive emotions arise, anxiety diminishes, stress is dissipated, symptoms of depression are reduced, and the chain of reparatory physiological effects is set in motion.

According to the theory of the five elements, the postures and movements relate to the organs (kidney, liver, heart, spleen and lungs) and the emotions (fear, anger, joy, sympathy, sorrow) which are associated with them. Simple belief, or unproven reality – the question remains. What is more certain is the benefit of *qigong* during the course of psychotherapy.[14] Thus a study of a group of patients addicted to heroin showed that daily practice of *qigong* speeded up the process of detoxification and reduced withdrawal symptoms and anxiety.[15] Moreover, a better awareness of their bodies stimulated the patients to a better respect for their limitations and needs. They learned to attend to the signals which their bodies produce in order to become able to avoid the imbalance provoked by stress, both physical and psychological.

Beneficial as *qigong* is to the health of the body and the mind, it is also the source of astonishing discoveries about oneself. In my own practice of the exercises, I receive great pleasure from feeling different parts of my own body vibrating as I explore the space outside and inside myself. Energy is then, all at once, not an abstract concept, it is a real perception. The fact of being fully present to oneself probably re-establishes sensory and motor connections between the brain and the rest of the organism. In any case, the concept of neuroplasticity allows us to think so. From this starting point *qigong* is a psychological and physical training the effects of which progressively establish themselves and are lasting. In time, the sensation of living becomes more and more intense, freedom of movement is more and more joyful: the peace experienced is exquisite.

The battle between the crane and the snake

Another form of energy training, *tai-chi* is distinguished from *qigong* by its slower and more continuous movements, essentially carried out in an upright position, the lower part of the body moving in a square and the upper in a series of circles. There is a legend that relates that this discipline was invented by a Taoist priest who watched a fight between a crane and a snake. Broad and circular, the movements of the snake allowed little chance of seizing hold of its adversary. By its suppleness and slowness, the crawling animal ended by defeating the bird.

Father of all martial arts, *tai-chi* is above all the inner task of achieving awareness of the different energies that infuse the body and the mind. It focuses on the *tan tien*: the centre of gravity set in the pelvis one or two centimetres lower than the navel; because of this, the sensation of being grounded and stable is strong. The major difficulty lies in slowing down one's way of moving. The extreme slowness of the movements allows one to detect the blockages and restrictions of the body and the mind. Here too one strives to feel: vibrations, heat, prickling, trembling. Sometimes emotions arise, old memories emerge. Deep breathing soothes and dissipates tension. Each in-breath and each out-breath are opportunities for regaining one's self-awareness in the here-and-now. Relaxation appears without effort. The mind is calm and alert at the same time. *Tai-chi* is a true meditation in movement.

Millions of Chinese practise it daily. In the West it is not rare to see groups of people devoted to it in public places. The spectacle is fascinating: strength and suppleness, slowness and precision, interior and exterior, the dynamic of *yin* and *yang* in action. It seems that practising in groups helps social integration, especially in the elderly who also find it a real pleasure. Moreover, a study has shown that they stick more easily to *tai-chi* than to other physical disciplines. The positive development of their health and the good mood when they have taken up the practice encourages them to devote themselves to it regularly.[16] I recall a cardiac patient who refused all forms of exercise despite repeated recommendations from his medical advisers. Six months after having at last agreed to take a course of *tai-chi*, he told me with enthusiasm: 'This is never boring; it is like dancing.'

Like *qigong*, *tai-chi* has a paradoxical effect: the body is at one and the same time stimulated and at ease, the mind is simultaneously alert and relaxed. This is especially helpful at the cardio-vascular level. A series of *tai-chi* movements are equivalent to an aerobic exercise like a walk at a good pace.[17] Its benefits are at the same time preventive and therapeutic: significant reduction of arterial pressure in the sedentary,[18] improvement of cardio-pulmonary function after coronary surgery,[19] quicker recovery after a myocardial infarction.[20] Compared with an aerobic exercise, such as an ergonomic bicycle, *tai-chi* provides a greater respiratory effect, probably because of the slow and deep mobilisation of the diaphragm.[21]

As in *qigong*, the process of developing balance, strength in the lower members, in the suppleness of the knees and the amplitude of the movements of the spinal column, *tai-chi* improves feelings of security in the elderly and reduces the frequency of falls.[22] The exercise stimulates bone growth and strengthens the connective tissues. That is why some physicians therefore do not hesitate to recommend a programme of *tai-chi* to replace medical treatment for osteoporosis, especially amongst menopausal women.[23]

Several studies provide evidence for the value of *tai-chi* in functional recovery following a cerebrovascular accident, after a neural trauma, or in cases of multiple sclerosis.[24] Regular practice also helps to reduce chronic pain, for example in rheumatoid arthritis.[25] Endorphin secretion in the course of the exercises is, no doubt, implicated in this effect.

The increase in parasympathetic tonus and the relaxation of tensions also contribute.

Amongst these numerous favourable effects, we find also improvement both in falling asleep and in the quality of sleep, to the point that some physicians consider *tai-chi* as an effective alternative to sleeping pills.[26]

Patients suffering from cancer can also draw benefit from *tai-chi*.[27] Because of its gentle nature, the approach can be recommended even to those who are very weakened. The relief is real. The meditational component improves the mobilisation of positive emotions, reduces stress and anxiety,[28] contributes to the activation of the immune reactions and stimulates the processes of repair of the organism.[29] The psycho-corporal integration is complete. *Qi* is balanced in all its forms.

THE MYSTERIES OF ACUPUNCTURE

An invisible anatomy

To think of *qi* as a metaphor for the sum total of the energies which drive us is rather reassuring for a mind formed in the scientific mould. A metaphor excuses us from having to prove the existence of a 'vital energy' that cannot be measured. Nonetheless, a question persists that is equally embarrassing: do the meridians described in traditional Chinese medicine really exist?

According to the texts, *qi* circulates in a series of channels of energy divided into 12 principal meridians – six *yin* meridians in the front of the body, six *yang* in the back – plus two central, and a network of secondary meridians. Each of these energy channels is related to an organ and each organ exercises a specific role in the conversion of air and food into vital substances: into blood and into *qi*. Classically, 365 points of contact with the energy that circulates in the meridians are described. Certain treatises number more than 2,000 such points. As in the postures and movements of *qigong*, the insertion of fine needles at the location of these points could balance the circulation of *qi* at the core of the network. The self-healing mechanisms of the body would be automatically set going and the various organs would harmonise their functions.

In practice, the choice of meridians and the points at which to treat is based upon detailed questioning. Guided by the theory of the five elements, the practitioner identifies the imbalances of the patient in discovering his tastes, his needs and his preferences: excellent indicators of what is missing and what is deficient. Attentive taking of the pulse, following a technique that is much more sophisticated than that of Western medicine, discloses the rhythm, the regularity, the strength, the depth and the quality of the pulsation: characteristics which, added to examination of the tongue, as well as detailed observation of posture and movements, are the vital elements in establishing a diagnosis.

Currently, there is no proof of the existence of such a network of energy channels. Nonetheless, a study carried out a few years ago by French researchers claimed the contrary: by injecting radioactive technetium at certain acupuncture points, the authors demonstrated a diffusion of the substance along the lines supposed to be the meridians, while an injection outside the acupuncture points produced only local diffusion.[30] As spectacular as they are unexpected, no one has as yet been able to replicate these observations, probably because it is illusory to hope to isolate such anatomical structures. If it exists, the network of meridians is likely to be of a functional nature.

Some research has shown a reduction of electrical resistance along the course of the supposed meridians, suggesting the presence of pathways of communication by electric current.[31] An increase in electrical conductance is also found at certain acupuncture points, especially in connection with a pathology of the organ to which it is related.[32] For example, the point 'liver number 8', situated at the level of the knee, had a conductance 18 times greater than normal in cases of cirrhosis or hepatitis. For James Oschman, who is interested in the properties of the 'living matrix' constituted by the connective tissues of the body, it seemed possible that a means of very primitive biological communication is hidden within the concept of the meridians.[34] The information could be conducted mechanically and electronically. Mechanically, we have seen how, following the principles of tensegrity, the least physical movement affects all the fascias around the most intimate structures of the body, and creates chemical and genetic changes at the heart of the cells of the entire organism (Chapter 8, pp. 123–124). Electronically, since the work of Albert Szent-Györgyi, awarded a Nobel prize in 1937 for his discovery of Vitamin C, we know that proteins have semiconductive properties.[35] On this basis, some researchers think that the connective tissues of the 'living matrix' constitute an electronic network of high velocity linking all the different structures of the body. Thus it seems that electronic circuits run throughout the body. Perhaps acupuncture influences their functioning.[36] Qi could then be compared with a chain of electronic exchanges which operate in the 'living matrix', a fundamental vector of information and energy. It must be clearly understood that this is only a working hypothesis: studies are needed to verify it.

The Western style of acupuncture

Although acupuncture has been practised in Europe since the end of the 17th century it did not appear in the Western media until 1971, when the journalist James Reston related the story of the misadventures he had experienced in the course of reporting Henry Kissinger's visit to China. The article, appearing in the *New York Times*, related how, when he had undergone an emergency operation for appendicitis in a hospital in Peking, his pain had been relieved by small needles inserted into his hands and feet.[37] The description was convincing. Nothing more was required to arouse the interest of the public. Many physicians, for their part, were reticent about their views of the rather esoteric theories of Chinese medicine. They endeavoured to free the technique from the beliefs that accompanied them in order to interest themselves solely in the physiological effects. 'Medical acupuncture' is therefore freed from the concepts and diagnostic techniques of traditional Chinese medicine. Lasers and electricity even replace the needles, and the number of points used is often reduced.

In this context, the American National Institutes of Health published a report in 1997 confirming that acupuncture is effective in relieving postoperative nausea, and vomiting related to pregnancy or following chemotherapy, and that it could be considered a complementary treatment for a number of other problems: postoperative pain, migraine, cramp associated with menstruation, muscular or joint pain, asthma, drug dependence and the sequelae of cerebrovascular accidents.[38] Three years later, the British Medical Association added more to this list of indications, notably chronic back pain.[39]

Acupuncture is used to relieve other pathologies. Nonetheless, well-conducted studies are lacking in those latter cases and it is impossible to recommend this intervention on a scientific basis. As the authors of a huge enquiry, carried out at the Centre for the Study of Complementary Medicine at the University of Münich in Germany reported, the fact that research on acupuncture cannot lead to any patent or commercialisation probably explains why the funds necessary for scientific study are so difficult to find.[40]

Acupuncture has nothing to sell – except wind, as some sceptics insist on thinking that this technique is only a descendant of shamanistic practices dating from prehistoric times. For these sceptics, it is nothing but the placebo effect. The reality is more subtle. In the case of chronic pain, for instance, imitation insertion of acupuncture needles, or their insertion outside the therapeutic zones ('sham' acupuncture), is effective in 30 to 50% of cases,[42] figures that are close to those obtained with placebo medication. An important placebo element explains perhaps why numerous writings from the Han Dynasty (first century BC) specified that those who did not believe in acupuncture should not use it.[43] '*I* am the first treatment needle,' I was told by a professor of acupuncture in Shanghai. However, when it is practised properly, acupuncture results in an improvement to the order of 55 to 85% of cases of pain. Inserting needles at acupuncture points has, therefore, a better effect than 'sham' treatment. The problem is that in the presence of a major placebo effect, establishment of statistical proof requires the recruitment of a large number of subjects. So far, no experiment has fulfilled the necessary conditions. However, a vast study, still current, has been launched, and is still in progress, in Germany, at the initiative of several health insurance companies and the Universities of Heidelberg, Bochum and Mannheim.[44]

Needles that stimulate the brain

Meanwhile, whether we are concerned with a placebo effect, or something that works in a quite different way, acupuncture produces effects in the brain that recent progress in imagery by magnetic resonance can objectify. For example, its analgesic and anti-inflammatory effects could be explained by the stimulation of the hypothalamus, responsible for the production of endorphins which inhibit pain, and of ACTH which leads to the production of cortisol in the adrenal glands.[45]

Some investigations done at Harvard showed that the stimulation of certain acupuncture points activated the nerve fibres which block pain, and de-activated the limbic zones in the brain that are involved in the subjective perception of pain. An important observation is that these phenomena are not produced by stimulation of 'sham' points.[46] It therefore appears that the action of the treatment is specific. Moreover, certain of the zones in the brain de-activated by acupuncture are stimulated in cocaine users: one can better understand, then, how these fine needles may help in weaning users from certain drugs and tobacco.[47]

Another study, carried out at the University of Pennsylvania with patients suffering from chronic pain in one side of the body, showed an asymmetry in the circulation of the blood around the thalamus, the part of the brain where the pain fibres lead. Treatment by acupuncture corrected this asymmetry.[48]

Obviously again, some of these observations could be the result of a placebo effect, because, as we have seen (Chapter 1, p. 14), the expectations of patients sometimes lead to cerebral changes that mimic the hoped-for therapeutic effects perfectly. Further investigations are necessary to clarify the specificity of the treatment.[49] In the meantime, the fact that we see real changes in cerebral areas involved in pain, makes us less incredulous of the Chinese statistics, which state that acupuncture can reduce by about 50% the doses of anaesthetics required for surgical interventions.[50]

In addition to the reduction in pain, the action of acupuncture on the limbic system probably explains some hormonal, immune, cardiovascular and gastro-intestinal effects. The rebalancing of the functions of the organs of the body could occur through the medium of the balance between the sympathetic and parasympathetic systems – *yin* and *yang* (see Chapter 2, p. 35.). At the digestive level, for instance, the same treatment can stimulate the contractions of the stomach in subjects where gastric motility is slow, but can also suppress peristalsis in those where motility is excessive.[51] It is also highly likely that the rebalancing of the autonomic system is at the root of certain anxiolytic and antidepressant effects of acupuncture.[52]

The discoveries achieved through cerebral imaging do not, however, stop here. In 1998, a study published in the *Proceedings of the National Academy of Sciences* by Zang-Hee Cho of the University of California, at Irvine, showed that the stimulation of acupuncture points intended to treat ocular problems increased the activity of the visual area of the cortex. On the other hand, stimulation of points sited several centimetres from the therapeutic points produced no change.[53] Subsequently, many researchers have obtained the same results, whether by the use of acupuncture needles or by laser stimulation.[54] It must be mentioned however, that, for reasons that are not understood, a study carried out by Isabel Gareus in 2002 at the University of Freiburg in Germany did not point in the same direction.[55]

This did not prevent Zang-Hee Cho from pursuing his research, stimulating this time the acupuncture points used in the treatment of auditory problems. One again, he found a correlation between the points stimulated and the activation of a specific area of the cortex – in this case, the auditory area.[56] These results really seemed to be too good to be true, although they seem to have been properly validated. Then in 2003 at the University of Hong Kong, Geng Li found that the stimulation of the two acupuncture points linked to language aroused activity in the cerebral zones relating to speech.[57] And in 2004 at Harvard, a team of researchers found that the stimulation of PC6 (point number 6 on the pericardial meridian) used in the treatment of nausea, activated the zones of the cerebellum implicated in the appearance of nausea.[58] Functional Magnetic Resonance Imaging is changing our understanding of acupuncture – and if the observed correlations are confirmed, we will have to admit that the body and the brain are connected by as yet unidentified nervous pathways.

A holographic body?

Personally, I think that if a cerebro-corporal connection exists outside the field of classical neurology, we must seek it in the study of embryology. We saw in Chapter 5 (pp. 81–82) that the various structures of the organism develop *in utero* according to a precise logic, starting with the three embryonic layers. We can then picture each part of the body as connected with a cerebral area following a pathway in which tissue is laid down in the course of the growth of the foetus. Thus the 'pathways' of dominant connections may become established through the 'living matrix' in accordance with a highly specific anatomy.

In the 1950s, the French physician-acupuncturist Paul Nogier made a discovery which leads in the direction of this hypothesis. In effect, he stated that stimulation at certain points of the ear aroused similar effects to those of classical acupuncture. His *Traité d'auriculothérapie*, published in 1957, describes the distribution of these points which schematically represents a human being in miniature – the image of a foetus, the head downwards in the uterine matrix configurated by the external ear. A troubling detail was that Nogier seemed to be ignorant of the fact that the description of 'a little man in the ear' had been established several thousand years earlier in the treatises on Chinese acupuncture. Auriculotherapy was shown to be as effective as classical acupuncture. For example, in a study carried out in 2003 at the Villejuif Hospital in France, on patients suffering from cancer-related pain which no medical treatment could ease, showed an overall diminution of complaints in 36% of patients treated by auriculotherapy, compared with 2% of those given a 'fake' treatment.[59]

The cartography of the ear presented by Nogier seems therefore to rest on the same bases as those of classical acupuncture. This is precisely the opinion of the psychobiologist Terence Oleson. In a study carried out to verify the correlations established by Nogier, he stated that a raised electric charge at the auricular points was an indication of pathology in the corresponding body part.[60] Intrigued by this, Oleson tells how one day he had noticed an abnormal scaly area of skin on the ear of a friend. This area was on a point related to the heart. He therefore advised his friend to undergo a medical check. The following day, a cardiologist diagnosed a serious problem and surgery was undertaken as a matter of urgency.[61]

To explain his observations, Nogier suggested the idea of an embryological connection between the auricular acupuncture points and the organs. Thus the centre of the ear seems to be related to the endoderm, the intermediate area to the mesoderm and the outer to the ectoderm, each of these three regions carrying the points linked to the organs in accordance with an upside-down configuration. It would certainly be a tedious task to verify this theory. However, this idea initiated what might be a new way of looking at the human anatomy, in which the body is thought of as a hologram – that is to say, a whole, of which each part contains the whole.

This concept of a hologram is well illustrated by taking the example of the cells of the organism, each one of which contains the genetic material necessary to the development of the whole body. Ralph Alan Dale, director of the Acupuncture Education Center in Miami, Florida, believes that there exist numerous 'microsystems of acupuncture', each reflecting the overall anatomy. This may be why Korean acupuncture of the hand or that of the scalp, seem to give results comparable to auriculotherapy, or the classical acupuncture practised on the whole of the body.[62]

Plantar reflexology was developed by the American, Eunice Ingham in the 1930s, and is founded on the same holographic principle: the whole of the body is represented on the sole of each foot. Deep massage of these areas stimulates the corresponding organs. A simple means of relaxation for some, reflexology is regarded as a true medicine by others. It is used to treat illnesses related to stress, as well as articulatory, muscular, cardiac, respiratory, digestive, gynaecological, hormonal and neurological problems. Even if its effectiveness remains controversial, reflexology produces unexpected effects. Thus in the course of her investigations concerning touch, Tiffany Field noticed that massage on the abdomen of pregnant women at about 20 weeks produced no reaction in the foetus, but massage of the feet immediately induced movements in the baby.[63] Such a link between a specific area of the body and the foetus has also been established in a study published in the (very serious) *Journal of the American Medical Association*: recourse to acupuncture can turn around a foetus with a breech presentation, within the uterus.[64] The fact is troubling, and remains unexplained.

The meridians and the emotions

Well before the use of needles, acupuncturists were probably 'accupressors'. A Japanese massage technique – *shiatsu* – consists still today in applying strong and prolonged pressure to stimulate a series of points – the *tsubo* – situated on the same lines as the meridians of acupuncture.[65]

Louisa, a patient with cancer of the ovaries to whom I had recommended that she should obtain massage between her courses of chemotherapy, told me how, during a session of *shiatsu* she suddenly felt terrified. Highly distressed, she told the therapist. 'Nothing surprising in that,' he replied, 'I am just now working on your kidneys, and the kidneys are the seat of fear.' What does that mean?

In fact, even if this is not the principal target, like all techniques using touch and relaxation of bodily tensions, *shiatsu* can provoke emotional discharges, the return of old memories, or the experience of unexpected emotions. However, there is no absolute proof of the correspondence between the emotions, the meridians and the organs – and for a good reason: it has never been studied.

A few years after Louisa had told me about her experience, I found myself facing the same question when I consulted an acupuncturist for the first time, encouraged to do so by a pain in my right shoulder. After thorough questioning, a very meticulous taking of my pulses and an examination of my tongue, the verdict of the practician was pronounced without any possible appeal: 'It is your liver!' The man seemed very sure of himself and added: 'Do you have a good reason to be angry?' Angry? I could not understand what he was getting at. Several needles were placed on the meridian of the liver, followed by a feeling of prickling, numbness in my right leg, and ten minutes later, a dull pain in my left side accompanied by an urgent desire to urinate. For a first contact with a medicine considered to be 'gentle', I have known better. All the same, I decided to follow the treatment recommended to the end. I therefore left having made another appointment.

The effects of my adventure might frighten anyone thinking of turning to this kind of care. For two days I suffered from violent colonic spasms and voided a large quantity of crystals in my urine. Chance, or a real connection of cause and effect – I could not know. It is, of course possible that a sympathetic/parasympathetic rebalancing was at the origin of a physiological chain-reaction the effects of which brought to an end the pain in my shoulder and – and this intrigued me enormously – released a profound anger. In a completely unexpected way, I became aware that I lacked space and time in my life. I wished to write the book you are at this moment reading and I was angry that I could not create for myself the opportunity of doing so.

Suggestion made by the question that the acupuncturist had asked me, or a real involvement of the liver meridian? It is altogether possible that, as with the examination grid for reading the psychocorporal symbolism, the emotional correlations of the Chinese system of beliefs had been for me the occasion of asking questions about my essential needs, in a crisis situation in which my tensions created pain in my shoulder (see Chapter 6, pp. 105–108). The relaxation produced by the acupuncture would then offer me the opportunity of getting in touch again with the repressed feelings. This explanation accords perfectly with the current state of scientific knowledge. At the same time, it is possible that some specific connections, currently uncorroborated, may function between certain parts of the body and the limbic areas of the brain where emotions are aroused. This would confirm the intuitions of those therapists for whom illnesses show themselves according to a precise emotional logic. Remember from Chapter 6 the case of Patricia, a young woman with an auto-immune hepatitis. Does there exist a link between her immense anger which had been denied expression and that part of the body where her disease occurred. Anger and the liver, kidneys and fear, the lungs and sadness: so many hypothetical relationships which the progress of neuroscience might verify in the future, hopefully not too far ahead. So many '*chinoiseries*' which will gain scientific confirmation or, on the contrary, perhaps remain poetic metaphors.

10
BEHIND THE INDIAN TRADITIONS

THE ASIATIC COUSINS

Far from being the prerogative of China, the energy concept of the human organism formed the origin of another great medical tradition: *ayurveda*. This 'science of life', born in India, is probably the oldest system of medicine still practised today. Its spread was immense, its influence extending as far as ancient Greece, China and Tibet, and for a long time it remained the principal system of medicine of the Indian subcontinent. Under the British occupation it was progressively abandoned in favour of the system imported from the West. For a time, this inestimable patrimony threatened to disappear, until 1980 when the National Congress of India rehabilitated *ayurveda* by giving it an official status. Since then, numerous *ayurveda* hospitals have been built around the country and a fruitful dialogue established with physicians trained in occidental medicine. In the same period, interest in Europe and the United States in *ayurveda* never stopped growing. Maharishi Mahesh Yogi, the Indian yogi who initiated the Beatles in transcendental meditation, and Deepak Chopra, the endocrinologist who founded the American Association of Ayurvedic Medicine, contributed greatly to that growth.

Amongst the similarities with its Chinese cousin, *ayurveda* also pictures the human being as a microcosm of the universe. Five elements combine to give birth to three fundamental forces, the *doshas*, – *vata*, *pitta*, *kapha* – the equilibrium between and the interactions amongst them which determine the nature of every individual on the physical, emotional, intellectual and spiritual planes (see Chapter 5, p. 84). Here the vital energy is not called *qi* but *prana*, and the channels in which it circulates are not meridians but *nadis*, constituting a vast network organised around the centres of energy called *chakras*.

As is the case with its Chinese cousin, Indian medicine is primarily concerned with prevention. Its purpose is to preserve the balance of the fundamental forces and the circulation of the vital energy. To do this, the Indian physicians have developed methods which closely resemble those used by their Chinese colleagues: diet, plant remedies, massage, meditation and physical exercises. Both Indian and Chinese medicines therefore represent real systems of integrated treatments:

perfect examples of holistic medicine. The individual is treated as a unity because he is thought of as such. And the common denominator of this globality is energy, an energy expressed as both physical and psychic.

Energy cooking

This concept of energy, unified and psychosomatic, influences all thought about health. From the dietary point of view, for example, the values attributed to food go well beyond that of obtaining calories. Nutrition is not solely qualified in terms of proteins, sugars, fats, vitamins and oligo elements. In Chinese medicine, every flavour (salty, sour, bitter, sweet, spicy) is connected with an organ (kidney, liver, heart, spleen, lungs) where it will compensate for any weakness. Each organ being the seat of an emotion (fear, anger, joy, sympathy, sadness), diet directly influences the behaviour of the individual. The energy of a foodstuff is therefore physical (its nutritive and calorific value), as well as emotional and intentional. The potential of this energy is defined in terms of its *yin* or *yang* charge. An excess of *yin* foods (sugar, alcohol, mushrooms, roots, fish, shellfish) can lead to lethargy, passivity, even depression. An overload of *yang* foods (salt, cheese, meat) leads to irritability, aggression and hyperactivity. Seeds, neutral foods, constitute the ideal basis of a balanced diet.

It is the same in India: six tastes (sweet, acid, salty, piquant, bitter, astringent) reduce or reinforce one or other of the three *doshas*. Individuals with a *vata* character, often hyperactive and versatile, need to eat nourishing meals, oily and sweet-and-sour, based on pastas, rice and meat. The *pitta* character, competitive, choleric and passionate, needs to avoid salt, oil and piquant sauces and to give preference to refreshing, bitter and astringent foods. The *kapha* character, robust, calm and affectionate, needs light meals based on fruit and raw vegetables. Three major categories of food – *sattvic*, *rajasic* and *tamasic* – influence spiritual development in precise ways. *Sattvic* foods (fruits and fresh vegetables, dried fruits, lentils, yoghurt, milk, cereals and whole rice) are considered to be pure and to foster kindness, intelligence, courage, discipline and sincerity. They should be used as the foundation of a diet because they contribute to well-being, preserve youthfulness and build up physical, psychological and spiritual health. *Rajasic* foods (potatoes, sugar, meat, fish, cheese, eggs) are rich in proteins and calories: they are stimulants and should, therefore, be eaten in moderation. They induce impatience, anxiety, excess, fickleness and egoism. Finally, the *tamasic* foods (cooked with preservatives, taste enhancers and alcohol) lead to physical, emotional and mental disorders: they are to be avoided.

It is clear that Chinese and Indian dietary principles are infinitely more detailed than those of Western medicine. In the East, for thousands of years, eating has been seen as a physical and psychological necessity *and* as a means of preserving the health of the body and the mind. This approach is developing in the West. The knowledge and experience accumulated by the Asiatic systems of medicine are able to provide an important contribution to scientific medicine, especially in managing the difficulties relating to ageing, an area in which Western medicine is poor in truly effective solutions. However, to achieve this, we need to consider the concept of energy in a wider perspective, physical and psychological, and, as we have seen concerning Chinese medicine, it is not always easy to translate metaphor into the language of modern science.

THE SACRED ANATOMY OF THE YOGIS

Ayurvedic concepts are more and more frequently referred to in Western media. Some patients who consulted me talked of their *chakras* as of something the reality of which had been scientifically proven. I was obliged to contradict them. Certainly, there are very sophisticated theories elaborated by researchers working in the great universities.[1] People speak of subtle energies, quantum physics, or thought fields. Numerous imaginative efforts try to create a correspondence between the theories of *ayurveda* and the developments of modern science. But in reality, whatever may be the hopes of these dreamers and popularisers, none of these theories has been formally demonstrated.

What on the other hand is certain, is that the drive towards proving everything exposes one to the danger of doing pseudo-science. Entire systems of reasoning are then founded on certainties which are in fact nothing but beliefs. The words of Raghubir Sangh, an Indian friend of mine trained in both ayurvedic and Western medicine, summarises the situation very well: 'Until the nature of *prana*, *nadis* and *chakras* is defined precisely, it would be illusory to wish to build the slightest theory validating an invisible anatomy of energy. Instead of inventing convoluted explanations, nourished on the imagination of science fiction, it would be better to read the theories of *ayurveda* in the light of what is actually known and unequivocally recognised by contemporary science. This would be enough to excite our curiosity and to convince us of the sound foundations of *ayurvedic* teaching.'

The balance between *Ida* and *Pingala*

Prudence dictates that we should not consider *prana* as a particular kind of energy but more like the sum of forces that are physical, emotional and intellectual – marshalled and regulated, amongst other things, by breathing. As with *qi*, *prana* seems to be the flux of information responsible for perfect coherence of body and mind. From this perspective, the *nadis* are probably not specific channels but simply circuits – nerves, lymphatic and blood vessels – which carry electrical and chemical information around the whole of the organism. As James Oschman suggested concerning the acupuncture meridians, it may be that the *nadis* correspond to pathways of electronic conduction in the heart of the 'living matrix'.[2]

According to Indian anatomy, three principal channels follow the course of the spinal column: *Sushumna* rises in the centre, from the coccyx to the top of the cranium, surrounded by *Ida* and *Pingala*, which, like two snakes, cross each other seven times. At each crossing a *chakra* emerges, a kind of 'energy wheel' where *prana* is metabolised. From the point of view of energies, *Ida* and *Pingala* perform the opposed and complementary functions of the Chinese *yin* and *yang*. Without trying to prove the existence of these channels, we are compelled to see a disconcerting analogy with the functioning of the autonomic nervous system. *Ida* is related to the feminine archetype of the moon; it is related to intuitive and emotional functions of the right hemisphere of the brain, associated with the parasympathetic system, which controls relaxation and loosening. On the other hand, *Pingala* is linked to the masculine archetype of the sun; it is related to the capacities for reasoning and logical analysis of the left hemisphere, corresponding perfectly to the sympathetic system, which sets in motion the reaction of flight or fight. Between them *Sushumna* represents the ideal balance, perfect homoeostasis, the necessary condition of good physical and mental health.

The psycho-neuro-endocrino-immunology of the *chakras*

The seven *chakras*, situated as they are at the meeting point between *Ida* and *Pingala*, correspond to the seven important neurological zones, the seven plexi where the sympathetic and parasympathetic nerves combine. The first *chakra*, located between the legs, seems to be linked to the nervous plexus of the coccyx; the second *chakra*, situated three to four centimetres below the navel, is at the sacral plexus; the third *chakra*, at the level of the stomach, at the solar plexus; the fourth *chakra*, at the level of the chest, at the cardiac plexus; the fifth *chakra*, at the level of the throat, at the pharyngeal and carotid plexi, as well as the cervical neural ganglia; the sixth *chakra*, between the eyes (at the site of the 'third eye'), the posterior part of the pituitary gland, directly linked to the hypothalamus; the seventh *chakra*, at the top of the cranium, linked to the cerebral cortex.

Described several millennia before our era, the system of the *chakras* would be the metaphorical representation of a neurological reality perceived in an entirely empirical and intuitive way by the Indian yogis.[3] The correlations seem relevant because the *chakras* are considered as wheels (that is the translation of the Sanskrit), transforming and redistributing the vital energy. So, according to the Vedic tradition, this energy acts upon the different organs, especially the related endocrine glands and immunological tissues: the adrenal glands for the first *chakra*; the testicles or ovaries for the second; the pancreas and spleen for the third; the heart and thymus for the fourth; the thyroid for the fifth; the anterior part of the pituitary gland for the sixth; the pineal gland for the seventh. In addition, according to the ancient texts, each *chakra* influences one stage in the psychological and spiritual evolution of the individual. New correlations can then be established between the actions of the hormones produced by the glands linked to the *chakras* and the behaviours foreseen by the Vedic theory. The logic of the system is astonishing: reviewing the *chakras* is enough to persuade us.

The first *chakra*, linked to the earth and the physical dimension, supports the survival of the individual. In fact, the adrenal glands to which it is attached produce both the adrenaline necessary for the reaction of 'flight or fight', and the cortisol secreted in the event of stress or danger.

Linked to the fluidity of water and the emotional life, the second *chakra* directs relationships with others, and especially sexuality. One cannot deny that the testicles and ovaries produce sexual hormones that influence mood, behaviour, personal relationships, and therefore the creativity of the individual, another aspect of the second *chakra*.

Related as it is to fire and the mind, the third *chakra* contributes to the development of the sense of self and gives rise to the ability to define the ego. We know that the pancreas and other digestive organs contribute to the assimilation of the foods that construct the individual, and the spleen stores the immune cells designed to defend the boundaries of the organism.

Thus the logic expressed by the first three *chakras* perfectly retraces the process of individuation of a human being: firstly to survive, then to relate to others and finally to define his identity. The analogy with the phylogenetic evolution of the instinctual, emotional and intellectual brain is sufficiently disconcerting (see Chapter 2, pp. 28–29). In fact, it is the instinct of the reptilian brain which secures survival; it is the emotions of the mammalian brain which regulate relationships with the outside world; and it is the cognitive faculties of the neocortex that develop self-awareness.

Related to air and love, the fourth *chakra* transforms the physical, emotional and intellectual aspects of the first three *chakras* into spiritual realities, pervaded by compassion and peace. It is love that enables unification of the self and communion with others. It is through the heart that the human being reaches the sublime. Even though its role is still poorly specified, we know that the thymus plays a first order part in the immune system, particularly through the T-lymphocytes; the heart secretes several hormones, including oxytocin, which aids attachment to others; and finally, there exists a regulatory loop between the cardiac plexus and the limbic brain, which, when activated, especially by a deep breath centred on the '*chakra* of the heart' and accompanied by positive thoughts, leads to emotional calming, consistent cardiac rhythm (called 'cardiac coherence'), a sympathetic/parasympathetic balance, optimalisation of cognitive faculties, strengthening of intuition and a tendency to empathy – effects demonstrated at the Institute of HeartMath in California.[4]

My friend Raghubir was right: re-reading the *ayurvedic* theories in the light of scientific discoveries is enough to convince one of the relevance of the thousand-year-old observations. It is impressive to note how, without knowing of the existence of hormones, the yogis understood how to translate their effects in terms of energy. We can, of course, continue the demonstration through the three next *chakras*.

The fifth *chakra* facilitates expression of the truth specific to each individual and allows him to define and fulfil his needs. The hormones secreted by the thyroid help this since they are regulators of metabolism and determinants of physical and mental development.

The sixth *chakra* is responsible for the higher intellectual functions. The anterior part of the pituitary gland to which is it related directs the whole endocrine system, while its posterior part regulates the sympathetic/parasympathetic balance of the hypothalamus. The neuro-endocrine balance thus obtained positively influences not only the physiology of the body but also the emotional state, reasoning and intuition of an individual.

Finally, the seventh *chakra* is linked to the spiritual feeling of oneness. It is interesting to note that recent research indicates that the pineal gland plays a co-ordinating and integrating function indispensable for maintaining the integrity of every individual. Thus the pineal gland transforms the information carried by light, temperature and magnetic fields into neuro-endocrine signals, especially melatonin, which regulate the whole physiology and influence the various rhythms of the body.[5] In this sense, it is by no means false to consider the seventh *chakra* as a door through which the individual is connected to the cosmos.

A psychosomatic tool

In his consultations, Raghubir uses the system of *chakras* as a model of 'mind–body unity'. 'It is a way of making patients aware of a reality that is described rather aridly by Western psycho-neuro-endocrino-immunology,' he commented with a big smile. 'The only thing that really counts,' he added, 'is to help patients to find peace of body and mind. Every zone of energy in the body, call it *chakra* if you like, can be the seat of disequilibria and blockages. Too much sympathetic tonus, not enough parasympathetic relaxation, and tensions become established, electrical and chemical information stagnates, the organs suffer and illnesses can arise. Explaining this to patients with the help of the theory of the *chakras*, enables them to recognise the reasons for their state of stress. They then have some keys for their healing.' This discourse would have pleased Wilhelm Reich or Alexander Lowen (see Chapter 5).

For Raghubir, the fear of revealing oneself or the inability to satisfy one's needs can promote the appearance of problems related to the fifth *chakra*, such as sore throat, respiratory infections or disturbances of the thyroid. He told me of the case of a woman patient who had to work beyond her strength to feed her family. For some years, she had suffered from hyperthyroidism, related, in her case, to the stress and necessity of being hyperactive. She suddenly became depressed. Blood analyses showed the development of hypothyroidism. The thyroid gland was exhausted, as was the patient – physically and psychologically.

Having myself used the interpretative grid of the *chakras* in my consultations, I noticed cases as eloquent as those described by Raghubir. Invariably schizophrenic patients whom I met turned their feet inwards, a position which betrayed the closing of the first *chakra* and thus a weak connection with tangible reality – a major problem in such patients. Similarly, I have treated a large number of patients suffering from gastric ulcers or diabetes in the context of romantic or professional set-backs responsible for a wound to the ego, typically associated with the third *chakra* and therefore the stomach and the pancreas. In addition, I often diagnosed a throat infection in patients who could not fulfil their essential needs or express their inner rage – a blockage that touches on the fifth *chakra*, or '*chakra* of the throat'. This reminds me of a study published in 1992 in *Biological Psychiatry* which showed that adolescents incapable of expressing their anger had a reduced level of immunity and an increase in the number of upper respiratory infections.[6] Apropos the 'throat *chakra*', linked to awareness of one's needs, a yogi told me that fatigue, hunger or boredom provoke a yawn which betrayed the need for sleep, food or change: 'Just because opening of the fifth *chakra* relaxes all the surrounding muscles. In this way, the body expresses its need,' he repeated with amusement, while yawning.

These observations merit being verified by rigorous studies, and as is the case with all interpretative patterns of the bodily symbology, it would be interesting to analyse the eventual impact of the theory of *chakras* on the appearance of illnesses, since, as we have seen in Chapter 6 (pp. 108–110), it is possible that a nocebo effect had suggested to the patients which pathology they could mobilise to express a malaise in a culture soaked in beliefs about the *chakras*. In the meantime, I remain confused because most of the patients in whom I have noticed a correlation between their illness and a psycho-spiritual disturbance associated with a particular *chakra*, had no appropriate vedic or esoteric knowledge. In all these cases, the theory of Wilhelm Reich was confirmed: a physical blockage or a psychological stress sets up contraction or 'closure' in a specific bodily zone (see Chapter 5, p. 85). The correlation between the relevant bodily zone and the theory of the *chakras* indicated to me which energetic disturbance was to be feared. I then found it sufficient to translate the concept of energy in terms of information. In the light of the laws of psycho-neuro-endocrino-immunology and the way of communication at the heart of the 'living matrix', I ended up understanding how the organs of the incriminated body part had become disturbed.

IN SEARCH OF UNITY

Science and tradition have been good partners for a long time in India. Thus in 1924, a biomedical research centre was set up at Lonavla in the State of Maharashtra near Bombay. The Kaivalyadhama Institute is exclusively committed to study the effects of yoga on health, is supported by the Indian government, and collaborates with researchers world-wide. The results of its work have greatly contributed to perpetuating the several-thousand-year-old tradition of the yogis.

Closely linked with Hinduism, and later Buddhism, yoga has been able to preserve its independence of all religious doctrine. This has certainly eased its spread in the West: today, if we look only at California, it is estimated that there are more yoga teachers there than in the whole of India.[7] Since quantity is not always synonymous with quality, the discipline is sometimes distorted. This is a pity because, far from being simple gymnastics with an exotic allure, yoga is above all an art of living: the philosophy at the heart of *ayurveda*. In this sense, it can be considered a true medicine, essentially preventive, sometimes curative.

Deriving from the root '*yug*' which means 'to re-unite', yoga resembles several practices intended to unify body and mind and to unite the individual with his environment. The principal goals are mental equilibrium and physical homoeostasis. As in the Chinese *qigong*, postures, breathing techniques and meditation make up the essentials of the practice. In the West, we often forget that in addition, it is necessary to respect a number of rules – of diet, habits and behaviour – just as important for health as the breathing exercises and physical postures. Yoga then becomes a pathway to personal development and the means of a profound understanding of oneself.

The sun meets the moon

The original *raja yoga*, a simple meditative technique carried out in a seated position, has evolved into a large number of postures or *asanas* which make up the *hatha yoga*. More physical, this form of yoga is the most widespread today. *Ha* means the sun and *tha* the moon: a meeting of opposites – day and night, masculine and feminine, tension and relaxation. Each posture involves an opportunity for stretching, flexion or turning, which favours the flexibility of the spinal column, makes the articulations supple, stimulates the circulation of the blood and the transmission of the nerve impulses, mobilises the organs and aligns the body in accordance with the principles of tensegrity. As in the Feldenkrais and Alexander techniques (see Chapter 8), it acts by never forcing, but progressively through becoming aware of tensions. Maintaining posture for a certain time trains the mind in perseverance and concentration, and is followed by a real meditative state. The breathing techniques, *pranayama*, increase the oxygenation of the blood, mobilise more energy and stimulate the parasympathetic system. The heart slows and the muscles relax. The fact of concentrating on the rhythm of breathing immediately promotes self-awareness. The mind is calmed and cleared. Positive emotions become dominant. One then learns to accept one's body as it is, shaped by one's history. The path that yoga offers is then that of listening and self-respect. It is also one of change because, in the course of practice, as rigidity gives way to fluidity, one discovers the astonishing plasticity of body and mind.

Often presented as a technique of relaxation, the practice of yoga reduces stress and anxiety, improves sleep patterns and fosters a feeling of well-being, as much in people who are well as in the sick.[9] A study carried out amongst medical students showed that those who practised yoga at examination time reported a significant reduction of stress, and better examination results.[10] Furthermore, for psychiatric patients, people undergoing detox, or patients with cancer, yoga forms a precious support. In addition to anti-depressant effects it can stimulate immunity and reduce pain.[11]

In 1998, Dean Ornish, director of the Preventive Medicine Institute at Sausalito and professor at the university of California at San

Francisco, published an article in the *Journal of the American Medical Association* which showed that a dietary regime associated with the practice of yoga could reduce narrowing of the coronary arteries and improve the circulation in the small peripheral arteries.[12] This raised a storm: that coronary disease could be reversible was unbelievable. Since then, numerous studies, notably in India, have shown that the practice of yoga reduces the level of harmful lipids in the arteries, as well as increasing the activity of antioxidants which protect against vascular lesions.[13] In addition, such practice often involves a change in dietary habits, stopping smoking, and a more relaxed way of life which, associated with a reduction in the sympathetic tonus and raised activity of the parasympathetic, lowers blood pressure.[14]

The demonstration of the positive effects of yoga is convincing: improvement of respiratory function, notably in asthmatic patients; increased flexibility in the tendons and improvement of muscle tone; and better irrigation of the organs and stimulation of the digestive tract, countering constipation.[15] Another study has even shown, in patients with irritable bowel syndrome, that yoga is more effective to treat the diarrhoea than the usual medicines.[16] We need no additional justification for introducing yoga into hospitals. At Columbia Presbyterian Medical Center in New York, the yoga teacher Robyn Ross set up a programme designed for cardiac patients who had undergone surgery. Practised in bed or wheel-chair, beginning the day after the operation, postures, breathing exercises and relaxation calmed the patients, improved their mood, eased their pain, gave them confidence in themselves and hastened their recovery.[17] When compared with classical physiotherapy, 'yoga is a gymnastic of the body and mind', I was told by a patient who had had a heart transplant and who had benefitted from this programme. 'One feels so energetic,' he added, 'as though one's breathing gives one great mental and physical strength, and at the same is very soothing.'

For each brain its own nostril

Yin and *yang*, *Ida* and *Pingala*, sympathetic and parasympathetic nervous systems; whatever the tradition, empirical or scientific, the human being feels that his happiness and health depend upon the balance between these two forces that act within him. Breathing is the most visible expression of this antagonism. Breathe in and out: the movements are opposite and complementary: they are the pulse of life.

However, we breathe badly. Often stressed, we are dominated by an upsurge of the sympathetic nerves. Our respiration is short, fast and shallow. Oxygenation of the red blood cells is mediocre, the circulation of the blood slows, and the amount of energy available to the cells of the organism is poor. The bodily suffering which follows increases our stress, and our breathing deteriorates again: a vicious circle is set up – but outside consciousness.

The Orient, having never separated mind from body, has effective techniques for breaking this negative cycle. Chinese or Indian, they all are concerned with breathing, and teach the mind to master the movements of the body, since breathing is the sole biological mechanism which can be either conscious or unconscious, automatic or voluntary. At first, an effort of attention brings tension into consciousness. Then a deep breath in is enough to raise the parasympathetic influx. The neural balance is re-established, oxygenation of the blood improves, cells increase the production of energy and the body relaxes, relieved.[18]

Carried out in full consciousness, perfect breathing consists of three phases: deep inspiration dilates the abdomen, opens the thoracic cage and allows air to penetrate right to the top of the lungs; then the relaxation of the rib cage pushes the air out of the lungs; finally, the contraction of the abdominal muscles completes expiration.

When I began to practise yoga, I learned to breathe out for twice as long as breathing in, in the classical manner. I remember my astonishment in noting the immediate effect of this '2/1 technique' on my stress. The explanation is simple: an imbalance in this direction between breathing in and out tilts the neurological balance towards the parasympathetic system. The relaxation obtained is then deep. More: the concentration required to maintain this rhythm plunges the mind into a very calming meditative state. To breathe in this way gave me a precious tool, especially in the operating theatre whenever I was faced with an especially difficult case.

Several years later when I was studying the influence of breathing on the emotional state, I once went to Franklin Park, near Princeton in New Jersey. There, in the middle of a green landscape, Sri Shyam-ji Bhatnagar, an Indian Master who had emigrated to the United States in the 1960s, taught the psychology of the *chakras*, healing by sounds and chanting, and, which intrigued me especially, the *swara yoga*, or 'yoga of breathing'[19]

According to *swara yoga*, each of the nostrils is connected with one of the energy channels, *Ida* or *Pingala*. Breathing through the left nostril activates *Ida*, breathing through the right nostril stimulates *Pingala*. As we have seen, *Ida* represents the parasympathetic system and *Pingala* is the equivalent to the sympathetic. After a brief theoretical introduction, Shyam-ji taught me how to manage a major stress simply by lying on my right side. In this position, mucus accumulates in the right nasal cavities, breathing takes place largely through the left nostril, *Ida* is stimulated and, after about 20 minutes, calm supervenes. The demonstration was convincing.

What was less so, were Shyam-ji's affirmations concerning which of the nostrils dominate breathing, by following an alternation influenced by the natural cycles of the organism and the movements of the planets. Intrigued, I went to Princeton University library to investigate this. To my great surprise, I found numerous studies demonstrating a cyclic alternation in nasal breathing. In conformity with the theory of *swara yoga*, these are produced in phase with natural ultradian rhythms which, every 90 minutes alternate the dominance of the cerebral hemispheres, induce hypovigilant phases during wakefulness, and lead to the periods of paradoxical sleep during which we dream.[20] EEG recordings show that the activation of the cerebral hemispheres is the opposite to the nostril used: when the air enters by the left nostril the right hemisphere is preferentially aroused; correspondingly, when the right nostril becomes predominant, it is the left hemisphere which is affected.[21] Forcing the passage of air through a congested nostril is then sufficient to bring about a change of cerebral dominance.[22]

The yogis do not therefore tell fantasies: it is possible to intervene in the functioning of the brain simply by modifying one's breathing. There is good reason for this: the nasal cavities are in close relationship with the hypothalamus, locus of the control of the autonomic system and central to the emotional brain. Further, each hemisphere is implicated in specific ways in the management of the emotions (see the work of Richard Davidson in Chapter 2, p. 32). Thus one can understand that a change in nasal dominance may modify cerebral dominance, and so influence the balance of the autonomic system, the emotional state and the functioning of the whole body.

In her doctoral thesis, the American psychologist Dorlene Osowiec showed that people who were serene and capable of positive self-realisation had a much more regular nasal cycle than those who were ill-adjusted and anxious, and who showed numerous symptoms of stress.[23] These results corroborate the ancient texts which link irregularity of the nasal cycle and prolonged dominance of one nostril with the emergence of physical diseases and psychological problems. For example, the yogis believe that if the respiration is exclusively through one nostril for more than three consecutive days, there is a risk of a mental, emotional or physical crisis. Nasal alternation seems therefore to be indispensable for the maintainance of good health, probably because it allows the establishment of regular parasympathetic phases, which above all are responsible for arousing the reparatory processes of the organism (see Chapter 2, p. 27).

Swara yoga could therefore have a number of therapeutic virtues, which would correspond to current neuro-physiological knowledge.[24] Some of them are easy to verify. In cases of fever, for instance, obstruction of the dominant nostril can lower the temperature. In cases of constipation, lying on one's left side before and after meals opens the right nostril, and therefore activates *Pingala*, which restarts the intestinal peristalsis. Stress, as we have seen, is reduced by the activation of *Ida* when lying on one's right side. The yogis of ancient times were not mistaken; the precision of their observations is impressive. The science that they passed down so wisely over the tens of centuries is a precious heritage. Can we have an openness of mind sufficient to explore even the strangest aspects of this? Such were the thoughts that accompanied me as I left the Princeton University library.

The relationships suggested here between *Ida* and *Pingala* on the one hand, and the two hemispheres of the brain and the autonomic system on the other, are wholly speculative. They are adumbrated in the hope of arousing interest in researchers so that they may be both tested and elaborated by scientific evaluation.

The rhythms of the body

As in traditional Chinese medicine, *ayurveda* and yoga emphasise the necessity of respecting the rhythms of the organism in accordance with the cycles of nature. For instance, the practice of *swara yoga* demands knowing the exact time of sunrise in order to synchronise opening the nostrils according to a precise calendar based on the positions of the sun and the moon. Western medicine, estranged for a long time from such ideas, has begun to become interested. Over the last 50 years, it has even invented a new discipline: chronobiology.

So far, one fact has been scientifically established: all living organisms have innate biological rhythms that are genetically programmed. In the human, the periodicity of these rhythms is defined by some kind of biological clocks – termed 'oscillators' – located at the level of the hypothalamus, the pineal gland, and in tissues as diverse as the retina, the skin, and the adrenal glands. A series of external 'synchronisers' exercise influence over these 'oscillators' in order to facilitate a perfect adaptation of the organism to its environment. Thus the light of day, climatic variations or fluctuations in the magnetic field control the temperature of the body, arterial pressure or hormonal secretions.[25]

This idea is not new, but it has taken a long time to become established. When Elliott Weitzman who, in 1971, discovered that the concentration of cortisol in the blood can be nil for a good while during the night, he did not dare to publish his findings because they appeared absurd. In the eyes of the majority of scientists, cortisol was a hormone that was too essential to be subject to such major fluctuations. Today we know that, with a very low level during the night, the secretion of cortisol is subject to a cycle that produces an increase in concentration around four o'clock in the morning, in anticipation of the individual waking up. Several studies have even shown that the rhythms of the adrenal glands are not only on a 24 hour cycle, but equally an annual one.

Thus the organism adapts its functioning with the help of the circadian rhythms with an approximately 24 hour period; the infradian rhythms, which is of more than 20 hours and may extend over several days; and the ultradian rhythms of less than 20 hours and which can reduce to a few seconds. The alternating breathing of *swara yoga* becomes part of the ultradian rhythms, as is the case of the periods of 90 minutes of paradoxical sleep and the states of hypovigilance which the psychobiologist Ernest Rossi compared with the phases of self-hypnosis necessary for learning and deep recuperation.[27]

The human being, synchronised in his relation with the environment, is programmed to live with the alternation of day and night and the progression of the seasons. Thus, over more than 600,000 years, subject to the cycles of agriculture, his physiology adapted to the need for activity in the summer and rest in the winter. Then the industrial revolution and massive urbanisation brusquely upset this harmonious synchronisation. The pattern of activity of modern man is therefore not in harmony with his own rhythms and often he lives dislocated from his relationship with the cycles of nature. For example, his choice of foodstuffs now depends less on the offers of the season than on the pressures of advertising. In the same way, it is also as well to remember that the 'summer holidays' come just when he has the least need for them.* Indeed, from a biological point of view, to rest in summer is an aberration. It is in winter that the body is fragile, its immunity diminished and the level of cortisol reduced. The tradition of summer holidays is not a biological necessity but above all is an historical error. In the past, the majority of children were released from the constraints of school during the summer months so that they could help with the work in the fields.[28]

The repercussions of such aberrations on health are still not well appreciated. Meanwhile, it would not be surprising if it were shown one day that there is a causal link between the chronobiological chaos in which we live and the appearance of illnesses such as Parkinson's or Alzheimer's, depression, and even cancer.

'The world is a complex network of events in which different kinds of connections interchange, overlap or combine, and influence the nature

---

* *Translator's note*: Perhaps it needs to be pointed out that in France and other continental countries, the whole of either July or August is the normal holiday.

of the whole,' stated Werner Heisenberg, Nobel prizewinner in 1939 for his discoveries in quantum physics. 'Each one of us is at the centre of a network of correlations,' said Ilya Prigogine, Nobel prizewinner for chemistry in 1977. From an understanding of these relationships will probably be born a new science, and then a new way of thinking about ourselves and the world.

11
BEHIND THE BELIEFS OF THE 'NEW AGE'

A RETURN TO THE SOURCES

'The crises of this age demand of the religions of the world that they formulate a new spirituality which would transcend all religious, cultural and national boundaries to promote a new consciousness of the unity of the human community. Stripped of all insularity, this new spirituality must be oriented towards a planetary awareness.' This declaration, published by the United Nations at their session in October 1975, summarises well the mental set from which arose the movement of 'The New Age'.[1]

Having appeared in the USA in the early 1970s, the hope for a 'new age' was without doubt a means of soothing the spiritual hunger which gnawed at a world stifled by the demands of material progress; a world which, faced with the uncertainties of a future dominated by technology, experienced a need to return to nature, to the essential values and solutions anchored in the traditions of the past. At the same time, some international exchanges built a bridge between the Orient and the Occident. A society lacking landmarks encountered a world still free of modernity onto which any projection was possible. Hinduism, Buddhism, Tantrism, Taoism – the possibilities satisfied the need. The ground was all the more favourable for the germination of new seeds because Eastern exoticism had fed the Western imagination throughout many centuries. Now there arose an overt hope of finding there the inner solutions the realisation of which had been prevented by material progress.

Thus the New Age nourished the purpose of a global civilisation built on the concept of unity in diversity. From then onward, all syncretism became permissible. Eastern and Western thought mingled, at risk of seeing their respective foundations distorted, completely altered, even simply forgotten. This desire for unification inevitably manifested itself in ideas about the nature of the human. The reconciliation of contrasting archetypes tended to harmonise the outer and the inner, man and woman, *yang* and *yin*, West and East, the material and the spiritual. It therefore seemed logical to see a concept of body–mind unity emerging: a global human in a global world. This echoed the macro- and microcosmic concepts of the Indian and Chinese traditions, extending equally to the theory of relativity and quantum physics: a global human being in a global world. Thus hope for the reconciliation between man and his environment became possible.

In this context, the energetic paradigm represented the ideal model, the indispensable link to explain the common nature of all things. As we have seen, the East, especially Asia, puts forward a series of concepts that are both ancient and full of common sense. From a medical point of view, the New Age has been largely inspired by the holistic thought of China and India. We can add others: several heritages – Amerindian, Soufi, Celtic and cabbalistic. Its ideals safeguard the beliefs in the power of healing in the terms of their Christian origins, which, from the Essenes to the kings of France, showed itself at the hands of many miracle workers.

The popularity of novels such as *The Celestine Prophecy* by James Redfield, or earlier, *The Third Eye* by Lobsang Rampa aka Cyril Hoskin, pretended Tibetan monk, inspired by the pseudo-Buddhist theories of the Theosophical Society of Helena Blavatsky, demonstrated how much the energy paradigm infused Occidental thought. Other concepts followed, such as the *chakras*, the astral body and telepathy, as well as spirits, spirit guides and the possibility of communicating with an unseen world – beliefs which, long before the dawn of the New Age, had belonged to esoteric and occult traditions, and before them to the primitive traditions of early Man.

THE NEW SORCERERS

A whole series of schools and practices grew out of this rag-bag, their promoters vaunting their merits with conviction. Surfing the Internet is sufficient to discover the extent of the commerce which develops around these 'new' practices that are inspired by the past. They all claim to reach an as yet unknown dimension, invisible and subtle, of the human being. None admit that the theories and explanations articulated are only cultural disguises, the trees that hid a forest of physiological effects which science could – or sometimes could not yet – explain. With campaigns of propaganda and registered trade marks, the sorcerers of the New Age end up by setting up a veritable commercial battlefield – a huge paradox as it comes from actors supposed to avoid opposition in order to allow diversity to co-exist with unity...

This esoteric-mystic-oriental folklore, apart from its sociological and anthropological interest, obviously has no credibility in the eyes of the scientific community. However, by refining these concepts, two approaches succeed in creating bridges with Western medicine. The first, identified as 'Therapeutic Touch' is purely a product of the West under the influence of the East. The second, *'reiki'*, originated in Japan under the influence of Christianity. Both are included in the list of alternative and complementary therapies, the study of which is encouraged by the National Institutes of Health in the United States (see the Introduction, p. 7).

A nurse meets a healer

'Therapeutic Touch' originated in 1972 through a meeting between two women: Dolores Krieger, nurse and professor at the University of New York, and Dora Kunz, a healer seduced by Theosophy. The doctrine of Theosophy, established in the 19th century by a group devoted to occultism, taught the existence of 'invisible masters', a 'vital energy' – comparable to *prana*, the *chakras* and energy fields – some kind of subtle networks which contain the physical, emotional and cognitive information that make up an individual. These notions can be seen as having been drawn from a fascination with Tibet which was considered magical and of which almost nothing was known, but which Helena Blavatsky, the founder of the Theosophical Society, claimed was peopled by lamas with extraordinary powers.[2]

Thanks to their greater rationality, the theory developed by Kunz and Krieger is less tainted with esotericism. It left no room for invisible beings who conferred special powers upon healers. In the eyes of these two women, anyone is capable of exerting 'spiritual' or 'energetic' healing on condition that they have developed sufficient sensitivity to the energy fields of their patients.[3] Contrary to what its name suggests, 'Therapeutic Touch' does not necessarily imply physical contact. The practician begins by centring himself, as is the case with every practitioner of *tai-chi* or *qigong*. This meditative state facilitates the perception of energy fields which radiate for some distance from the body. Large movements of the hands release 'congested' zones, relieve 'blockages' and 'reharmonise' the energy fields by projecting thoughts, colours or sounds.

For a mind habituated to reasoning from the basis of concrete facts, such procedures seem closer to delusions than to real techniques of treatment. Nevertheless, an increasing number of nurses and other health professionals seek training in touch therapy. Taught within some schools of nursing, this approach is more and more frequently practised at the bedside of the sick in some hospitals in the USA as well as in some other countries.[4]

A study published in 1998 in the *Journal of the American Medical Association* tried to establish whether the practitioners of Therapeutic

Touch were really capable of detecting the energy fields of a patient or not. Only 44% of the 280 tests carried out appeared conclusive. 'This is an irrefutable proof and there is no doubt that "Therapeutic Touch" is without foundation and its professional use is unjustified,' was the verdict of the authors of that article.[5] The controversy is not yet closed though, because, apart from the fact that the study has a number of methodological weaknesses, it does not permit exclusion of the efficacy of the approach, since this latter has simply not been evaluated. As Eric Leskowitz, psychiatrist at the faculty of medicine at Harvard has pointed out, the only conclusion to be drawn from these results is that it is impossible to detect in a reproducible way the presence of a possible human energy field.[6]

Patients themselves say that they feel pricking, vibrations, a feeling of heat or of cold or the circulation of energy through their body. This is the kind of experience to which I can testify having repeatedly submitted to the care of 'energy healers'. Suggestion, or reality? These sensations are not necessarily either surprising or unexpected. In effect, the simple fact of being taken into the care of another person often stimulates a true relaxation. As in massage, the parasympathetic nervous system is stimulated and vasomotor reactions at the level of the skin can explain the sensations reported by patients. Such profound relaxation is perhaps the root of the positive results recorded in cases of stress and anxiety.[7] It explains similarly the improvements noted in pain and the immune system.[8] However, we must not indulge in dreams: rigorous studies are badly lacking. An enquiry carried out by the Center of Research in Complementary and Alternative Medicine at the University of Michigan, showed that in 82 studies of 'Therapeutic Touch' only 18 were carried out according to criteria that would allow a sound evaluation of the results. From the summary of the report, it appeared that the technique is moderately effective in the management of anxiety.[9] The results were confirmed by another survey of studies, published in 2000 in the highly respected review, the *Annals of Internal Medicine*.[10] For all other indications, proofs are lacking. According to many specialists, it is the methods of the studies on energy treatments which should be examined. Indeed, the exclusion of a possible placebo effect demands the addition of a control condition of fake or pretend sessions. However, according to the practitioners it is their *intention* that is the key element of their work: intention which no fake session could possibly exclude.

Letting the universal energy flow

Another approach of energy healing in which intention occupies an essential role is *reiki*, a Japanese word that identifies the universal (*rei*) energy (*ki*). Brought into the light of day at the beginning of the 20th century by Mikao Usui, this method seems to have its origin in ancient Indian texts written in Sanskrit, the circumstances of their discovery being unclear. The identity of Mikao Usui is shrouded in legend: a Christian theologian who sought to understand the miracles of Christ, or a Buddhist monk, close to a Japanese scholar who had converted to Christianity? His research on Christ led him once to the United States, before he turned to the stories of healing practised by the Buddha. In fact, it seems that the story was altered towards the end of the 1930s by Hawayo Takata, a Japanese woman who lived in Hawaii. Having escaped an episode of surgery in Japan thanks to the healing effects of *reiki*, the young woman decided to teach this technique in the West. The Christian references involved probably eased her task, and for good reason: healing by the imposition of hands is more strongly attached to Western culture than to the Eastern traditions. One finds traces of it in the *tantras* of Tibetan Buddhism or in the *Vedas* of Hinduism, but none in medical systems – whether Tibetan or Ayurvedic – which do not use practices of this kind.

Free of all religious dogma, *reiki* distances itself from the healing practices of certain Christian churches. Nonetheless, the initiation rituals required give it an esoteric character. Detractors of the technique emphasise this point, pointing out the substantial sums that the candidate therapist must spend in order to gain access to mastery of the art.

Once again, centring himself plunges the practician into a meditative state, being at the same time relaxed and alert. This is necessary to allow him to 'channel' the universal energy, which penetrates the body and the energy fields of the patient, relieving certain 'blockages', whether physical, emotional or intellectual. During this period, the practician has nothing other to do except 'letting go' and becoming an instrument of healing. With humility and confidence, he allows the intelligence of the vital energy to work towards the re-establishment of fluidity and balance. His hands are placed at different points over the body of the patient, particularly at the position of the *chakras*. Visualising certain symbols or an organ bathed in a 'golden light of healing', helps him to remain concentrated, in contact with the patient, with the intention of promoting a return to full health, physical, emotional and spiritual. Remaining aware of himself and the other constitutes the actual secret of this practice.

These therapists will say that a session of *reiki* confers as much benefit to him who 'gives' as to him who 'receives'. Having experimented in both situations, I can confirm this: as in the case of massage, the touching of *reiki* creates a real sense of well-being in him who touches as well as in him who is touched (see Chapter 7, p. 117). What is even more astonishing is that the same effects of soothing and relaxation appear even when the treatment is carried out at a distance from the body.

As with other bodily therapies, emotions are aroused, tears may appear, and insights may arise in a completely unexpected manner. In addition, prickling, impressions of cold, shivering, yawning and muscular relaxation are such as what one may consider to be the results of parasympathetic stimulation. A study carried out at the University of South Glasgow, in Scotland, showed a greater diminution in arterial pressure and heart frequency in subjects receiving a session of *reiki*, than in those who simply relaxed, or in those whose treatment was administered by a practician who had not been initiated. The parasympathetic effect of *reiki* seems then to be specific and especially intense.[11]

At the University of Texas at Houston, an evaluation of the effects of *reiki* revealed a significant reduction in anxiety, a lowering of blood pressure and an increase in salivary IgA, no doubt in relation to parasympathetic stimulation and the resultant immunological cascade.[12] Other studies showed a favourable effect on some chronic pain, migraines, postoperative suffering, the formation of scar tissue on wounds, asthma, digestive problems and in the support of the dying. The normalisation of glycaemia has even been reported in patients whose blood sugar was excessively high.[13] Unfortunately again, weaknesses in the methodology of the greater part of these studies make definitive conclusions impossible.[14]

Sangeeta Singg, of Indian origin, is professor of psychology at the Angelo State University in Texas. Frustrated by the lack of well-conducted studies, she undertook a programme of researches in collaboration with Linda Dressen, a '*reiki* master'.[15] They investigated the effects of ten sessions of *reiki*, with a frequency of two a week, on a group of patients suffering from chronic illnesses. Compared with a control group who received treatment from a non-initiated practitioner, those patients who had received the 'real *reiki*' showed a clear reduction in their pain, their anxiety and their depressive symptoms, a small improvement in their self-esteem and a degree of spiritual lightening. Pain reduction was always present when a check was carried out, and remained three months after the end of treatment.[16]

It seems, therefore, that the fact of being truly initiated as a *reiki* healer does make a difference. Placing hands where indicated by the theory is not enough: it is necessary that the practitioner is in a state that will be 'favourable to letting the universal energy run naturally between him and the patient'. One might think that by distinguishing between the true *reiki* 'masters' and the false, the patients set in train a placebo effect which would explain the difference in efficacy of the two types of treatment. A study carried out at the University of Saskatchewan in Canada showed however, that the patients did not actually recognise the difference between the fake and the real *reiki* sessions.[17]

Such results probably justify the infatuation felt by some nurses and even certain doctors. Just like Touch Therapy, *reiki* has made an entry into hospitals. Since 1997 for instance, the surgeons at Columbia/HCA Portsmouth Hospital propose such a session before operations.[18] Some '*reiki* masters' are admitted to centres as prestigious as the Memorial Sloane Ketering Hospital in New York, the Tucson Medical Center in Arizona and the University of Michigan in Ann Arbor.[19] In Columbia Presbyterian Medical Center, New York, Mehmet Oz, professor of surgery and director of integrative medicine invited Julie Motz, a *reiki* practitioner, to carry out *reiki* on cardiac transplant patients. In an astonishing way, the patients had very little postoperative pain, showed none of the depressive symptoms which normally accompany the aftermath of this kind of intervention, and later did not show any rejection of the transplanted organ.[20] Placebo or no, *reiki* is gaining ground. In Canada and in Europe I know many physiotherapists and nurses, who, quite unostentatiously, practise it daily at their patients' bedsides.

An esoteric physicist

Intrigued by the healers of the New Age, I decided in 1999 to undertake training at the Barbara Brennan School of Healing in Miami, Florida. Founded in the early 1980s, this school had received official recognition by the State of Florida. At the end of a programme copied from those of any and all other colleges, it provided certificates of professional competence and even bachelor degrees. Nothing really very special, were it not for the topics taught: a solid training in psychotherapy centred on the body, apprenticeship to various energy therapies, and in contrast to Therapeutic Touch and *reiki*, a highly developed system of beliefs involving auras, *chakras*, collaboration with spirit guides and communication with the invisible in the course of 'channelling'. The whole panoply of New Age practice is therefore taught in the strictest legality.[21]

A physicist by training, Barbara Ann Brennan had left her post at NASA to undertake a course of personal development: psychotherapy, bioenergetic analysis, various energy disciplines, and spiritual research in the heart of the Pathwork Community. Twenty years later, this eclectic path resulted in an original teaching programme, followed by several hundred students, who travelled to Florida from all over the world five times a year for training over four years. An adventure.

At first I had to become familiar with all of these intangible concepts without ever considering them in a pejorative way, since they were necessary to me as a therapeutic framework and as tools. Then I had to learn the technique of 'letting go', and the quality of 'presence' required for the successful unfolding of the 'healings', or sessions of 'energy therapy' – an unusual procedure for a surgeon like me, accustomed to being totally in control.

Set between the non-directive work of *reiki* and the active re-harmonisations of Therapeutic Touch, Brennan's approach consisted of a well-ordered series of techniques – a sophisticated 'science' based on a number of heterogeneous beliefs, largely influenced by the theosophy of Helena Blavatsky. After a while I understood that the processes I had been taught allowed me to better focus my attention – it was a means of sharpening my concentration. Thus, in a meditative state, the mind empty, centred on the present moment, I was plunged into a kind of trance, induced by the breathing exercises based on *tai-chi* and *qigong*. Immediately, my senses opened in an astonishing manner. At that moment I became able to 'see', to 'feel', or simply have an intuition of a physical or psychological disorder in the patient lying on the treatment table. This is what Barbara Brennan called 'the high sense of perception'.

I remember the case of Elsa. Aged about 50, she consulted me because she had heard that the energy therapies such as *reiki* or 'healings' helped one to relax. After the period of centring by means of breathing, I put my hands on the patient's feet and immediately smelt a strong odour of urine. Having learned not to allow my state of concentration be disturbed by asking questions, I continued the session. The smell of urine continuing, I directed my gaze towards the abdomen of the patient, and there I 'saw' a dark patch around her right ovary. 'See' is a word which is not at all appropriate for the experience that I am describing, but I know none more appropriate. At the end of the session, careful not to alarm Elsa, I asked if she was seeing a gynaecologist. She replied that she regularly consulted her gynaecologist because she had a cyst on her right ovary. Surprised by the match of my 'vision', I recommended that she should have another check very soon, because the energy seemed 'not to circulate properly in the region of that ovary'. Three months later, Elsa telephoned me to say that a tumour of 12 centimetres in diameter had been found on the right ovary!

My perceptions in the course of this session reminded me of observations published some years ago in *The Lancet*, that dogs could detect cancers of the skin, the lungs or the breast, simply because their olfactory sense is so well-developed that they can detect the volatile substances produced by the tumours.[22] A study that appeared in the

British Medical Journal in 2004 even showed that some dogs are trained to recognise the urine of patients suffering from cancer of the bladder.[23] Is it therefore possible that a human, in certain states of consciousness, might be able to perceive information normally inaccessible to the senses because inhibited by the constant activity of the cerebral cortex? Are there circumstances when, in place of thinking and informing the outside world, we allow ourselves to be wholly informed by it? Intuition appears above all a bodily process: in an unceasing way, the brain records information which awakens emotional feelings at a physical level. Decoding these sensations is then a source of information vital for making a decision. One might then imagine, in facilitating feeling, the act of centring by a healer allows the development of his intuition. It remains meanwhile necessary to pay attention to identifying the eventual projections which may distort the value of the perceived information.

Such an experience leads one to think of the 'energy work' in terms of information (see Chapter 9, pp. 139–140). That which some people call 'communication between one unconscious and another unconscious' may depend quite simply on an extremely sensitive perception of reality. Most of the time, this phenomenon occurs in an unconscious way. The skill of certain psychotherapists, psychoanalysts and healers is to make this experience more conscious. In this sense, the Brennan training is a very powerful tool in relationships.

As in *reiki*, healing sessions create emotional changes, insights and calming which help patients in their psychological evolution. After a period of 'integration', which may last from a few hours to several days, the beneficiaries of this kind of treatment often declare that they 'see things differently': pay more attention to their body and feel more spiritual. Specific effects of the treatment, or simple consequences of a wish for a more general change in the process of having recourse to such practices? It is difficult to judge. Nevertheless, it seems obvious that, before receiving their first session, most of those seeking energy therapies are already in search of personal and spiritual development.

Numerous psychologists and psychiatrists turn to *reiki* or 'healing' to speed up the therapeutic process of their patients.[24] I have myself noted the beneficial effects of this way of working. However, one cannot recommend too strongly the use of caution because the metaphorical images used by certain practitioners can impress themselves on a patient's mind to the extent of making these concepts primary, when they ought to be of secondary, or even tertiary importance. For example, the practice of 'channelling' and the search for spiritual guidance provided by the invisible beings must be analysed in the light of the beliefs of Western mythology. It may not be a matter of chance, since most Master Healers of the 'New Age' declare themselves to be inspired by external revelation. Such belief in a 'revelation' has led in the past to Moses, Jesus, Mahomet or even Joseph Smith, founder of the Mormon Church. The 'revealed truths' from a 'higher intelligence' can become dogmas imposed on others in the name of that superiority. It is then not difficult to imagine the manipulation, conscious or not, that could be exercised on those who have not understood that the messages of gurus of the New Age are nothing but products of their own imagination, an imagination that is not always enlightened or kindly.

VITALISTS VERSUS MECHANISTS

The need to convince

The practices of the New Age are not at all new. On the contrary. Every period in history and every culture has invented rituals during which a spiritual authority obtains therapeutic effects linked to a state of trance, which we now describe as hypnotic. A simple gesture, a touch or a glance may suffice. The smell of incense, the rhythms of drums, songs, dances, or more simply, magical passes enacted around the patient, create conditions which mobilise the power of his own autosuggestion, his own wish for healing. The forces of the unconscious may express themselves in archetypal images: angels and demons, good or evil spirits.

Before the birth of the scientific culture, suggestion was at the core of a large number of therapies, and since the human mind is never short of efforts of the imagination in order to calm its distresses, numerous metaphors have been used to explain the inexplicable. Then, in the 17th and 18th centuries, great discoveries in physics and chemistry revealed a tangible reality. Immediately the language of healers had to adapt to the dominant discourse. Thus when in 1779, the German physician Franz Anton Mesmer attempted to explain the 'miraculous' effects of healing sessions, it was in his *Mémoire sur la découverte du magnétisme animal* (Memorandum on the Discovery of Animal Magnetism) that he did so. What could be more obvious, in an epoch when electricity had just been discovered? To describe suggestion as a process in which a magnetic fluid operated between a healer and his patient would provide the scientific credibility required by the medical community. This was, however, without taking account of the perspicacity of savants like Benjamin Franklin and Antoine Laurent de Lavoisier, members of the commission appointed by Louis XVI to examine the theories of Mesmer. Their conclusion was irrefutable: 'The fluid alone, without suggestion, is impotent; imagination without the fluid can produce the effects which are attributed to the fluid.' Magnetism or 'mesmerism' was therefore placed within the category of charlatanry.

Some years ago, I read with interest a series of studies published by Daniel Wirth, about the influence of Therapeutic Touching on the healing of skin wounds. The results were convincing, since the treatment speeded up healing of the lesions.[25] It remained to be explained how such treatment might act. Was it the consequence of the action on a possible energy field, as the practitioners of Therapeutic Touch proclaimed, or rather the result of a hypnotic suggestion that triggered off the neuro-endocrino-immunological cascade? A study carried out at Ohio State University by Janice Kiecolt-Glaser showed a slowing of skin wound healing in people who were under stress from Alzheimer's disease in their spouse (see Chapter 3, p. 41). Carol Ginandes, a psychologist at Harvard, proposes arguments in favour of hypnotic effects. In a study carried out on patients immobilised by a fracture of the ankle and treated by a weekly session of hypnosis over a period of 12 weeks, she noted a significant shortening of healing time.[26] In order to evaluate whether psychological treatment was the sole cause of the results, she carried out another study in women having undergone a mammary reduction, divided into three groups: the first receiving no postoperative treatment at all, the second receiving eight session of psychotherapy, and the third receiving eight sessions of hypnosis focused on wound healing. The results favoured the specific action of suggestion, since the patients receiving hypnotic treatment showed significantly faster healing than the other two groups.[27]

The results obtained by Daniel Wirth could therefore also be explained by a hypnotic process, and by suggestion – if indeed the results were real, since I was stupefied to find when I checked my sources that Wirth was not a physician as he claimed. More seriously still, he had taken part in a fraudulent study claiming to show that prayer had a positive influence on *in vitro* fertilisation.[28] This study, published in a respected scientific review, was the subject of an enquiry, at the end of which Bruce Flamm, professor of gynaecology at the University of California at Irvine, revealed the scandalous past of Wirth.[29] False identities, numerous swindles and criminal connections: his compromising *curriculum vitae* would not qualify his name to appear in this book were it not to illustrate how the desire to convince blinded the promoters of a theory which had escaped all scientific validation.

Waves and fields

One can understand the general mistrust since evinced towards researchers in the field of 'energy medicine'. All the more the desire to prove the existence of a force different from those described by modern physics relaunches the old debate which, for 400 years has set at odds the vitalists and the mechanists. The quarrel is passionate: on the one side the mechanists affirm that reality is exclusively material and that science can or will describe everything with the aid of the laws of physics and chemistry; on the other, the vitalists consider this reductionism unacceptable because it does not take account of the 'vital force' which acts behind the mechanisms identified by materialist science. Strengthened in their beliefs by the discovery of electromagnetism, the vitalists describe the 'vital force' as a group of 'fields' which interact at a distance. Their fingers burnt by such pseudo-scientific demonstrations in the manner of Mesmer, the mechanists distrust and suspect the vitalists of wishing to prove the existence of the divine. The debate is, therefore, not only philosophic, but also religious.

It is not always easy, in this context, to discern the influence exerted by the beliefs of the researchers on the interpretation of the phenomena being observed. One fact is nevertheless well-established: there are fields of energy produced by the activity of the human body. A familiar example: the calorific field. Created by cellular metabolism, this field is given off outside the limits of the skin and one can perceive the warmth at some distance from the individual. Another example: the magnetic fields generated by the electrical activity of the muscles and organs. This phenomenon appears more mysterious, yet it is entirely physiological. In effect, since the beginning of the 19th century, we have known that an electric current passing through a conductive material creates a magnetic field capable of diverting the magnetic needle of a compass. Now electricity is the basis of nervous, muscular and cardiac functioning. In the heart, for example, each beat begins with an electrical impulse; the circulatory system being a good conductor, the cardiac electrical flux is propagated throughout the organism, and inevitably, a magnetic field appears around the body. Some measurements made by an extremely sensitive magnetometer – the SQUID (Superconducting Quantum Interference Device) – shows that the field extends infinitely in space, its intensity diminishing progressively until it becomes undetectable within the context of other electromagnetic fields produced in the environment.[30] This phenomenon can be observed for all organs. Nevertheless, since the cardiac electric activity is the most intense of those produced by the body, the cardiac biomagnetic field is much stronger than the others – around 5,000 times more than the magnetic fields produced, for example, by the brain.[31]

For a long time, the electrical and magnetic fields produced by the body were considered to be epiphenomena: simple derivatives of the physiological activity of the cells. They were used only for the diagnosis of certain pathologies: muscular (electromyogram), ocular (oculogram), cardiac (electrocardiogram or magnetocardiogram) and cerebral (electroencephalogram). Today there are more and more arguments for thinking that biomagnetism plays an important part in the regulation of biological processes,[32] probably through the intermediation of the 'living matrix'. As we saw in Chapter 9 (p. 146), the perineurial, perivascular, perilymphatic, perimuscular connective tissue, and the periosteum make up an excellent network to conduct information. Thus, by being propagated throughout the 'living matrix', electrical and magnetic fields may act on every cell in the body down to the level of the DNA. This mode of communication is likely to be older than the conduction of electric current by the nervous system.

Certain researchers did not consider it necessary to wait to understand the conductive properties of the 'living matrix' before exploiting the central controlling role that electrical and magnetic fields demonstrate, for therapeutic purposes. Already in the 19th century needles were planted in the areas over fractured bones in order to pass an electric current believed to stimulate healing. Considered to be 'without foundation', this practice was banned in the early 20th century. All the same, the phenomenon is entirely explicable: the magnetic fields so produced, induced an electrical activity in the bone of the same kind as that produced by muscular movements; by that very fact, bone growth is automatically stimulated. Nowadays magnetic fields are applied with success in activating the healing of bony fractures, sometimes several decades after the process of bone regeneration had been interrupted.[33] Subsequent research has shown that a field with a frequency of 2 hertz is especially well adapted to neural regeneration, 7 hertz for bone growth, 10 hertz for the healing of ligaments and 20 hertz for the proliferation of blood vessels and the fibroblasts which repair tissues.[34]

A healing energy?

Whether one is a vitalist or a mechanist, there remains a question: are electric and magnetic fields implicated in Therapeutic Touch, *reiki*, or other 'healings'? In other words, do energy healings work by other mechanisms than suggestion and relaxation?

To answer this question, John Zimmerman at the University of Colorado, Denver, by means of a SQUID magnetometer, recorded the biomagnetic fields emitted by the hands of practitioners of the 'Therapeutic Touch' while at work.[35] Similar tests have been carried out in Japan on the hands of people practising *qigong*, *yoga* or meditation.[36] In both studies, the biomagnetic fields emitted by the practitioners' hands were very intense, up to a thousand times stronger than those produced by the heart and a million times stronger than those of the brain. The frequencies of these fields varied between 0.3 and 30 hertz with an average around 7 to 8 hertz. This is worrying; as we have just seen, these frequencies have been shown to be effective in healing damaged tissues. One may therefore be tempted to see a connection. However, none of these studies sought to establish whether the fields recorded had produced any improvement in the health of the people who underwent this treatment.

Another troubling fact: the frequency of 7 to 8 hertz corresponds to the alpha rhythm of the brain, characteristic of meditative states and relaxation. Now alpha waves have been recorded by the electroencephalograms (EEG) of healers of different traditions in the course of their healing sessions.[37] Further, the frequency of 7 to 8 hertz is close to that of the 'geomagnetic resonance' of Schumann, a phenomenon arising from the 200 lightning flashes which split the sky every second and generate electromagnetic waves whose trajectory around the planet rebounds ceaselessly between the Earth and the ionosphere.[38] In the opinion of some biologists, this conjunction could be at the origin of the sensitivity of living organisms to variations of the Earth's magnetic field.[39] It could also explain how the hands of healers produce such powerful biomagnetic fields, the frequency of which is aligned to that of Schumann. In his book *Energy Medicine: The Scientific Basis* James Oschman clearly shows how meditation or other calming practices cause one zone of the hypothalamus, which controls the electrical activity of the brain, to quieten. The disconnection of this 'cerebral pacemaker' could allow the geomagnetic pulses to co-ordinate the brain waves by a mechanism no doubt implicating some receptors in the pineal gland that are sensitive to magnetic impulses. In this way, the cerebral waves could align themselves to the Schumann frequency, adopting a frequency of 7 to 8 hertz, close to the alpha rhythm. In penetrating the 'living matrix', these waves could produce biomagnetic fields whose strength, dictated by the Schumann frequency, becomes amplified. This could be sufficient to confer on them a therapeutic potential.[40] Delirium, or a hypothesis to explore? The response depends on whether one accepts the concept of such an interdependence between the organism and its environment.

THE UNSEEN CONNECTIONS

The phenomena of leading and resonance of vibrations similar to those that we find in Oschman's hypothesis is rather like what happens when two identical clocks are hung on the same wall, they eventually match each other's movements. Or when one sounds the strings of a guitar, the strings of another nearby begin to vibrate at the same frequency.

An identical mechanism is probably at the root of the synchronisation observed between human beings, such as when women live under the same roof they frequently menstruate eventually at the same time. In the 1930s, Harold Saxton Burr, professor at Yale, noticed that ovulation caused modifications of an electric field, the detection of which at the fingers enabled one to predict the fertility of women.[41] Thus one might imagine that an invisible communication is established between cohabiting women through their electrical and magnetic fields, ending in the synchronisation of their menstrual cycles.

When the heart talks to the brain

Communication between individuals is an extremely complex process. It implies a very subtle series of interactions: the signals expressed by the body (facial expressions, quality of the voice, gestures, postures); the physico-chemical signals projected in space (sounds, heat, odours, pheronomes); and perhaps, electromagnetic signals that remain totally unconscious. At any rate, this is the suggestion of researchers at the Institute of HeartMath, who are exploring the role of cardiac biomagnetic fields on the internal coherence of the functioning of every organism and on the external coherence of the links between individuals.

A series of tests were conducted on pairs of subjects placed facing each other without physical contact. The results showed that the electrocardiac signals emitted by the heart of one of the two could be detected in the electroencephalogram (EEG) recording the cerebral activity of the other person, while neither of the two subjects were aware of the purpose of the experiment. From this, Rolin McCraty, Research Director of the Institute of HeartMath, supposes that direct communication is set up between the heart of one and the brain of the other.[42] This is also the view of Gary Schwartz and Linda Russek, who obtained the same kind of results in their experiments conducted at the University of Arizona.[43]

This heart–brain communication seems to be better when the subjects being tested visualise positive thoughts and breathe deeply while focusing attention on their hearts – a technique advocated by the Institute of HeartMath to stabilise variability in cardiac rhythm (see Chapter 4, p. 70). According to McCraty, the emotional balance and physiological harmony created by 'cardiac coherence' produce more structured biomagnetic fields. The difference in 'vibratory' quality could be automatically perceived by others. This may be especially the case if the latter are themselves in this state of coherence which, according to McCraty, renders them more sensitive to the decoding of the information contained in the fields produced by their interlocutor.[44]

Thus it seems as though the heart and the body together function as transmitting and receiving antennae for very subtle communication.

I remember an Indian swami who taught 'listening with the heart'. His advice was simple: 'Breathe deeply in stretching the chest, picture the wheel of your fourth *chakra* opening to allow a rose to blossom, feel the empathy toward your interlocutor, and allow yourself to be filled with positive feelings' – a technique very close to that described by the researchers at the Institute of HeartMath to bring about 'cardiac coherence'. When used in my consultations, this creates an easy and warm communication with my patients. A profound understanding develops between them and myself without a word having been spoken.

Real cardioelectromagnetic communication, or simple perception of an empathic attitude amongst the small signs analysed by the brain in an unconscious way? The answer is not clear. There are indeed many studies which have proved the existence of a physiological synchronisation between patients and their therapist, between husband and wife, or between humans and their pets.[45] Is this science, or pseudoscience? A new avenue for research, or a utopian desire to translate the metaphor of 'heart love' into scientific terms? The spectre of the 'New Age' is perhaps not far away. There is a risk of taking short-cuts and of drawing hasty conclusions: therefore we need to be careful.

The intention in question

Prudence and curiosity do not always make good partners. What should one think of those experiments, more and more numerous, done in laboratories in order to test the effects of a 'healing energy' on living cells or micro-organisms? A joint work entitled *Healing, Intention, and Energy Medicine*, published in 2003 at the initiative of Wayne Jonas and Cindy Crawford, researchers at the Samueli Institute for Information Biology, gathered together a series of results that are, to say the least, surprising. Under the influence of healers, cancerous cells were inhibited; white blood cells proliferated if they were normal, or on the contrary, stopped growth if they were malignant; the activity of the NK cells of the immune system increased; the DNA and other molecules changed their structure.[46] One study even allows one to think that the *intention* of the healer caused the growth or diminution of proliferation of bacteria in petri cultures.[47]

Inevitably such investigations arouse scepticism. 'Nevertheless, a little daring often allows development in our ways of thinking,' said a biologist at the Institute of HeartMath. That is probably why there is a growing number of researchers with prestigious backgrounds, gathering together at the heart of various independent institutions – in the United States for instance, the Institute of HeartMath, the Samueli Institute for Information Biology and the Institute of Noetic Sciences – which collaborate with particular universities and sometimes even with the Ministries of Health and Defence. The influence of the mind on material; power of intention; 'remote viewing'; 'non-local' consciousness: the titles of some protocols of research make one smile. That is of little importance: the curiosity of committed researchers is unlimited. At the Engineering Anomalies Research Laboratory (PEAR Lab) at Princeton University for example, an international research programme has been initiated in order to study the influence of collective consciousness on random number generators.[48]

All these projects seem to pursue the same dream. Consciously or not, they speak of encounters, of contacts, of relationships and of love – so many things badly lacking in our technological societies. Patients, therapists and researchers show this need clearly in their craze for the energy therapies. As Alan, a fellow orthopaedic surgeon to whom I had given a session of healing therapy, said to me: 'Whether one believes or not, and unimportant as is the explanation when one human puts his hand with love on another human, something passes between them without words. In this process, suddenly they become one. It creates a bond.'

'Relationships are the cement of life. Without them, nothing takes shape. Relationships are the framework of the tissue that is life. Without them, no shape makes sense. They are the Essence.' These words, spoken to me by my friend Raghubir, reminded me of a question that had been asked of me by Arnulfo – you remember, the Mexican healer of whom I spoke in Chapter 1: 'Between you and me, who is the most important?' My immediate reaction was 'me', but I felt a little ashamed to admit it. My hesitation amused the sorcerer because the answer he had expected was neither 'me' nor 'you'. It was 'both': the link. 'This is what is important,' commented Arnulfo. 'It is the link between the body and the mind that creates the unity of the human being. The link between individuals creates the unity of humanity. The link between humanity and the Earth that makes the unity of the world.' New Age or no: the idea is beautiful.

CONCLUSION
A MEDICINE OF THE HUMAN POTENTIAL FOR LIFE IN THE 21st CENTURY

> *Utopia is visible only to the inner eye*
> Jorge Luis Borges

When we began this book, we had our sights fixed on the target of clarifying the still obscure landscape of alternative and complementary medicines. We immediately discovered that 'unconventional' approaches acted at the level of the essential connections that exist between thought and matter, culture and biology, mind and body.

At the level of mind, we have grasped the importance of metaphors, suggestion and the 'effect of meaning' in the processes of healing; we have seen how positive emotions, hope and humour set in motion the reparatory mechanisms of the body; and we have surveyed the effectiveness of visualisation, meditation and hypnosis in the treatment of suffering, both physical and psychological.

At the level of body, we have noted the damage done by the repression of emotions; we have learned how the release of tension restores the fluidity and coherence that are indispensable to the preservation of health; we came to understand the necessity of maintaining a balanced posture and moving harmoniously; we have evaluated the benefits of touch, massage and muscular and skeletal manipulations, and we have discovered the relevance of exploring the intricacies of body–mind memory and its transgenerational roots.

Between these two, we have emphasised the relevance of oriental metaphors where energy represents the substratum common to the mind and the body; and, beyond some exotic or esoteric practices, we have followed new pathways towards understanding how it is possible to help someone to heal the entirety of his being.

Phenomena such as the neuroplasticity of the brain, the psycho-neuro-endocrino-immunological chain reactions, electronic and vibrational communication at the core of the connecting tissues of the 'living matrix', bio-electro-magnetic interactions between individuals: our enquiry has been focused on the scientific arguments to do with the controversial nature of alternative and complementary medicines. It is apparent that every individual possesses inside himself important resources for the prevention of disorders and for healing. Aldous Huxley, author of *Brave New World*, called this 'the human potential': in itself, it does not represent a new discovery. Many people have intuitive recourse to it. Nonetheless, demonstrating its existence scientifically raises the question whether it is absolutely necessary to have immediate recourse to external remedies.

SOME CLARIFICATIONS

Responsible but not guilty

'To make people believe that they possess the capacity to protect and to heal themselves is a hateful way of making them feel guilty,' a rheumatologist colleague of mine said to me one day. This remark reveals a misunderstanding which poisons Western medicine. First and foremost, we are not concerned with 'making people believe' in the existence of these internal resources. They exist for good or bad, as the scientific work reported in these pages witnesses. Therefore it is not a question of 'making people feel guilty' but simply one of giving an individual a sense of responsibility for his own health.

I have a feeling that this confusion between guilt and responsibility concerning health, is the heritage of a remote religious past where good, evil, and error or sin terrorised our minds. How can one recognise simple responsibility if one dreads to be also judged guilty? Many ill people, preferring the status of victims, consider themselves to be powerless, without resources and compelled to submit. They are convinced that the solutions to their problems can come only from outside.

This is one way of thinking, but not the only way. Replacing judgment with calm analysis makes it possible to identify the facts, the causes and the results. It is then possible to choose which causes to implement in order to obtain which results. This is where self-interest becomes responsibility for oneself.

When applied to medicine, this principle is sometimes difficult to explain, as much to patients as to some practitioners. However, if we examine diseases and their development carefully, we can often identify those causes which the patient is in a position to tackle himself. It may then seem obvious that if a patient accepts his part of 'response-ability' in the process that led to the illness, he will automatically be led to find appropriate responses. From victim, he becomes actor in the preservation of his health and author of the healing of his state.

Take a simple and frequent example: influenza. Obviously, no one can be blamed for being exposed to infection by the influenza virus. On the other hand, one is often responsible for certain factors that favour this contamination. As we saw in Chapter 3, fatigue, overwork, and stress are factors that predispose towards this disease. But even though it is impossible to prevent the virus from being around, everyone can look after his general state and develop a sufficiently strong degree of immunity to avoid being contaminated – or if it is too late, to help his organism eliminate the virus more quickly.

In my experience, the principle of responsibility can be applied to the treatment of many illnesses, even cancers and congenital malformations. This is not to say that patients with such pathologies can act upon the hereditary, toxic or viral causes which create them. It simply means that the way in which they react when faced with such pathologies profoundly influences the development of these pathologies. I recall here Arthur, a small boy handicapped with psychomotor problems. For some years he had suffered from terrible epileptic seizures. No treatment had succeeded in relieving the condition, until one day a paediatrician advised his parents to consult a therapist – 'a kind of healer who massaged him, taught him to breathe and made him properly aware of his own body'. Results were not long in appearing: Arthur became more relaxed, the seizures occurred less frequently and when they did, were experienced as much less painful. 'He's a different child,' his mother told me, 'and the fact that he has changed, changed the whole family. Or maybe it was our changing that allowed Arthur to become different....' Because Arthur's parents had themselves entered psychotherapy and, having become conscious of their bodily tensions, they took up the practice of *tai-chi*.

Beware of the fantasy of omnipotence!

The idea of responsibility in the face of the chain reaction of cause and effect threatening to create imbalances and illness is close to the oriental concept of *karma*. This notion emphasises the possibility of changing causes in order to avoid the repetition of the same effects. Without necessarily believing in reincarnation, more and more Westerners have the intuitive feeling that they are actors in, even creators of, their ills. The emphasis that is placed on the prevention of illnesses is a good example of this, as is interest in psychosomatic symbolism. More significant still is the emergence of transgenerational psychology, which teaches that the chain reaction of cause and effect surpasses the individual and is engraved in a form of transmission at the centre of an evolutionary process. Here too there is no guilt to feel. However, even if the past inevitably escapes our control, the present belongs to him who lives. Thus, in understanding his responsibility in the maintenance of the beliefs, habits and loyalties of his ancestors, anyone can avoid establishing the elements necessary for the appearance of a symptom (see Chapter 6, p. 103).

This way of thinking might make some patients believe that it is possible to control the course of their illness by an act of will, resolving certain emotional conflicts, healing unconscious memories inherited from previous generations and mobilising the mechanisms of self-healing. To think in such a way would be an error, a lack of humility and an illusion of omnipotence: we must never underestimate the complexity of the human being nor ignore the laws of nature.

This is what Mary, a young woman with pancreatic cancer, had experienced during her illness. In tandem with chemotherapy, she undertook psychotherapy, learned *qigong*, and was regularly massaged by a Master of *shiatsu*. She had healed old emotional wounds, and relaxed deep muscle tensions. 'Oddly enough, I have never felt as well in my head and in my body,' she told me. Nevertheless, the cancer progressed. Disappointed, she felt she was guilty. 'Perhaps I did not go far enough in psychotherapy. I should have taken better care of my body. I have not yet developed enough fluidity and coherence between my body and my mind,' she accused herself. She was wrong because, even if we have within ourselves the means of self-healing, we must accept that sometimes the process of the disease is irreversible. It is a fact: no one is guilty; nature can act in this way. A few days after we had discussed all this, Mary telephoned me. 'I am healed,' she told me in a very calm voice. 'My body may not have cast off the tumour, but my being is freed: I am relieved of an immense weight. I understand the meaning of my life, or at least, I can give it meaning. I am at peace.' Mary's desire for omnipotence and her feeling of guilt had then given way to humility and wisdom. Two weeks later, she died.

The desire for omnipotence leads to magical thinking, comparable to that which animates the fantasies of childhood. The danger is that one may easily lose contact with reality. I frequently meet patients who are convinced that they can cause a malignant tumour to reabsorb by visualisation, meditation or comprehending the 'message' of their disease. They talk to me about opening *chakras*, explain that they *know* it is possible to be healed without either surgery or chemotherapy, and demand that I help them by putting my hands on their bodies as the sorcerers with whom I had worked used to do. The hope they feel is certainly helpful for their healing, but in the Western context in which I had been trained and in which I work, I am invariably moved to reply that *my* sorcery could be summed up as making people aware of their own multiple dimensions. If they have a tumour embedded in their physical body, I recommend that they use physical means to treat it. Nowadays surgery, radiotherapy and chemotherapy are what biomedical science has found to be the best way to intervene. These procedures are not perfect and they have adverse side-effects, but at the same time they render appreciable services. I add here, however, that in view of all we have explored together in this book, that is not enough. In addition to physical methods and conventional medicine there is a whole series of complementary approaches which help the organism to recover more easily, and stimulate the processes of self-healing. Furthermore, in order that an individual should become able to heal the whole of his being, it is necessary to encourage him to explore his psychological and emotional suffering, to encourage him to free himself from the conditioning of his past, and to show him the possibility of *his* choosing his future.

Freeing the person

Becoming aware of one's potential for the prevention of illness and for healing helps one to maintain the strength to face up to an illness and to preserve a degree of autonomy in the relationship with those who are providing treatment. This is important because, as much in the context of conventional medicine as in alternative and complementary approaches, there is a risk of a dependence being established between the patient and those treating him. It is important not to delude oneself as this can show itself in two ways: the patient adopts the behaviour of a child by demanding help, and those treating him find him a source of psychological and financial comfort. The trap is real; to frustrate this, the therapist must behave like a good father who values the capacities of his child.

This aspect of treatment is vital because, as we have seen, self-confidence sows positive emotions and a cascade of physiological processes which participate in healing. From inner confidence arises the desire to take care of oneself and play an active role in re-establishing health. The majority of books on alternative and complementary medicines emphasise this point: to heal an individual is to give treatment or prescribe a remedy; to heal a person is to give him access to this confidence and inner certainty. The act of therapy is then an act of love.

Instead of this, without actually being conscious of it, many physicians and therapists consider their patients simply as consumers of remedies and treatments. This is a pity because there is probably no more rewarding an action than to help another to believe in himself and encourage him to explore and exploit his inner resources. 'That is a utopia,' I was told by the director of a pharmaceutical company at a lunch arranged to launch a new 'anti-ageing' product. 'There are always strong or weak people; those who invent solutions and those who consume them,' he said without the slightest shadow of hesitation in his voice.

Such ideas reveal the cynicism which one sometimes encounters in the world of commerce. During the same meal, my interlocutor tried to convince me that ageing is an illness against which one must fight at all cost. 'The old are a huge market, with millions of consumers,' he told me with a greedy smile. I allowed myself to remark that, thanks to scientific proofs, we know that the best way of ageing well is to learn to relax, eat correctly, develop positive feelings and to have regular exercise: inner answers that do not cost much and respect the individual's freedom. 'All that is out of date,' he replied. 'Science has made progress, technology gives us new answers. One must live in the present. Be modern!'

Nobody wants to seem out-of-date, nor to seem to be in the 'camp of weaklings'. Nevertheless, I persist in thinking that if the strong invent solutions for the weak, they have a duty to remind all human beings that they have powerful solutions inside themselves, more than they can imagine. That is certainly the best way in which the weak can feel stronger, even if as a consequence the strong lose a little of their advantage. The idea is probably not very modern: it may well be in advance of its time.

UNDERSTANDING MODERNITY

Too many external solutions

A short history is probably worth more than a long one. Catherine was 52 years old. For about 15 years she had suffered from very painful rheumatoid arthritis. In the course of inflammatory swellings, her shoulders had frozen and her fingers were deformed. A divorced mother of three children, she had followed a brilliant career in an important Swiss company. 'I don't have a moment to myself,' she told me with a kind of pride in her voice, 'but I am on the verge of depression,' she added, with a glance full of anxiety. 'Luckily I take Omega-3. Without that, I could not carry on.'

The list of pills that Catherine swallowed was impressive: one medicine for arterial hypertension, another to reduce her level of cholesterol, methotrexate and an anti-inflammatory for her polyarthritis, an antacid for gastric ulcer, hormone replacement because of her menopause, DHEA to help her remain young, thyroxin supplement because her daytime vitality was poor, a sleeping pill to get peace at night, and the

Omega-3 which she took instead of antidepressants, which her general practitioner wanted to prescribe.

This seemed totally absurd to me. Did Catherine not know that her fatigue, her sleep problems, hypertension, raised cholesterol level, peptic ulcer and probably many of the symptoms associated with polyarthritis, could be reduced, or even cured, by a hygiene of life better respecting her essential needs, and especially by taking up regular exercise? 'Yoga, *tai-chi* or *qigong*? You don't think that!' she said to me. 'I don't have the time, I have responsibilities, I have to earn my living. And it doesn't work as well as the medications!' Wrong: the studies quoted in this book prove it.

Thoroughly doped with the thyroid hormones, the DHEA (also a hormone) and the Omega-3, Catherine took no account of the stress under which she lived. Did she not know that hormones constitute an extremely subtle communication in which it is not without danger to interfere? The increased risk of breast cancer has been well shown in women taking hormone replacement after the menopause.[1] 'The human being behaves like an apprentice sorcerer,' said Arnulfo, the Mexican healer. 'How to repair a machine is not always obvious, even to the engineer who designed it. So how can one believe anything different for the doctor, who can only attempt to decipher plans of such complexity when he is not the creator?'

Apropos sorcerers, has Catherine thought how a placebo effect could be the source of the benefits accruing from her consumption of DHEA or Omega-3? (Studies showing the influence of publicity on the efficacy of medicines are noted in Chapter 1, p. 16.) This is the more probable still because the level of publicity in the media adds a real power of suggestion. 'Placebo or not, if they do me good, why should I deny myself?' she replied. It is obvious. It should always be on condition that she does not lose sight of the necessity of changing her way of life and her eating habits. In compensating for deficiencies, one never heals the causes which provoke them. In the case of Omega-3, for instance, their consumption in capsules should not exempt us from seeking a diet that is naturally provided with it – and if, as David Servan-Schreiber, author of a book on the subject,[2] told me, there are not sufficient fish farmed in conditions capable of providing as much as we need, we must campaign to change this situation.

The influence of fear

It is a constant factor in Western medicine: patients take too many medicines and use too much technology. One could also say that doctors prescribe too many pills and too many examinations. But the important point is not to identify the guilty; it would be better to understand how this situation occurs.

It is collective beliefs that determine the behaviour of individuals within a society. So now in the West, a catalogue of beliefs stemming from the Age of Enlightenment in the 17th and 18th centuries is deeply embedded in our minds: the world is dangerous; the human being is insufficiently rich in his own resources to defend himself; we must invent, produce and consume to protect and heal ourselves. In this context, progress is associated with the accumulation of sophisticated devices aimed at countering the threats of the environment; science is placed before nature, which it considers an enemy; and fear is the motor of what we call modernity.[3]

Western civilisation is thus organised around the dogma of the absolute necessity of having recourse to external remedies. Production and consumption are the core of economic activity. The logic of growth encourages research, demands the invention of new technologies, and depends on the creation of new needs. Security and happiness depend essentially on the capacity to act, to produce and to own. To *be* has become less important than to *do*. Consequently, modern man is less interested in his internal potential than in his external production.

A veritable spur for the survival instinct, fear is a motor for all humans. It is therefore not surprising to see the promises of contemporary ideologies succeed everywhere they reach. Rich or poor, Western or Eastern, we are all afraid of being alone, separated, abandoned, unable to get what we need. We all dread losing control of the world around us. We are all afraid to die. 'And we all kill ourselves in trying to escape death,' a yogi said to me in a bantering tone when I met him at Mahabalipuram in southern India.

It is true that the price of this frenzied progress to sophistication is high: denial of the essential needs of the individual leads to exaggerated stress, impoverishment of the environment, pollution of the infrastructure of life. The logic of growth crushes everything in its path. Ecological catastrophes, poverty and murderous conflicts. Depressions, illnesses linked to stress, and cancers. Never in our history has the survival of the human species appeared so threatened. No matter: the system looks inwards on itself, convinced that it has found the ideal solution for the existential fear that haunts the collective unconscious.

Recognising the contradictions

In common with many physicians and therapists, I note the extent of the ill-being of my contemporaries. Every day I meet people who are exhausted and who tell me they need rest, trying to justify the obligation of working beyond their limits in order to be able to pay for their holidays. They forget that the remedy for their fatigue is not to be found in a stay at the seaside, even less in swallowing stimulants or sedatives. Only a change in their every-day attitudes can resolve the problem at its roots in an effective and definitive way. This presupposes that they define their priorities, identify their essential needs, and respect the sensitivity of their bodies. Instead, many people prefer to justify their contradictions by blaming society and the laws of the modern world. They continue to swallow their medication, dream of the couple of weeks of rest that they offer themselves each year, or smoke and/or drink to forget their discomfort.

In the year 2000 the three top causes of death in the United States were tobacco (435,000 deaths, i.e. 18.1% of total deaths); poor eating habits and lack of exercise (400,000, 16.6%); and the consumption of alcohol (85,000, 3.5%).[4] What system of health care can justify the invention of expensive and polluting remedies to treat pathologies due to avoidable behaviours? An answer is not easy to find because, as the American economist Jeremy Rifkin emphasised, the costs of the poor health of the population are included in the calculation of the Gross National Product of the United States – regarded as an indicator of economic well-being.[5] It is the same with the costs of waging war, dealing with crime, and an entire series of destructive economic activities. The whole economic system therefore depends on the misfortune of the many for the greater happiness of the few.

Beliefs are often blind, and the logic underpinning them appalling. The strategies of great industrial organisations prevent any questioning of the dogma of the absolute necessity of recourse to external remedies. Some pharmaceutical companies for example, manufacture remedies against cancer; sponsor campaigns on prevention in which they make no mention of the carcinogenic substances produced by the group to which they belong; own cancer treatment centres where the medications they manufacture are prescribed; and fund university departments where the politics of health are developed and taught.[6] It must be said that in these times when civilisation is seeking a way forward, conflicts of interest are not lacking.

CHOOSING THE FUTURE

Taking part in sustainable development

'We cannot solve problems by using the same kind of thinking we used when we created them,' wrote Albert Einstein. Medicine is in a privileged position to stimulate other ways of thinking about the human being, his relationships with himself and his environment. The emergence of alternative and complementary medicines gives us new questions to ask and new answers to find. Without denying the need for drugs and technological methods, an 'integrative medicine' would bring hope of diminishing our recourse to external remedies in favour of methods capable of mobilising the natural defences of the organism. In time, this development would contribute to slowing the expansion of production and consumption, and at the same time, help us to escape from the vicious circle of pollution.

Such a change of attitude would certainly have repercussions on every sector of Western society. But we must not dream too far, or too quickly. Such a proposal to exploit the inner resources of the individual would seem to be a very obsolete solution to those pure unrelenting modernists who see in disease and their treatments the opportunity to feed the economic system. From time to time they promote this or that approach intended to mobilise the human potential, but very quickly exploit it like any other consumable and in so doing, distort the message of liberty and responsibility which could transform the attitude of individuals towards their own health. We must never underestimate the power of an ideology.

A realistic analysis of the situation obliges us equally to take account of the pendulum swing which is growing between the East and the West. In effect, if in Western countries the limitations of existing medical practices become better and better recognised, this is not the case in other countries, where Western modernity is, with difficulty, beginning to be employed. It is thus that in the United States, Canada, and Europe voices are raised to denounce a medical system that is exclusively based on the consumption of medication and the use of technology, while at the same time in India and China the importance of the potential of self-healing and the principles of prevention inherited from their ancestral holistic medicine, are forgotten in favour of complete acceptance of the materialist fantasies of the modern West. This phenomenon is paradoxical but seems inescapable. Let us hope that in the end, the international community of medicine will draw on the best of both approaches – Oriental and Occidental, traditional and modern – and, between the extremes of this continuum, will invent a medicine where the patient will have the last word.

To help patients exploit their own resources would certainly be beneficial both for their health and for the ecology of the planet. At the same time, it would involve important changes in their way of life. The structure of society would be disturbed. Much employment would be lost, not only in the commercial exploitation of products that are prejudicial to health, but also in the pharmaceutical industry, current technologies, research and even in hospitals. The running of the economic system would be fundamentally disturbed and the foundations of our civilisation shaken. The whole structure of the modern world would be threatened with collapse. We can understand why there is so much opposition to change – but can we avoid it?

More and more people believe that we cannot. A huge enquiry published in 2000 led by the sociologist Paul Ray at the University of Michigan, and the psychologist Sherry Ruth Anderson at the University of Toronto, showed that 24% of Americans – a quarter of the population, more than 50 million people – no longer lead their lives according to this modern model. They have abandoned their individualistic, capitalistic and hedonistic ideas in order to adopt new ways of behaviour, centred on ecology, solidarity, more peaceful principles and the hope of an inner awakening.[7] A similar survey commissioned by the Prospective Unit of the European Commission in 1997 showed similar results: tens of millions of Europeans are changing their paradigm.[8] They fight for the protection of the environment, wish to eat healthily and avoid useless consumption. For them, a coherent attitude is the inescapable condition for the pursuit of human experience because, they say: 'One cannot hope for healing while continuing to make oneself ill.' Their target is plain: it is to anchor globalisation in sustainable development.

Thus a new culture is emerging. Born in the 1960s, it is occupying a more and more important position. For the actors in this transformation, the battle between the modernists, in which they feel as children, and the traditionalist reactionaries who reject the acquisitions of modernity, is no longer topical. They know that evolution is never achieved by wiping the past clean. They seek therefore to unite the whole of their heritage. And surprisingly, as happens with every important cultural change, the old system does not understand what is happening. Blinded by its own logic, it cannot detect the signs of transformation. Most of the politicians and media are blind to what probably constitutes the beginning of postmodern civilisation.

Postmodern medicine

In the light of what we have explored together in this book, one can perhaps have some hope that the medicine of this new culture will develop around a unified picture of the human body and mind which will foster better use of the inner potentials of the individual: that it will focus as much on prevention as on cure and will become integrated in an ethical development, in which individual responsibility will be proof of a real commitment to the preservation of life on Earth.

To promote this, orthodox physicians must ally themselves with the practitioners of alternative and complementary medicines in order to share their experiences, question their own beliefs and widen the scope of their investigations, because these two approaches have a great deal to contribute to each other.

The time is come when the practitioners of alternative and complementary medicines must commit themselves to biomedical research. Biology has the virtue of describing phenomena beyond their psychological, philosophical or mythical interpretations; it is anchored in material reality which enables it to put forward concrete answers to the major problems of mankind; its precise language can be used by all cultures on the planet. Therefore it seems vital that these practitioners unite in professional associations in order to develop their research and organise their training in the same spirit of rigour, quality and effectiveness that has been developed by conventional medicine. It seems equally essential that beyond their sectarian disputes, they open up profound reflection on the principles held in common by their different therapies. They can then identify the conceptual and practical contributions which could transform the medicine of the future. This is one of the great principles of postmodernity: the future does not lie in competition; it lies in co-operation.

On their side, conventional physicians will have to integrate the new paradigm of 'body–mind unity' into their thinking, interest themselves more in the preservation of health, and exchange their role of users of technology and prescribers of medication for the more noble one of revealing potentials and teaching health. Few physicians are really aware of the economic subtexts of their profession. This is regrettable since the exercise of medicine risks being rapidly transformed into an immense commercial process where the ignorance of doctors and their patients becomes a guarantee of profit. The medical profession has far greater gifts to offer the world than economic growth. One of its roles could be to point out the road to wisdom that leads to life and supports the survival of the human species. This implies that it must stand aside from the world of the merchant and devote its efforts to humanising the relationship between patients and physicians. As Joël de Rosnay wrote in his book *The Symbiotic Man*, 'the greatest challenge of the future is not technological; it is human'.[9]

A new medicine will not see the light of day unless the training of physicians changes. In the mid 1990s, Andrew Weil, professor of medicine at the University of Arizona pleaded for a profound reorganisation of the medical curriculum.[10] He suggested reducing the teaching of unnecessary detail of theory in order to allow more time for future physicians to open their minds and hearts and to become more aware of their own bodies. From this perspective, teaching the philosophy of science, the history of medicine, and the various systems of health to be found throughout the world would develop the critical sense of the students and provide them with the keys required to select the way in which they will exercise the 'art of healing'. A profound examination of human potential, an understanding of the connections between body and mind, as well as a thorough knowledge of psychology, would allow them to approach both the disease and the diseased in a broader and more respectful way. Made aware of the emotional dimension of human relationships, future physicians would need to be introduced to the arts of communication: questioning and reassuring patients. Touching, massaging and consoling would no longer frighten them because their own sufferings will have been tamed and their boundaries defined unambiguously. Convinced of the influence of mental processes on bodily health, they would learn to exploit the placebo effect, they would guard against arousing stress in their patients and the nocebo effect which can be triggered by some of the things they say. Aware of the multifactorial origin of most diseases, they would apply themselves to treat all the causes involved. Their intimate knowledge of human nature – physical, psychological, spiritual – would be at least as important as their scientific knowledge. In this way, they would not be only physician-technicians but would become physician-healers. Informed in the principles of balanced nutrition, initiated in the practice of relaxation or meditation, and habituated to move their own bodies harmoniously, they would present a model of personal development to the patient. Finally, trained in – or at least informed about – various presently non-conventional practices, they would be in a position to direct their patients towards other therapists, sometimes better qualified to help them, or quite simply better adapted to their particular culture. They would then be respecting the co-operation advocated by postmodernity.

When I describe this ideal programme to medical students, I can see a gleam of hope appear in their eyes. 'The hope of getting back some sense of life in my studies, and later in my practice,' said a young woman who was aiming at gynaecology. It is true. It is enough to read a medical treatise or more simply, follow a course in cardiology or surgery to be convinced of it: scientific reductionism has drained medicine of life. Now, as Linus Pauling, awarded the Nobel Prize for Chemistry in 1954 and the Nobel Peace Prize in 1963, remarked: 'Life does not reside in molecules, but in the relationships they establish amongst themselves.' Life does not exist except through links and exchanges, in multiplicity and diversity, fluidity and movement, spontaneity and vivacity, imagination and creativity. Postmodern physicians need to possess all these essential qualities if they desire to safeguard life.

From this mutation in medical science would certainly develop a different way of approaching research. Nourished by a pluricultural and multidisciplinary attitude, postmodern physicians would put the impact of their discoveries in perspective, and so would remain more open to new ideas. This is exactly what is happening currently in genetics. The fact is sufficiently important to be underlined. Remember that in the year 2000 the scientific community announced triumphantly that the sequencing of the human genome had been achieved. The 20th century ended with a resounding success, all therapeutic hopes were reinforced, and the supremacy of gene therapy seemed unshakeable. Five years later, biologists had become disenchanted. 'We have teased out the puzzle,' declared Professor Denis Noble of the University of Oxford; 'we must now work out how to put it back together.'[11] Genetic reductionism is now out of fashion; biology changes its paradigm; physicists, mathematicians and specialists in information technology unite in their efforts to understand the dynamic that governs the destiny of the living.[12] Arrogance has given way to humility.

The same thing can be seen in the neurosciences. Some researchers responsible for spectacular advances recall that the role played by glial cells is almost completely unknown although these form 90% of the cells in the brain. For a long time they had been thought to be exclusively concerned with the support, nourishment and protection of neurones. Now we know that they play a part in the handling of information, the construction of memory, and the mechanisms of the neuroplasticity of the brain.[13] Enquiring minds of the 21st century have more fine discoveries to make.

What will the postmodern physicians find when they question their patients about their maladies? What will they understand about the influences of hope and positive emotions when these parameters are systematically included in the evaluation of the results of therapy? Will we not find that psychological factors are responsible for differences in the success rates of healing, once serious research is carried out to answer that question? Will we still be convinced of the primacy of conventional treatments when we have the curiosity to ask patients if they have had recourse to other therapies in addition? Who can declare that certain practices such as *tai-chi* or yoga do not influence the development of certain diseases, cancer included? Meditation, breathing, laughter or simply movement – are they not essential to healing? Questions of this kind can seem silly, and yet a study published by researchers at Harvard in May 2005 in the *Journal of the American Medical Association* proves that it is useful to ask them. Who would have believed that women with breast cancer have a 50% less risk of dying of that disease if they take care to keep up a physical activity as simple as walking three to five hours a week?[14]

By insisting on mobilising the help of the inner resources of the individual for prevention as well as cure of diseases, the physicians of the postmodern era could influence the policy of payments by the insurance companies. New professions in health care could be created because it is better to inform than to treat. Physician-teachers could go into schools to explain to children how to protect the precious treasure which is life for all of us. Responsibility and self-discipline could become the keys to a happy life. And in university lecture rooms it will be shown that the English philosopher John Locke was wrong when, in the 17th century, he suggested that 'the negation of nature is the way to happiness'.[15]

Reconciled to nature and aware of being a part of it, the people of the third millennium will probably wish to be reconciled with themselves. Humankind will inevitably ask questions about the need to flee forwards towards ever more technology, production and consumption. And unstoppably, they will wish to love, to laugh and to dance, simply because they will be aware that the best means of preserving their health and that of the planet on which they live, is to create balance and the wholeness of mind and body.

Utopia, or the reality of the future? No one can say. But in waiting for an answer, what can we do other than endeavour to understand the nature of things the better, in order one day, to respect better the things of nature?

ACKNOWLEDGEMENTS

This book is the result of a reconciliation between a surgeon and a psychotherapist, a physician and a healer, a scientist and a poet, who all live inside me. It comes from a lengthy labour which would not have been possible save for the support of a little clan who helped me disperse my fears and my doubts. So I thank François Marcq, the uncontested chief of this clan, as well as Caroline Francq, Olivier Roquigny, Natacha Severin, Nissim and Patsy Israël, Daniel Frachon, Emile Mahy, Anita Vaxelaire, Neyde Nunes Ferreira Sperandio, Gilles Fontugne, Valérie Lelièvre, Pascale Renaux, Guillemette Jooris, Matthieu Vanham, Dominique Guetta, John van Cauwenberghe, Alain Matheï, Christophe Vaessen, Geneviève Fink, Larbi Ourhiagli, Caroline Mijnssen, Henri Baeyens, Carine and Dominique Derwa, Anja Ulhig, Kimberley Hirsch, Clovis Marques, and my parents, Colette and Georges Janssen.

I thank also all those who, in one way or another, through a meeting or an exchange of letters at certain critical moments of writing, sharpened my thinking and made my work more precise: Elisabeth Kübler-Ross (who died at the time I began editing this work), Arthur Janov, Daniel Moerman, Ghislain Devroed, Sri Shyam-ji Bathnagar, James Oschman, Fred Gallo, David Isaacs, Barbara Ann Brennan, Pnina Polishook, Enrique Arellano, Matthieu Ricard, Jacques Lefèvre, Dominique Thommen, Nicole Lattès, Nathalie Le Breton, David Servan-Schreiber, Yuichi Kawada, Danièle Rousseau, Antoine Valabregue, Marc Luyckx Ghisi, Thierry Gaudin and Elise Roy (who read the manuscript with care). I will not forget two unusual personalities, virtual mirrors of my consciousness: Raghubir Sangh and Arnulfo Olivares.

I will not forget either the many researchers, physicians, therapists, healers and sorcerers whom I met on my journey. I do not quote their names so that I can be sure not to forget anyone. But like all the others, if they remember having met me, let them be assured of my recognition of their teaching, the inspirations and the questions that they revealed to me. Without them, this book would not exist. It would not exist either without the patients who put their confidence in me. They find here witness of my gratitude and an expression of my profound respect.

Finally, recognition of the godparents of *The Solution Lies Within*: Abel Gerschenfeld, editor of my earlier books and the first to encourage me to write this one; Jean-Philippe de Tonnac, whose generous confidence lives on in the pages of this work; and Henri Trubert, in whom I found the enthusiasm, the sensitivity, the culture and the intelligence indispensable for the maturation of this project. It was his precious qualities that led me to confide the destiny of this text to the good care of the Fayard Publishing House.

A special thanks also to Hellmut Karle and Trevor Brown who made it possible for this book to be published in English translation by Free Association Books.

Thierry Janssen

Translator's note

The translator wishes to acknowledge the invaluable and generous help given by Thierry Janssen in preparing this translation.

NOTES

INTRODUCTION

1. Barnes P., Powell-Griner E., McFann K., Nahin R., 'Complementary and alternative medicine use among adults', *CDC Advance Data Report # 343*, USA, 2002 (27 May 2004).
2. Inquête sur la santé des collectivités canadiennes, *Statistique Canada*, www.statcan.ca.
3. Tzu Chi Institute, 'Statut et contexte des approches complementaires et parallèles en santé au Quebec', *Résau canadien de la Santé*, 2003.
4. Fisher P., Ward A., 'Complementary medicine in Europe', *British Medical Journal*, 1994, 309, pp. 107–111.
5. Maclennan A.H., Wilson D.H., Taylor A.W., 'Prevalence and costs of alternative medicine in Australia', *Lancet*, 1996, 347, pp. 569–573.
6. Suzuki N., 'Complementary and alternative medicine: a Japanese perspective', *Evidence-based Complementary and Alternative Medicine*, on-line eCAM 2004, http://ecam.oxfordjournals.org/content/vol1/issue2/index.dtl.
7. Louis C., 'Thérapies alternatives: à travers le monde, la science du XXIe ciècle tente de comprendre, voir de s'approprier, les savoirs ancestraux', *Le Figaro*, 3 August 2004, p. 8.
8. Gordon J.S., 'The White House Commission on Complementary and Alternative Medicine Policy and the Future of Health', in Schlitz M., Amorok T., Micozzi M.S. (eds) *Consciousness and Healing. Integral Approaches to Mind–Body Medicine*, St Louis MO, Elsevier Churchill Livingstone, 2005, pp. 489–498.
9. Barzansky B., Jonas H.S., Etzel S.I., 'Educational program in US medical schools, 1999–2000', *Journal of the American Medical Association*, 2000, 284, pp. 1114–1120.
10. Wetzel M.S., Kaptchuk T.J., Haramati A., Eisenberg D.M., 'Complementary and alternative medical therapies: implications for medical education', *Annals of Internal Medicine*, 2003, 138, pp. 191–196.
11. Jonas W.B., 'Researching alternative medicine', *Nature Medicine*, 1997, 3, pp. 824–882.
12. World Health Organisation, *Traditional Medicine*, Washington DC, WHO Publications, 1978.
13. Weil A., 'The body's healing systems: the future of medical education', *Journal of Alternative and Complementary Therapies*, 1995, 1, pp. 305–309.
14. Eisenberg D.M., Davis R.B., Ettner S.J. et al., 'Trends in alternative medicine use in the United States 1990–1997: results of a follow-up national survey', *Journal of the American Medical Association*, 1998, 280, pp. 1569–1575.
15. Kamohara S. in *Alternative Medicine*, Tokyo, Tyuou Kouron Shinsha, 2002, 1st edition, pp. 30–35.
16. Visser G.L., Peters L., Rasker J.J., 'Rheumatologists and their patients who seek alternative care', *British Journal of Rheumatology*, 1992, 31, pp. 485–490.
17. Astin J.A. et al., 'A review of the incorporation of CAM by mainstream physicians', *Archives of Internal Medicine*, 1998, 158, pp. 2303–2310.

18. Verhoef M.J., Sutherland L.R., 'Alternative medicine and general practitioners', *Canadian Family Physician*, 1995, 41, pp. 1005–1011.
19. Perlman A. (ed.), 'Complementary and alternative medicine', *The Medical Clinics of North America*, January 2002, 86(1).
20. *Evidence-Based Complementary and Alternative Medicine (eCAM)*, Oxford University Press, http://ecam.oxfordjournals.org.
21. Tada T., 'Towards the philosophy of CAM: super-system and epimedical sciences', *Evidence-Based Complementary and Alternative Medicine*, on-line: eCAM, 2004, http://ecam.oxfordjournals.org/content/vol1/issue1/index.dtl.
22. This list is published on the National Center for Complementary and Alternative Medicine site: http://nccam.nih.gov.
23. Chaitow L., 'Les cliniques de médécines intégrées', interview held on 14 May 2004 and published on-line on www.reseauproteus.net.

CHAPTER 1   EMBARRASSING: THE PLACEBO EFFECT

1. Cannon W., '"Voodoo" death', *Psychosomatic Medicine*, 1957, 19, pp. 182–190.
2. Beecher H.K., 'The powerful placebo', *Journal of the American Medical Association*, 1955, 159, pp. 1602–1606.
3. Amanzio M., Pollo A., Maggi G., Benedetti F., 'Response variability to analgesics: a role for non-specific activation of endogenous opioids', *Pain*, 2001, 90, pp. 205–215.
4. Petrovic P., Kalso E., Petersson K.M., Ingvar M., 'Placebo and opioid analgesia – imaging a shared neuronal network', *Science*, 2002, 295, pp. 1737–1740.
5. Wager T.D., Rilling J.K., Smith E.E., Sokolik A.S., Casey K.L., Davidson R.J., Kosslyn S.M., Rose R.M., Cohen J.D., 'Placebo-induced changes in fMRI in the anticipation and experience of pain', *Science*, 2004, 303, pp. 1162–1166.
6. Arstein P., 'The Placebo Effect', in Leskowitz E.D. (ed.) *Complementary and Alternative Medicine in Rehabilitation*, New York, Churchill Livingstone, 2003.
7. Kienle G.S., Kiene H., 'A critical re-analysis of the concept, magnitude and existence of placebo effects', in Peters D. (ed.) *Understanding the Placebo Effect in Complementary Medicine*, Edinburgh, Churchill Livingstone, 2001.
8. Turner J.A., Deyo R.A., Loeser J.D. *et al.*, 'The importance of placebo effects in pain treatment and research', *Journal of the American Medical Association*, 1994, 271, pp. 1609–1614; De Craen A.J.M., Lampe-Schoenmaeckers A.J.E.M., Kleijnen J., 'Non specific factors in randomized clinical trials: some methodological considerations', in Peters D. (ed.) *Understanding the Placebo Effect in Complementary Medicine*, Edinburgh, Churchill Livingstone, 2001.
9. Benson H., Epstein M.D., 'The placebo effect: a neglected asset in the care of patients', *Journal of the American Medical Association*, 1975, 232, pp. 1225–1227.
10. Moerman D., *Meaning, Medicine and the 'Placebo Effect'*, Cambridge, Cambridge University Press, 2002.
11. Moerman D., 'Cultural variations in the placebo effect: ulcers, anxiety and blood pressure', *Medical Anthropology Quarterly*, 2000, 14, pp. 1–22.
12. Graceley R.H., Dubner R., Deeter W.R. *et al.*, 'Clinicians' expectations influence placebo analgesia', *Lancet*, 1985, 331, p. 43.
13. Braithwaite A., Cooper P., 'Analgesic effects of branding in treatment of headaches', *British Medical Journal (Clinical Research Ed.)*, 1981, 282, no. 6276, pp. 1576–1578.
14. Nathan T., Stengers I., *Médécins et Sorciers*, Paris, Les Empêcheurs de penser en rond, 1999.
15. This expression was coined by Alexandro Jodorowsky.

16. Lévi-Strauss C., 'The sorcerer and his magic', in *Structural Anthropology*, Garden City NY, Anchor Books, 1967, pp. 180–201.
17. Cobb L.A., Thomas G.I., Dillard D.H. *et al.*, 'An evaluation of internal-mammary-artery-ligation by a double-blind technique', *New England Journal of Medicine*, 1959, 260, pp. 1115–1118; Dimond E.G., Kittle C.F., Crockett J.E., 'Comparison of internal mammary ligation and sham operation for angina pectoris', *American Journal of Cardiology*, 1960, 5, pp. 483–486.
18. Moseley J.B., O'Malley K., Peterson N.J. *et al.*, 'A controlled trial of arthroscopic treatment of osteoarthritis of the knee', *New England Journal of Medicine*, 2002, 347, p. 81.
19. McRae C., *Archives of General Psychiatry*, April 2004.
20. Helman C.J., 'Placebos and nocebos: the cultural construction of belief', in Peters D. (ed.) *Understanding the Placebo Effect in Complementary Medicine*, Edinburgh, Churchill Livingstone, 2001.
21. Long J., Gillilan R., Lee S.G., Kim C.R., 'White coat hypertension: detection and evaluation', *Maryland Medical Journal*, 1990, 39, pp. 555–559; Campbell L.V., Ashwell S.M., Borkman M., Chisholm D., 'White coat hyperglycaemia: disparity between diabetes clinic and home blood glucose concentrations', *British Medical Journal*, 1992, 305, pp. 1194–1196.
22. Groopman J., *The Anatomy of Hope*, New York, Random House, 2004.
23. Barsky A.J., Saintfort R., Rogers M.P., Borus J.F., 'Non-specific medication side-effects and nocebo phenomenon', *Journal of the American Medical Association*, 2002, 287, pp. 622–627.
24. Eaker E., Pinsky L., Castelli W.P., 'Myocardial infarction and coronary death among women: psychosocial predictors from a 20-year follow-up of women in the Framingham Study', *American Journal of Epidemiology*, 1992, 135, pp. 854–864.
25. Hahn R.A., 'The nocebo phenomenon: scope and foundations', in Harrington A. (ed.) *The Placebo Effect. An Interdisciplinary Exploration*, Cambridge MA, Harvard University Press, 1997, pp. 56–76.
26. Peterson C., Bossio L., 'Healthy attitudes: optimism, hope and control', in *Mind Body Medicine*, Consumer Reports Books, 1993, pp. 351–366.
27. Maruta T., Colligan R.C., Maclinchoc M., Offord K.P., 'Optimism-pessimism assessed in the 1960s and self-reported health status 30 years later', *Mayo Clinic proceedings*, 2002, 77, pp. 748–753.
28. Danner D., Snowden D., Friesen W., 'Positive emotion in early life and longevity', *Journal of Personality and Social Psychology*, 2001, 8, p. 84.
29. Fenwick P., 'Psychoneuroimmunology: the mind-brain connection', in Peters D. (ed.) *Understanding the Placebo Effect in Complementary Medicine*, Edinburgh, Churchill Livingstone, 2001.
30. Kamen-Sigel L., Rodin J., Seligman M., Dwyer J., 'Explanatory style and cell mediated immunity in elderly men and women', *Health Psychology*, 1991, 10, pp. 229–235.
31. Buchannan G.M., Seligman M.E.P., *Explanatory Style*, Hillsdale, NJ, Lawrence Erlbaum Associates, 1995, p. 303.
32. Levi S., Herberman R., Lippmann M., D'Angelo T., Lee J., 'Immunological and psychological predictors of disease. Recurrence in patients with early stage breast cancer', *Behavioural Medicine*, 1991, 17, pp. 67–75.

CHAPTER 2   CLARIFYING: PSYCHO-NEURO-IMMUNOLOGY

1. Jung C.G., *Collected Works of C.G. Jung*, 2nd ed. vol. 2, Princeton NJ, Princeton University Press, 1972.

2. Mackenzie J.N., 'The production of so-called "rose cold" by means of an artificial rose', *American Journal of Medical Science*, 1895, 91, pp. 47–57.
3. Hill L.E., *Philosophy of a Biologist*, London, Arnold, 1930.
4. Ader R., Cohen N., 'Behaviourally conditioned immunosuppression', *Psychosomatic Medicine*, 1975, 37, pp. 333–340.
5. Felten D., Felten S., Carson S., Olschowka J., Livnat S., 'Noradrenergic and peptidergic innervation of lymphoid tissue', *The Journal of Immunology*, 1985, 135, pp. 755–765.
6. Ader R., Cohen N., Felten D.L., 'Psychoneuroimmunology: interactions between the nervous system and the immune system', *Lancet*, 1995, 345, pp. 99–103; Cardinali D.P., Cutrera R.A., Esquifino A.I., 'Psychoimmune neuroendocrine integrative mechanisms revisited', *Biological Signals and Receptors*, 2000, 9, pp. 215–230.
7. Pert C.B., *Molecules of Emotion*, New York, Touchstone, 1997.
8. Stonier T., *Information and the Internal Structure of the Universe*, New York, Springer-Verlag, 1990.
9. Sperry R., 'The great cerebral commissure', *Scientific American*, 1964, 210, pp. 42–52.
10. Gazzaniga M., *The Social Brain: Discovering the Networks of the Mind*, New York, Basic Books, 1985.
11. Mazziotta J., Phelps M., Carson R., Kuhl D., 'Tomographic mapping of human cerebral metabolism: auditory stimulation', *Neurology*, 1982, 32, pp. 921–937.
12. Janov A., *The Biology of Love*, New York, Prometheus Books, 2000.
13. LeDoux J., *The Emotional Brain*, New York, Simon and Schuster, 1996.
14. Works cited in Fredrickson B.L., 'L'importance du bonheur', *Cerveau & Psycho*, June–August 2004, 6, p. 44.
15. Fredrickson B.L., 'The role of positive emotions in positive psychology: the broaden-and-build theory of positive emotions', *American Psychologist*, 2001, 56, p. 218.
16. Davidson R.J., Sutton S.K., 'Affective neuroscience: the emergence of a discipline', *Current Opinion in Neurobiology*, 1995, 5, pp. 217–224.
17. Tomarken A.J., Davidson R.J., 'Frontal brain activation in repressors and non-repressors', *Journal of Abnormal Psychology*, 1994, 103, pp. 339–349.
18. Wheeler R.E., Davidson R.J., Tomarken A.J., 'Frontal brain asymmetry and emotional reactivity: a biological substrate and affective style', *Psychophysiology*, 1993, 30, pp. 820–829.
19. Rossi G.F., Rosadini G., 'Experimental analysis of cerebral dominance in man', in *Brain: Mechanisms Underlying Speech and Language*, New York, Grune and Stratton, 1967.
20. Barnoud P., Le Moal M., Neveu P., 'Asymmetrical distribution of monoamines in left and right handed mice', *Brain Research*, 1990, 520, pp. 317–321.
21. Kang D.H., Davidson R.J., Coe C., Wheeler R.E., Tomarken A.J., Ershler W.B., 'Frontal brain asymmetry and immune function', *Behavioral Neuroscience*, 1991, 105, pp. 860–869.
22. Rosenkrantz M.A., Jackson D.C., Dalton K.M., Dolski I., Ryff C.D., Singer B.H., Muller D., Kalin N.H., Davidson R.J., 'Affective Style and *in vivo* immune response: neurobehavioral mechanisms', *Proceedings of the National Academy of Sciences*, 2003, 100, pp. 11148–11152; Meador K.J., Lecuona J.M., Helman S.W., Loring D.W., 'Differential immunologic effects of language-dominant and non-dominant cerebral resections', *Neurology*, 1999, 53, pp. 1183–1187.
23. Clerici M., Shearer G.M., 'The Th1-Th2 hypothesis of HIV infection: new insights', *Immunology Today*, 1994, 15, pp. 575–581.

24. Gruzelier J., Burgess A., Baldewig T. et al., 'Prospective associations between lateralised brain function and immune status in HIV infection: analysis of EEG, cognition and mood over 30 months', *International Journal of Psychophysiology*, 1996, 23, pp. 215–224.
25. Martin I., 'Human electroencephalographic (EEG) response to olfactory stimulation: two experiments using the aroma of food', *International Journal of Psychophysiology*, 1998, 30, pp. 287–302; Clow A., 'Behavioral conditioning of immune system', in Peters D. (ed.) *Understanding the Placebo Effect in Complementary Medicine*, Edinburgh, Churchill Livingstone, 2001.
26. Oppenheimer S., Gelb A., Girvin J., Hachinski V., 'Cardiovascular effects of human insular cortex stimulation', *Neurology*, 1992, 42, pp. 1727–1732.
27. Selye H., *The Stress of Life*, New York, McGraw-Hill, 1978.
28. Elenkov I.J., Chrousos G.P., 'Stress Hormones pro-inflammatory and anti-inflammatory cytokins and autoimmunity', *Annals of the New York Academy of Sciences*, 2002, 966, pp. 290–303.
29. Levenstein S., 'Psychosocial factors in peptic ulcer and inflammatory bowel disease', *Journal of Consulting and Clinical Psychology*, 2002, 70, pp. 739–750.
30. Zautra A.J., Hamilton M.A., Potter P., Smith B., 'Field research on the relationship between stress and disease activity in rheumatoid arthritis', *Annals of the New York Academy of Sciences*, 1999, 876, pp. 397–412.
31. Walsh J.H., Peterson W.L., 'The treatment of helicobacter pylori infection in the management of peptic ulcer disease', *New England Journal of Medicine*, 1995, 333, pp. 984–991.
32. Epel D., Lapidus R., McEwen B., Brownell K., 'Stress may add bite to appetite in women: a laboratory study of stress-induced cortisol and eating behavior', *Psychoneuroendocrinology*, 2000, 26, pp. 37–49.
33. De Quervain D.J.F., Roozendaal B., McGaugh J.L., 'Stress and glucocorticoids impair retrieval of long-term spatial memory', *Nature*, 1998, 394, pp. 787–790; Sheline Y.I., Sanghavi M., Mintun M.A., Gado M.H., 'Depression duration but not age predicts hippocampal volume loss in medically healthy women with recurrent major depression', *Journal of Neuroscience*, 1999, 19, pp. 5034–5043.
34. Starkman M., Schteingart D., 'Neuropsychiatric manifestations of patients with Cushing's syndrome', *Journal of Clinical Psychiatry*, 1981, 141, pp. 215–219.

CHAPTER 3   DISTURBING: THE DANGERS OF STRESS

1. www.stress.org.
2. Cohen S., Tyrrel D.A.J., Smith A.P., 'Psychological stress and susceptibility to the common cold', *New England Journal of Medicine*, 1991, 325, pp. 606–611.
3. Cohen S., Doyle W.J., Skoner D.P., 'Psychological stress, cytokine production and severity of upper respiratory illness', *Psychsomatic Medicine*, 1999, 61, pp. 175–180.
4. Cohen S., Frank E., Doyle W.J., Skoner D.P., Rabin B.S., Gwaltney J.M., 'Types of stressors that increase susceptbility to the common cold in healthy adults', *Health Psychology*, 1998, 17, pp. 214–223.
5. Selye H., 'The evolution of the stress concept', *American Science*, 1973, 61, pp. 692–699; Segerstrom S.C., Miller G.E., 'Psychological stress and the human immune system: a meta-analytic study of 30 years of enquiry', *Psychological Bulletin*, 2004, 130, pp. 601–630.
6. Kasl S.V., Evans A.S., Niederman J.C., 'Psychological risk factors in the development of infectious mononucleosis', *Psychosomatic Medicine*, 1979, 41, pp. 445–466.

7. Luborsky L., Brightman V.J., Katcher A.H., 'Herpes simplex virus and mood: a longtitudinal study', *Journal of Psychosomatic Research*, 1976, 20, pp. 543–548.
8. Kiecolt-Glaser J.K., Glaser R. *et al.*, 'Modulation of cellular immunity in medical students', *Journal of Behavioral Medicine*, 1986, 9, pp. 5–21; Jemmot J.B., Borysenko J.Z., Borysenko M., 'Academic stress, power motivation and decrease in secretion rate of immunoglobulin A', *Lancet*, 1983, pp. 1400–1402.
9. Arnetz B.B., Wasserman J., Petrini B. *et al.*, 'Immune function in unemployed women', *Psychosomatic Medicine*, 1987, 49, pp. 3–12; Marriott D., Kirwood B.J., Stough C., 'Immunological effects of unemployment', *Lancet*, 1994, 344, pp. 26–27.
10. Pressman S.D., Chen S., Miller G.E., Barkin A., Rabin B.S., Treanor J.J., 'Loneliness, social network size, immune response to influenza vaccination in college freshmen', *Health Psychology*, 2005, 24, pp. 297–306.
11. Janov A., *The Biology of Love*, New York, Prometheus Books, 2000.
12. Rosenthal M.J., 'Psychosomatic study of infantile eczema', *Pediatrics*, 1952, 10, pp. 581–593; Saint-Mézard P., Chavagnac C., Bosset S., Ionescu M., Peyron E., Kaiserlian D., Nicholas J.F., Bérard F., 'Psychological stress exerts an adjuvant effect on skin dendritic cells', *The Journal of Immunology*, 2003, 171, pp. 4073–4080.
13. Bartrop R.W., Keller S.E. *et al.*, 'Depressed lymphocyte function after bereavement', *Lancet*, 1977, 1, pp. 834–836.
14. Irwin M., Daniels M., Risch C. *et al.*, 'Plasma cortisol and natural killer cell activity during bereavement', *Biological Psychiatry*, 1988, 24, pp. 173–178.
15. Kiecolt-Glaser J.K., Fisher L., Ogrocki P., Sout J., Speicher C., Glaser R., 'Marital quality, marital disruption and immune function', *Psychosomatic Medicine*, 1987, 49, pp. 13–53.
16. Kiecolt-Glaser J.K., Glaser R., Cacioppo J.T., Malarkey W.B., 'Marital stress: immunological, neuro-endocrine and autonomic correlates', *Annals of the New York Academy of Sciences*, 1998, 840, pp. 656–663.
17. Vedhara K., Cox N.H.M., Wilcock G.K. *et al.*, 'Chronic stress in elderly carers of dementia patients and antibody response to influenza vaccination', *Lancet*, 1999, 353, pp. 627–631.
18. Kiecolt-Glaser J.K., Preacher K.J., MacCallum R.C., Atkinson C., Malarkey W.B., Glaser R., 'Chronic stress and age-related increases in the pro-inflammatory cytokin39e IL-6', *Proceedings of the National Academy of Sciences*, 2003, 100, pp. 9090–9095.
19. Kiecolt-Glaser J.K., Marucha P.T., Malarkey W.B., Mercadio A.M., Glaser R., 'Slowing of wound healing by psychological stress', *Lancet*, 1995, 346, pp. 1194–1196.
20. Glaser R., Robles T.F., Sheridan J., Malarkey W.B., Kiecolt-Glaser J., 'Mild depressive symptoms are associated with amplified and prolonged inflammatory responses after influenza virus vaccination in older adults', *Archives of General Psychiatry*, 2003, 60, pp. 1009–1014; Rosenkranz M.A., Jackson D.C., Dalton K.M., Dolski I., Riff C.D., Singer B.H., Muller D., Kalin H., Davidson R.J., 'Affective style and in vivo immune response: neurobehavioral mechanisms', *Proceedings of the National Academy of Sciences*, 2003, 100, pp. 11148–11152.
21. Solomon G., Moos R., 'Psychological aspects of response to treatment in rheumatoid arthritis', *General Practitioner*, 1965, 32, pp. 113–119.
22. Zautra A.J., Hamilton M.A., Potter P., Smith B., 'Field research on the relationship between stress and disease activity in rheumatoid arthritis', *Annals of the New York Academy of Sciences*, 1999, 876, pp. 397–412.
23. Sternberg E.M., 'The stress response and the regulation of inflammatory disease', *Annals of Internal Medicine*, 1992, 117, pp. 854–866.

24. Qui B.S., Vallance B.A., Blennerhassett P.A., Collins S.M., 'The role of CD4+ lymphocytes in the susceptibility of mice to stress-induced reactivation of experimental colitis', *Nature*, 1999, 5, pp. 1178–1182.
25. Aoyama N., Kinoshita Y., Fujimoto S. *et al.*, 'Peptic ulcers after the Hanshin-Awaji earthquake increased incidence of bleeding gastric ulcers', *American Journal of Gastroenterology*, 1998, 93, pp. 311–316.
26. Walsh J.H., Peterson W.L., 'The treatment of helicobacter pylori infection in the management of peptic ulcer disease', *New England Journal of Medicine*, 1995, 333, pp. 984–991.
27. Levenstein S., 'Stress and peptic ulcer. Life beyond Helicobacter', *British Medical Journal*, 1998, 316, pp. 538–541; Levenstein S., 'The very model of a modern etiology: a biopsychosocial view of peptic ulcer', *Psychosomatic Medicine*, 2000, 62, pp. 176–185.
28. Miller G.E., Freedland K.E., Carney R.M., Stetler C.A., Banks W.A., 'Cynical hostility, depressive symptoms and the expression of inflammatory risk markers for coronary heart disease', *Journal of Behavioral Medicine*, 2003, 26, pp. 501–515.
29. Miller G.E., Friedland K.E., Carney R.M., Stetler C.A., Banks W.A., 'Pathways linking depression, adiposity and inflammatory markers in healthy young adults', *Brain, Behavior and Immunity*, 2003, 17, pp. 276–285.
30. Baghurst K.I., Baghurst P.A., Record S.J., 'Public perceptions of the role of dietary and other environmental factors in cancer causation or prevention', *Journal of Epidemiology and Community Health*, 1992, 46, pp. 120–126.
31. Chen C.C., David A.S., Nunnerly H., Michell M., Dawson J.L., Berry H., Dobbs J., Fahy T., 'Adverse life events and breast cancer: case control study', *British Medical Journal*, 1995, 311, pp. 1527–1530; Lillberg K., Verkasalo P.K., Kaprio J., Teppo L., Helenius H., Koskenvuo M., 'Stressful life events and risk of breast cancer in 10,808 women: a cohort study', *American Journal of Epidemiology*, 2003, 157, pp. 415–423.
32. Protheroe D., Turvey K., Horgan K., Benson E., Bowers D., House A., 'Stressful life events and difficulties and onset of breast cancer: case-control study', *British Medical Journal*, 1999, 319, pp. 1027–1030.
33. Schernhammer E.S., Hankinson S.E., Rosner B., Kroenke C.H., Willet W.C., Colditz G.A., Kawachi I., 'Job stress and breast cancer risk', *American Journal of Epidemiology*, 2004, 160, pp. 1079–1086; Kroenke C.H., Hankinson S.E., Schernhammer S.E., Colditz G.A., Kawachi I., Holmes M.D., 'Care-giving stress, steroid hormone levels and breast cancer incidence', *American Journal of Epidemiology*, 2004, 159, pp. 1019–1027.
34. Fenwick P., 'Psychoneuroimmunology: the mind–brain connection', in Peters D. (ed.) *Understanding the Placebo Effect in Complementary Medicine*, Edinburgh, Churchill Livingstone, 2001.
35. Persky V.W., Kempthorne J., Shekelle R.B., 'Personality and risk of cancer: 20 years follow-up of the Western Electric Study', *Psychosomatic Medicine*, 1987, 49, pp. 435–449.
36. Perrin L., *Le psychism, le stress et l'immunité. La santé est en nous*, Paris, Odile Jacob, 2003; Zonderman A.B., Costa P.T., McCrae R.R., 'Depression as a risk for cancer morbidity and mortality in a nationally representative sample', *Journal of the American Medical Association*, 1989, 262, pp. 1191–1195; Caplan G.A., Reynolds P., 'Depression and cancer mortality and morbidity, prospective evidence from the Alameda County Study', *Journal of Behavioral Medicine*, 1988, 11, pp. 1–13; Hahn R.C., Petitti D.B., 'Minnesota Multiphasic Personality Inventory-rated depression and the incidence of breast cancer', *Cancer*, 1988, 61, pp. 845–848.

37. Tomei L.D., Kiecolt-Glaser J.K., Kennedy S., Glaser R., 'Psychological stress and phorbol ester inhibition of radiation-induced apoptosis in human PBLs', *Psychiatric Research*, 1990, 33, pp. 59–71; Kiecolt-Glaser J.K., Stephen R.E., Lipitz P.D., Speicher C.E., Glaser R., 'Distress and DNA repair in human lymphocytes', *Journal of Behavioral Medicine*, 1985, 8, pp. 311–320; Glaser R., Thorn B.E., Tarr K.L., Kiecolt-Glaser J.K., D'Ambrosio S.M., 'Effects of stress on methyltransferase synthesis: an important DNA repair enzyme', *Health Psychology*, 1985, 4, pp. 403–412.
38. Epel E.S., Blackburn E.H., Lin J., Dhabhar F.S., Adler N.E., Morrow J.D., Cawthon R.M., 'Accelerated telomere shortening in response to life stress', *Proceedings of the National Academy of Sciences*, 2004, 101, pp. 17312–17315.
39. Vulliamy T., Marrone A., Goldman F., Dearlove A., Bessler M., Mason P.J., Dokal I., 'The RNA component of telomerase is mutated in autosomal dominant dyskeratosis congenita', *Nature*, 2001, 413, pp. 432–435; Cawthon R., Smith K., O'Brien E., Sivatchenko A., Kerber R., 'Association between telomere length in blood and mortality in people aged 60 years and older', *Lancet*, 2003, 361, pp. 393–395; Brouilette S., Singh R.K., Thompson J.R., Goodall A.H., Samani N.J., 'White cell telomere length and risk of premature myocardial infarction', *Arteriosclerosis, Thrombosis and Vascular Biology*, 2003, 23, pp. 842–846.
40. Jung W., Irwin M., 'Reduction of natural killer cytotoxic activity in major depression: interaction between depression and cigarette smoking', *Psychosomatic Medicine*, 1999, 61, pp. 263–270.
41. Linkins R.W., Comstock G.W., 'Depressed mood and development of cancer', *American Journal of Epidemiology*, 1990, 132, pp. 962–972.
42. Kiecolt-Glaser J.K., Glaser R., 'Psychoneuroimmunology and immunotoxicology: implications for carcinogenesis', *Psychosomatic Medicine*, 1999, 61, pp. 271–272.
43. Visintainer M., Volpicelli J., Seligman M., 'Tumour rejection in rats after inescapable or escapable shock', *Science*, 1982, 216, pp. 437–439.
44. Riley V., 'Psychoneuroendocrine influence on immunocompetence and neoplasia', *Science*, 1981, 212, p. 110.
45. Friedman M., Rosenman R., *Type A Behaviour and Your Heart*, New York, Knopf, 1974; Friedman M., 'Type A behaviour: its diagnosis, cardiovascular relation and the effects of its modification on recurrence of coronary artery disease', *American Journal of Cardiology*, 1989, 64, pp. 12–19.
46. 'Reflections in 2001', by Elaine Woo, journalist on the *Los Angeles Times*.
47. McCormick C.M., Smythe J.W., Sharma S., Meany M.J., 'Sex-specific effects of pre-natal stress on hypothalamic-pituitary-adrenal responses to stress and brain glucocorticoid receptor density in adult rats', *Brain Research. Developmental Brain Research*, 1995, 84, pp. 55–61.
48. Maccari S., Darnaudéry M., Van Reeth O., 'Hormonal and behavioral abnormalities induced by stress "in utero": an animal model for depression', *Stress*, 2001, pp. 12–23.
49. Morley-Fletcher S., Rea M., Maccari S., Laviola G., 'Environmental enrichment during adolescence reverses the effects of prenatal stress on play behaviour and HPA reactivity in rats', *European Journal of Neuroscience*, 2003, 18, pp. 1–8.
50. Lesage J., Del-Favero F., Leonhardt M., Louvart H., Maccari S., Vieau D., Darnaudéry M., 'Prenatal stress induces intrauterine growth restriction and programs insulin resistance and feeding behavior disturbance in the aged rat', *Journal of Endocrinology*, 2004, 181, pp. 291–296.
51. Kofman O., 'The role of pre-natal stress in the etiology of developmental behavioral disorders', *Neuroscience and Biobehavioral Reviews*, 2002, 26, pp. 457–470.

52. Huizink A.C., Robles de Medina P.J., Mulder E.J., Visser G.H., Buitelaar J.K., 'Psychological measures of prenatal stress as predictors of infant temperament', *Journal of the American Academy of Child and Adolescent Psychiatry*, 2002, 41, pp. 1078–1085; Buitelaar J.K., Huizink A.C., Mulder E.J., Robles de Medina P.G., Visser G.H., 'Prenatal stress and cognitive development and temperament in infants', *Neurobiology of Ageing*, 2003, 24, pp. S53–S60.
53. Poggi Davis E., Snidman M., Wadhwa P.D., Glynn L.M., Schetter C.D., Sandman C.A., 'Prenatal maternal anxiety and depression predict negative behavioral reactivity in infancy', *Infancy*, 2004, 6, pp. 319–331.
54. Linnet K.M., Dalsgaard S., Obel C., Wisborg K., Henriksen T.B., Rodriguez A., Kotimaa A., Moilanen I., Thomsen P.H., Olsen J., Jarvelin M-R., 'Maternal lifestyle factors in pregnancy risk of attention deficit disorder and associated behaviors: review of current evidence', *American Journal of Psychiatry*, 2003, 160, pp. 1028–1040.
55. Kippin T.E., Cain S.W., Masum Z., Ralph M.R., 'Neural stem cells show bidirectional experience-dependent plasticity in the perinatal mammalian brain', *The Journal of Neuroscience*, 2004, 24, pp. 2832–2836.
56. Kandle E.R., 'Cellular mechanisms of learning and the biological basis of individuality', in *Principles of Neural Science*, New York, McGraw-Hill, 2000.

CHAPTER 4   REASSURING: THE POWER OF THE MIND

1. Seligman M.E.P., *Authentic Happiness*, New York, The Free Press, Simon and Schuster, 2002.
2. This expression is borrowed from Matthieu Ricard: *Le Moine et le Philosophe*, Paris, Nil Editions, 1977.
3. Davidson R.J., 'Affective style, psychopathology and resilience: brain mechanisms and plasticity', *American Psychologist*, 2000, 55, pp. 1196–1214.
4. Csikszentmihalyi M., *Flow: The Psychology of Optimal Experience*, New York, Harper and Row, 1990.
5. Fredrickson B.L., 'The role of positive emotions in positive psychology: the broaden-and-build theory of positive emotions', *American Psychologist*, 2001, 56, p. 218.
6. Cousins N., 'Anatomy of an illness (as perceived by the patient)', *New England Journal of Medicine*, 1976, 295, pp. 1458–1463.
7. Berk L.S., Felten D.L., Tan S.A., Bittman B.B., Westengard J., 'Modulation of neuroimmune parameters during the eustress of humour-associated mirthful laughter', *Alternative Therapies*, 2001, 7, pp. 62–76.
8. Tan S.A., Tan L.G., Berk L.S., Lukman S.T., Lukman L.F., 'Mirthful laughter an effective adjunct in cardiac rehabilitation', *Canadian Journal of Cardiology*, 1997, 13, (suppl. B) p. 190.
9. Kimata H., 'Effect of humor on allergen-induced wheal reactions', *Journal of the American Medical Association*, 2001, 285, p. 738.
10. Yoshino S., Fujimori J., Kohda M., 'Effects of mirthful laughter on neuroendocrine and immune systems in patients with rheumatoid arthritis', *Journal of Rheumatology*, 1996, 23, pp. 793–794.
11. Pennebaker J.W., *Opening Up. The Healing Power of Confiding in Others*, New York, W.M. Morrox & Co., 1990.
12. Petrie K.J., Booth R.J., Pennebaker J.W., Davison K.P., Thomas M.G., 'Disclosure of trauma and immune response to hepatitis B vaccination program', *Journal of Consulting and Clinical Psychology*, 1995, 63, pp. 787–792.

13. Smyth J.M., Stone A.A., Hurwitz A., Kaell A., 'Effects of writing about stressful experiences on symptom reduction in patients with asthma or rheumatoid arthritis. A randomised trial', *Journal of the American Medical Association*, 1999, 281, pp. 1304–1309; Spiegel D., 'Healing words. Emotional expression and disease outcome', *Journal of the American Medical Association*, 1999, 281, pp. 1328–1329.
14. Hirschberg C., Barasch M.I., *Remarkable Recovery*, New York, Riverhead Books, 1995.
15. Visintainer M., Volpicelli J., Seligman M., 'Tumour rejection in rats after inescapable or escapable shock', *Science*, 1982, 216, pp. 437–439; *Science*, 1983, 221, pp. 568–570.
16. Cole S.W., Kemeny M.E., Taylor B.R. et al., 'Elevated physical health risk among gay men who conceal their homosexual identity', *Health Psychology*, 1996, 15, pp. 243–251.
17. Cole S.W., Kemeny M.E., Taylor B.R. et al., 'Accelerated course of human immunodeficiency virus infection in gay men who conceal their homosexual identity', *Psychosomatic Medicine*, 1996, 58, pp. 219–231.
18. Cole S.W., Naliboff B.D., Kemeny M.E. et al., 'Impaired response to HAART in patients with high autonomic nervous system activity', *Proceedings of the National Academy of Sciences*, 2001, 98, pp. 12695–12700.
19. Spiegel D., Bloom J.R., Kraemer H., Gottheil E., 'Effect of psychosocial treatment on survival of patients with metastatic breast cancer', *Lancet*, 1989, 50, pp. 681–689.
20. Fawzy F.I., Fawzy N.W., Hyun C.S., Elashoff R., Guthrie D., Fahey J.L., Morton D.L., 'Malignant melanoma: effects of an early structured psychiatric intervention, coping and affective state on recurrence and survival 6 years later', *Archives of General Psychiatry*, 1993, 50, pp. 681–689.
21. Goodwin P.J., Leszcz M., Ennis M. et al., 'The effect of group psychosocial support on survival in metastatic breast cancer', *New England Journal of Medicine*, 2001, 345, pp. 1719–1726.
22. Riley V., 'Psychoneuroendocrine influence on immunocompetence and neoplasia', *Science*, 1981, 212, p. 110.
23. Andersen B.L., Farrar W.B., Golden-Kreutz D. et al., 'Stress and immune responses after surgical treatment for regional breast cancer', *Journal of the National Cancer Institute*, 1998, 90, pp. 30–36.
24. Andersen B.L., Farrar W.B. et al., 'Psychological, behavioral and immune changes after a psychological intervention: a clinical trial', *Journal of Clinical Oncology*, 2004, 22, pp. 3570–3580.
25. Spiegel D., Sephton S.E., Terr A.I., Stites D.P., 'Effects of psychosocial treatment in prolonging cancer survival may be mediated by neuroimmune pathways', *Annals of the New York Academy of Sciences*, 1998, 840, pp. 674–683.
26. Luborsky L., Singer B., Luborsky L., 'Comparative studies of psychotherapies. Is it true that "Everyone has won and all must have prizes"?', *Archives of General Psychiatry*, 1975, 32, pp. 995–1008; Smith M.L., Glass G.V., 'Meta-analysis of psychotherapy outcome studies', *American Psychologist*, 1977, 32, pp. 752–760; Landman J.T., Dawes R.M., 'Psychotherapy outcome. Smith and Glass's conclusions stand up under scrutiny', *American Psychologist*, 1982, 37, pp. 504–516.
27. Strupp H.H., Hadley S.W., 'Specific vs non-specific factors in psychotherapy. A controlled study of outcome', *Archives of General Psychiatry*, 1979, 36, pp. 1125–1136.
28. Moerman D., *Meaning, Medicine and the 'Placebo Effect'*, Cambridge, Cambridge University Press, 2002.

29. Lévi-Strauss C., 'The effectiveness of symbols', in *Structural Anthropology*, Garden City, New York, Anchor Books, 1967.
30. Benson H., Alexander S., Feldman C.L., 'Decreased premature ventricular contractions through use of the relaxation response in patients with stable ischaemic heart disease', *Lancet*, 1975, 2, pp. 380–382.
31. Benson H., *The Relaxation Response*, New York, Morrow, 1975.
32. Kiecolt-Glaser J.K., Glaser R., Wiliger D. et al., 'Psychosocial enhancement of immunocompetence in a geriatric population', *Health Psychology*, 1985, 4, pp. 25–41; Cacioppo J.T., Bernston G.G., Malarkey W.B., Kiecolt-Glaser J. et al., 'Autonomic, neuroendocrine and immune responses to psychological stress: the reactivity hypothesis', *Annals of the New York Academy of Sciences*, 1998, 840, pp. 664–673.
33. Bernadi L., Sleight P., Bandinelli G. et al., 'Effect of rosary prayer and yoga mantras on autonomic cardiovascular rhythms: comparative study', *British Medical Journal*, 2001, 323, pp. 1446–1449.
34. Ernst E., Rand J.I., Stevinson C., 'Complementary therapies for depression: an overview', *Archives of General Psychiatry*, 1998, 55, pp. 1026–1032.
35. Teesdale J., Williams J., Soulsby J. et al., 'Prevention of relapse/recurrence in major depression of mindfulness-based cognitive therapy', *Journal of Consulting and Clinical Psychology*, 2000, 68, pp. 615–623; Miller J., Fletcher K., Kabat-Zinn J., 'Three year follow-up and clinical implications of a mindfulness meditation-based stress-reduction intervention in the treatment of anxiety disorders', *General Hospital Psychiatry*, 1995, 17, pp. 192–200.
36. Castillo-Richmond A. et al., 'Effects of stress reduction on carotid atherosclerosis in hypertensive African Americans', *Stroke*, 2000, 31, pp. 568–573.
37. Barnes V.A., Treiber F.A., Johnson M.H., 'Impact of transcendental meditation on ambulatory blood pressure in African American adolescents', *American Journal of Hypertension*, 2004, 17, pp. 366–369.
38. Davidson R.G., Kabat-Zinn J., Schumacher J., Rosenkrantz M. et al., 'Alterations in brain and immune function produced by mindfulness meditation', *Psychosomatic Medicine*, 2003, 65, pp. 564–570.
39. Lutz A., Greischar L.L., Rawlings N.B., Ricard M., Davidson R.J., 'Long-term meditators self-induce high amplitude gamma synchrony during mental practice', *Proceedings of the National Academy of Sciences*, 2004, 101, pp. 16369–16373.
40. Begley S., 'Scans of monks' brains show meditation alters structure, functioning', *The Wall Street Journal*, 5 November 2004.
41. Simonton C.O., Matthews-Simonton S., Creighton J., *Getting Well Again*, New York, Bantam, 1978.
42. Bakke A.C., Purtzer M.Z., Newton P., 'The effect of hypnotic guided imagery on psychological well-being and immune function in patients with prior breast cancer', *Journal of Psychosomatic Research*, 2002, 53, pp. 1131–1137.
43. Mundy E.A., DuHamel K.N., Montgomery G.H., 'The efficacy of behavioral interventions for cancer treatment-related side effects', *Seminars in Clinical Neuropsychiatry*, 2003, 8, pp. 253–275.
44. Ranganathan V.K., Siemionow V., Liu J.Z., Sahgal V., Yue G.H., 'From mental power to muscle power. Gaining strength by using the mind', *Neuropsychologia*, 2004, 42, pp. 944–956.
45. Warner L., McNeill M.E., 'Mental imagery and its potential for physical therapy', *Physical Therapy*, 1988, 68, pp. 516–521.

46. Morganti F., Gaggioli A., Castelnuovo G., Bulla D. et al., 'The use of technology-supported mental imagery in neurological rehabilitation: a research protocol', *Cyberpsychology & Behavior*, 2003, 6, pp. 421–427.
47. Lehrer P.M., Vaschillo E. et al., 'Biofeedback treatment for asthma', *Chest*, 2004, 126, pp. 352–361.
48. McCraty R., *Science of the Heart: Exploring the Role of the Heart in Human Performance*, Boulder Creek CA, Institute of HeartMath 2001. (Available to order from www.heartmath.org.)
49. Lang E.V., Benotsch E.G., Fick L.J. et al., 'Adjunctive non-pharmacological analgesia for invasive medical procedures: a randomized trial', *Lancet*, 2000, 355, pp. 1486–1490; Lang E.V., Rosen M.P., 'Cost analysis of adjunct hypnosis with sedation during outpatient interventional radiologic procedures', *Radiology*, 2002, 222, pp. 375–382.
50. Setter F., Kupper S., 'Autonomic training: a meta-analysis of clinical outcome studies', *Applied Psychophysiology and Biofeedback*, 2002, 27, pp. 45–98.
51. Black S., Humphrey J.H., Niven J.S.F., 'Inhibition of Mantoux reaction by direct suggestion under hypnosis', *British Medical Journal*, 1963, pp. 1649–1652.
52. Spiegel D., *Psychiatric Clinics of North America*, 12 June 1989.
53. Lang E.V., Benotsch E.G., Fick L.J. et al., 'Adjunctive non-pharmacological analgesia for invasive medical procedures: a randomised trial', *Lancet*, 2000, 355, pp. 1486–1490.
54. Spiegel H., Spiegel D., *Trance and Treatment: Clinical Uses of Hypnosis*, Washington DC, American Psychiatric Press Inc., 1978.
55. Rainville P., Hofbauer R.K., Paus T., Duncan G.H., Bushnell M.C., Price D.D., 'Cerebral mechanisms of hypnotic induction and suggestion', *Journal of Cognitive Neuroscience*, 1999, 11, pp. 110–125; Rainville P., Carrier B., Hofbauer R.K., Bushnell M.C., Duncan G.H., 'Dissociation of sensory and affective dimensions of pain using hypnotic modulation', *Pain*, 1999, 82, pp. 159–171.
56. Faymonville M-E., Meurisse M., Fissette J., 'Hypnosedation: a valuable alternative to traditional anaesthetic techniques', *Acta Chirugia Belgica*, 1999, 99, pp. 141–146.
57. Horton J.E., Crawford H.J., Harrington G. et al., 'Increased anterior corpus callosum size associated positively with hypnotisability and the ability to control pain', *Brain*, 2004, 127, pp. 1741–1747.
58. Faymonville M-E., Roediger L., Del Fiore G. et al., 'Increased cerebral functional connectivity underlying the antinociceptive effects of hypnosis', *Cognitive Brain Research*, 2003, 17, pp. 255–262.
59. Rainville P., Hofbauer R.K., Bushnell M.C., Duncan G.H., Price D.D., 'Hypnosis modulates activity in brain structures involved in the regulation of consciousness', *Journal of Cognitive Neuroscience*, 2002, 14, pp. 887–901.
60. Hoffman H.G., Patterson D.R., Carrougher G.J., 'Use of virtual reality for adjunctive treatment of adult burn pain during physical therapy: a controlled study', *Clinical Journal of Pain*, 2000, 16, pp. 244–250.
61. Hoffman H.G., Richards T., Coda B., Richards A., Sharar S.R., 'The illusion of presence in immersive virtual reality during an fMRI Brain Scan', *Cyberpsychology & Behaviour*, 2003, 6, pp. 127–131.

CHAPTER 5 OBSERVING THE BODY THAT SUFFERS

1. Sheldon W.H., *The Varieties of Temperament*, New York, Harper and Brothers Publishers, 1942.

2. Epel E.S., McEwen B., Seeman T., Matthews K., Castellazzo G., Brownell K.D., Bell J., Ickovics J.R., 'Stress and body shape: stress-induced cortisol secretion is consistently greater among women with central fat', *Psychosomatic Medicine*, 2000, 62, pp. 623–632.
3. Svoboda R., Lade A., *Tao and Dharma: Chinese Medicine and Ayurveda*, Twin Lakes WI, Lotus Press, 1995; Frawley D., *Ayurveda and the Mind*, Twin Lakes WI, Lotus Press, 1997.
4. Olson J.M., Vernon P.A., Aitken Harris J., 'The heritability of attitudes: a study of twins', *Journal of Personality and Social Psychology*, 2001, 80, pp. 845–860.
5. Reich W., *Character Analysis*, New York, Touchstone, 1972.

CHAPTER 6 INTERROGATING THE BODY THAT REMEMBERS

1. Extract from a letter sent by Sigmund Freud to his friend, Wilhelm Fliess, 13 March 1895. In Masson J. (ed.) *The Complete Letters of Sigmund Freud to Wilhelm Fliess*, Harvard MA, Belknap, 1985, p. 120.
2. Eiden B., 'Application of post-Reichian body psychotherapy: a Chiron perspective', in Staunton T. (ed.) *Body Psychotherapy*, Hove UK, Brunner-Routledge, 2002.
3. Lowen A., *Bioenergetics*, New York, Penguin Books, 1975; Lowen A., *The Language of the Body*, New York, Macmillan, 1971 (originally published under the title: *Physical Dynamics of Character Structure*, New York, Grune and Stratton, 1958); Lowen A., *The Vibrant Way to Health: A Manual of Exercises*, New York, Harper and Row, 1977.
4. James W., *The Principles of Psychology*, Cambridge MA, Harvard University Press, 1981 (original edition: 1890).
5. Rosenberg M.B., *Nonviolent Communication: A Language of Compassion*, Del Mar CA, PuddleDancer Press, 1999.
6. Berthoz S., Artiges E., Van der Moortele P-F., Poline J.B., Rouquette S., Consoli S.M., Martinot J-L., 'Effect of impaired recognition and expression of emotions on frontocingulate cortices: an fMRI study of men with alexithymia', *American Journal of Psychiatry*, 2002, 159, pp. 961–967.
7. Rolf I.P., *Rolfing: The Integration of Human Structures*, Santa Monica CA, Dennis-Landmann, 1977.
8. The case of Jeannine is very similar to that experienced by the Child Psychiatrist Joëlle Coron described in Coron J., 'La mémoire altérée', in Ferragut E. (ed.) *Emotion et mémoire. Le corps et la souffrance*, Paris, Masson, 2004.
9. Janov A., *Why You Get Sick and How You Get Well*, West Hollywood CA, Dove Books, 1996.
10. Janov A., *The Biology of Love*, New York, Prometheus Books, 2000.
11. Ferragut, *Emotion et mémoire*.
12. Janov, *Why You Get Sick and How You Get Well*.
13. Damasio A.R., *Descarte's Error: Emotion, Reason and the Human Brain*, New York, Avon Books, 1994.
14. Devroede G., *Ce que les maux de ventre disent de notre passé*, Paris, Payot 2003.
15. Ibid., p. 133.
16. Kisilevsky B.S., Hains S.M.J., Lee K., Xie X., Huang H., Ye H.H., Zhang K., Wang Z., 'Effects of experience on fetal voice recognition', *Psychological Science*, 2003, 14, pp. 220–224.
17. Ancelin Schützenberger A., *Aïe, mes aïeux*, Paris, Desclée de Brouwer, 1993.
18. Some statistical studies on the 'anniversary syndrome' were carried out between 1952 and 1957 by Josephine Hilgard on 8,680 patients admitted to two Californian

hospitality. These studies are discussed by Anne Ancelin Schützenberger in her book *Aïe, mes aïeux*.
19. Abraham N., Török M., *'L'ecorce et le noyau*, Paris, Aubier-Flammarion, 1987, p. 431.
20. Gampel Y., *Ces parents qui vivent à travers moi*, Paris, Fayard, 2005, p. 84.
21. Ancelin Schützenberger A., Devroede G., *Ces enfants malades de leurs parents*, Paris, Payot, 2003, p. 123.
22. Zajde N., *Souffle sur tous ces morts et qu'ils vivent!* Grenoble, La Pensée sauvage, 1993.
23. Van Eersel P., Maillard C., *J'ai mal à mes ancêtres. La psychogenealogie aujourd'hui*, Paris, Albin Michel, 2002, p. 87.
24. Hamer R.G., *Fondement de la Médecine nouvelle*, Chambéry, ASAC, 1993.
25. Dransart P., *La maladie cherche à me guerir*, Grenoble, Le Mercure dauphinois, 1999; Flèche C., *Mon corps pour me guerir: décodage psychobiologique des maladies*, Barrett-le Bas, Le Souffle d'or, 2000; Martel J., *Le Grand Dictionnaire des malaises et des maladies*, Aubagne, Editions Quintessence, 1998; Sellam S., *Origines et préventions des maladies*, Aubagne, Editions Quintessence, 2000.
26. Souzenelle A. de, *Le Symbolisme du corps humain*, Paris, Albin Michel, 1991; Odoul M., *Dis-moi où tu as mal, je te dirai pourquoi*, Paris, Albin Michel, 2002.
27. Shapiro D., *Your Body Speaks Your Mind*, London, Judy Piatkus Pub., 1996.
28. Siegel B.S., *Peace, Love and Healing*, New York, Harper and Row, 1989.
29. Payer L., *Medicine and Culture*, New York, Holt, 1988.
30. Harrington A., *The Placebo Effect. An Interdisciplinary Exploration*, Cambridge MA, Harvard University Press, 1997.

CHAPTER 7   TOUCHING THE BODY THAT RELAXES

1. Freud S., Breuer J., *Studies on Hysteria*, 1885, in *Penguin Freud Library*, vol. 3, Harmondsworth, Penguin, 1974.
2. Montagu A., *Touching. The Human Significance of the Skin*, New York, Harper and Row, 1986, p. 204.
3. Crusco A., Wetzel C.G., 'Touch', *Journal of Personality and Social Psychology*, 1973, 10, pp. 21–29.
4. Fisher J.A., Rytting M., Heslin R., 'Affective and evaluative effects of an interpersonal touch', *Sociometry*, 1976, 39, pp. 416–421.
5. Juhan D., *Job's Body: A Handbook for Bodywork*, New York, Station Hill Press, 1987.
6. Field T., *Touch*, Cambridge MA, MIT Press, 2001.
7. Harlow H., Zimmerman R.R., 'The development of affectional responses in infant monkeys', *Science*, 1959, 130, pp. 421–423; Harlow H.F., Harlow M.K., Dodsworth R.O., Arling G.L., 'Maternal behavior of rhesus monkeys deprived of mothering and peer associations in infancy', *Proceedings of the American Philosophical Society*, 1966, 110, pp. 58–66.
8. Suomi S.J., 'Touch and the immune system in rhesus monkeys', in Field T. (ed.) *Touch in Early Development*, Mahwah NJ, Lawrence Erlbaum Associates, 1995.
9. Spitz R., 'An enquiry into the genesis of psychiatric conditions in early childhood', *Psychoanalytic Study of the Child*, 1945, 1, pp. 53–74.
10. Field T., 'Young children's adaptations to repeated separations from their mothers', *Child Development*, 1991, 62, pp. 539–547.
11. Rosenthal M.J., 'Psychosomatic study of infantile eczema', *Pediatrics*, 1952, 10, pp. 581–593.

12. Montagu, *Touching*, p. 282.
13. Field T., 'Preschoolers in America are touched less and are more aggressive than preschoolers in France', *Early Child Development and Care*, 1999, 151, pp. 11–17.
14. Field T., 'American adolescents touch each other less and are more aggressive towards their peers as compared with French adolescents', *Adolescence*, 1999, 34, pp. 753–758.
15. Field T., Quintino O., Hernandez-Reif M., Koslovsky G., 'Adolescents with attention deficit hyperactivity disorder benefit from massage therapy', *Adolescence*, 1998, 33, pp. 103–108.
16. Nathan B., 'Philosophical notes on osteopathic theory. Part II: on persons, bodies, touching and inherent self-healing capacity', *British Osteopathic Journal*, 1995, 15, pp. 15–19.
17. Gellhorn E., 'Motion and emotion: the role of proprioception in the physiology and pathophysiology of emotions', *Psychological Review*, 1964, 71, pp. 457–472.
18. Lynch J.J. *et al.*, 'Effects of human contact on the heart activity of curarized patients in a shock-trauma unit', *American Heart Journal*, 1974, 88, pp. 160–169.
19. Veldman F., *Haptonomie, amour et raison*, Paris, PUF, 2004.
20. Triplett J., Arneson S., 'The use of verbal and tactile comfort to alleviate distress in young hospitalised children', *Research in Nursing and Health*, 1979, 2, p. 22.
21. Penny K.S., 'Postpartum perceptions of touch received during labour', *Research in Nursing and Health*, 1979, 2, pp. 9–16.
22. Field T.M., Hernandez-Reif M., Quintino O., Schanberg S., Kuhn C., 'Elder retired volunteers benefit from giving massage therapy to infants', *Journal of Applied Gerontology*, 1998, 17, pp. 229–239.
23. Field T., Schanberg S.M., Scadifi F. *et al.*, 'Tactile/kinaesthetic stimulation effects on pre-term neonates', *Pediatrics*, 1986, 77, pp. 654–658.
24. Uvnas Moberg K., 'Role of efferent and afferent vagal nerve activity during reproduction: integrating function of oxytocin metabolism and behavior', *Psychoendocrinology*, 1994, 19, pp. 687–695.
25. Field T., Morrow C., Valdeon C. *et al.*, 'Massage reduces anxiety in child and adolescent psychiatric patients', *Journal of the American Academy of Child and Adolescent Psychiatry*, 1992, 31, pp. 125–131.
26. Hart S., Field T., Hernandez-Reif M. *et al.*, 'Anorexia nervosa symptoms are reduced by massage therapy', *Eating Disorders. The Journal of Treatment and Prevention*, 2001, 9, pp. 217–228.
27. Jones N.A., Field T., 'Right frontal EEG asymmetry is attenuated by massage and music therapy', *Adolescence*, 1999, 34, pp. 529–534.
28. Hernandez-Reif M., Dieter J., Field T. *et al.*, 'Migraine headaches are reduced by massage therapy', *International Journal of Neuroscience*, 1998, 96, pp. 1–11.
29. Sunshine W., Field T., Quintino O. *et al.*, 'Fibromyalgia benefits from massage therapy and transcutaneous electrical stimulation', *Journal of Clinical Rheumatology*, 1996, 2, pp. 18–22; Field T. *et al.*, 'Burn injuries benefit from massage therapy', *Journal of Burn Care and Rehabilitation*, 1998, 19, pp. 241–244; Post-White J., Kinney M.E., 'The effects of therapeutic massage and healing touch on cancer patients', presented at the 1st International Symposium on Science of Touch, May 2002, Montreal, Quebec (reported by Kahn J.) 'Therapeutic massage in rehabilitation', in Davis C.M. (ed.) *Complementary Therapies in Rehabilitation: Evidence for Efficacy in Therapy, Prevention and Wellness*, Thorofare NJ, Slack Inc., 2004.
30. Field T., Presentation at the First International Symposium on Science of Touch, May 2002, Montreal, Quebec.

31. Ironson G., Field T., Scafidi F. et al., 'Massage therapy is associated with enhancement of the immune system's cytotoxic capacity', *International Journal of Neuroscience*, 1996, 84, pp. 205–217.
32. Diego M.A., Hernandez-Reif M., Field T. et al., 'Massage therapy effects on immune function in adolescents with HIV', *International Journal of Neuroscience*, 2001, 106, pp. 35–45.
33. Hernandez-Reif M., Ironson G., Field T. et al., 'Breast cancer patients have improved immune functions following massage therapy', study mentioned in the article by Field T., 'Massage therapy', in 'Complementary and alternative medicine', *The Medical Clinics of North America*, January 2002, 86 (1), pp. 163–171.
34. Field T., Hernandez-Reif M., Quintino O. et al., 'Elder retired volunteers benefit from giving massage therapy to infants', *Journal of Applied Gerontology*, 1998, 17, pp. 229–239.
35. Field T., Hernandez-Reif M., LaGreca A. et al., 'Massage therapy lowers blood glucose levels in children with diabetes', *Diabetes Spectrum*, 1997, 10, pp. 237–239.
36. Shulman K.R., Jones G.E., 'The effectiveness of massage therapy intervention on reducing anxiety in the workplace', *Journal of Applied Behavioral Science*, 1996, 32 (2), pp. 160–173.
37. Hodge M. et al., 'Employee outcomes following work-site acupressure and massage', in Rich G.J. (ed.) *Massage Therapy: The Evidence for Practice*, Saint Louis, Mosby, 2002.
38. Field T. et al., 'Massage therapy reduces anxiety and enhances EEG pattern of alertness and math computations', *International Journal of Neuroscience*, 1996, 86 (3–4), pp. 197–205.

CHAPTER 8 ALIGNING THE BODY THAT BALANCES ITSELF

1. Robbie D.L., 'Tensional forces in the human body', *Orthopaedic Review*, 1977, 6, pp. 45–48.
2. Myers T.W., 'The "anatomy trains"', *Journal of Bodywork and Movement Therapies*, 1997, 1, pp. 134–145.
3. Rolf I.P., 'Structural integration. Gravity: an unexplored factor in a more human use of human beings', *Journal of the Institute for the Comparative Study of History, Philosophy and the Sciences*, 1962, 1, pp. 3–20; Rolf I.P., *Rolfing: The Integration of Human Structures*, Santa Monica CA, Dennis-Landman, 1977.
4. Goldthwait J.E., *Body Mechanics in the Study and Treatment of Disease*, Philadelphia, J.B. Lippincott, 1934.
5. Strait L.A., Inman V.T., Ralston H.J., 'Sample illustrations of physical principles selected from physiology and medicine', *American Journal of Physiology*, 1947, 15, pp. 375–382; Hellebrandt F.A., Franseen E.B., 'Physiological study of the vertical stance of man', *Physiological Review*, 1943, 23, pp. 220–255.
6. Tanaka T., 'Gels', *Scientific American*, 1981, 244, pp. 124–138.
7. Rolf, *Rolfing*.
8. Wang J.Y., Butler J.P., Ingber D.E., 'Mechanotransduction across the cell surface and through the cytoskeleton', *Science*, 1993, 260, pp. 1124–1127.
9. Ingber D.E., 'The architecture of life', *Scientific American*, 1998, 278 (1), pp. 48–57; Ingber D.E., 'Cellular tensegrity: defining new rules of biological design that govern the cytoskeleton', *Journal of Cell Science*, 1993, 104, pp. 613–627.
10. Chen C.S., Mrksich M., Huang S., Whitesides G.M., Ingber D.E., 'Geometric control of cell life and death', *Science*, 1993, 276, pp. 1425–1428.

11. Oschman J.L., *Energy Medicine: The Scientific Basis*, Edinburgh, Churchill Livingstone, 2000.
12. Alexander F.M., *Man's Supreme Inheritance*, Long Beach, Centerline Press, 1984.
13. Alexander F.M., *The Use of the Self and Conscious Constructive Control of the Individual*, Long Beach, Centerline Press 1984.
14. Tinbergen N., 'Ethology and stress diseases', *Science*, 1974, 185, pp. 20–27.
15. Batson G., 'The Alexander technique', in Wainapel S.F., Fast A. (eds) *Alternative Medicine and Rehabilitation: A Guide for Practitioners*, New York, Demos, 2003; Dennis R.J., 'Functional reach improvement in normal older women after Alexander Technique instruction', *Journals of Gerontology. Series A, Biological Sciences and Medical Sciences*, 1999, 54, pp. 8–11; Austin J.H., Ausubel P., 'Enhanced respiratory muscular function in normal adults after lessons in proprioceptive musculoskeletal education without exercises', *Chest*, 1992, 102, pp. 486–490.
16. Stallibrass C., Sissons P., Chalmers C., 'Randomized controlled trial of the Alexander Technique for idiopathic Parkinson's disease', *Clinical Rehabilitation*, 2002, 16, pp. 695–708.
17. Feldenkrais M., *The Potent Self. A Guide to Spontaneity*, San Francisco, Harper and Row, 1985.
18. Feldenkrais M., *Body Awareness as Healing Therapy: The case of Nora*, Berkeley, Frog Ltd, 1993; Kaas J.H., 'Plasticity of sensory and motor maps in adult mammals', *Annual Review of Neuroscience*, 1991, 14, pp. 137–167; Nudo R.J., Milliken G.W., Jenkins W.M., Merzenich M.M., 'Use-dependent alterations of movement representations in primary motor cortex of adult squirrel monkeys', *Journal of Neuroscience*, 1996, 16, pp. 785–807; Nudo R.J., Friel K.M., 'Cortical plasticity after stroke: implications for rehabilitation', *Revue Neurologique (Paris)*, 1999, 155, pp. 713–717.
19. Damasio A.R., *Descartes' Error: Emotion, Reason and the Human Brain*, New York, Avon Books, 1994.
20. Bertherat T., *Le corps a ses raisons: autoguérison et anti-gymnastique*, Paris, Seuil, 1976; Bertherat T., *Les saisons du corps: garder et regarder la forme*, Paris, Albin Michel, 1985.
21. Pilates J.H., *Return to Life Through Contrology*, New York, J.J. Augustin, 1945.
22. Kudlas M.J., 'Chiropractic', in Leskowitz E.D. (ed.) *Complementary and Alternative Medicine in Rehabilitation*, New York, Churchill Livingstone, 2003; Fietchtner J.J., Brodeur R.R., 'Manual and manipulation techniques for rheumatic disease', *The Medical Clinics of North America*, January 2002, 86 (1), pp. 91–103.
23. Haldeman S., 'Neurological effects of the adjustment', *Journal of Manipulative and Physiological Therapeutics*, 2000, 23, pp. 112–114; Nelson C.F., 'The subluxation question', *Journal of Chiropractic Humanities*, 1997, 7, pp. 46–55; Hestbaek L., Leboef-Yde C., 'Are chiropractic tests for lumbo-pelvic spine reliable and valid? A systematic critical literature review', *Journal of Manipulative and Physiological Therapeutics*, 2000, 23, pp. 258–275.
24. Assendelft W.J. et al., 'The relationship between methodological quality and conclusions in reviews of spinal manipulation', *Journal of the American Medical Association*, 1995, 274, pp. 1942–1948.
25. Ernst E., Harkness E., 'Spinal manipulation: a systematic review of sham-controlled, double-blind, randomized clinical trials', *Journal of Pain and Symptom Management*, 2001, 22, pp. 879–889.
26. Bronfort G., Assendelft W.J., Bouter L., 'Efficacy of spinal manipulative therapies for conditions other than neck and back pain: a systematic review and best evidence synthesis', *Proceedings of the International Conference on Spinal Manipulation*,

1996, Bournemouth UK, Brookline MA, Foundation for Chiropractic Education and Research, 1996, pp. 105–106.
27. Kaptchuk T.J., Eisenberg D.M., 'Chiropractic: origins, controversies and contributions', *Archives of Internal Medicine*, 1998, 158, pp. 2215–2224; Morley J., Rosner A.L., Redwood D., 'A case study of misrepresentation of the scientific literature: recent reviews of chiropractic', *Journal of Alternative and Complementary Medicine* 2001, 7, pp. 65–78; Cooper R.A., McKee H.J., 'Chiropractic in the United States: trends and issues', *Millbank Q*, 2003, 81, pp. 107–138; Assendelft W.J. *et al.*, 'Spinal manipulative therapy for low back pain', *Annals of Internal Medicine*, 2003, 138, pp. 871–881.
28. Cherkin D.C. *et al.*, 'A comparison of physical therapy, chiropractic manipulation and provision of an educational booklet for treatment of patients with low back pain', *New England Journal of Medicine*, 1998, 339, pp. 1021–1029.
29. Ramey D.W., Rollin B.E., *Complementary and Alternative Veterinary Medicine Considered*, Ames IA, Iowa State Press, 2004.
30. Ibid., p. 132.
31. Oschman J.L., *Energy Medicine: The Scientific Basis*, Edinburgh, Churchill Livingstone, 2000.
32. Still A.T., *Autobiography with a History of the Discovery and Development of the Science of Osteopathy*, New York, Arno Press, 1972.
33. Ramey, Rollin, *Complementary and Alternative Veterinary Medicine Considered*.
34. Oschman, *Energy Medicine*.
35. Burton A.K., Tillotson K.M., Cleary J., 'Single blind randomized controlled trial of chemonucleolysis and manipulation in the treatment of symptomatic lumbar disc herniation', *European Spine Journal*, 2000, 9, pp. 202–207; Jarski R.W., Loniewski E.G., William J. *et al.*, 'The effectiveness of osteopathic manipulative treatment as a complementary therapy following surgery: a prospective match-controlled outcome study', *Alternative Therapies in Health and Medicine*, 2000, 6, pp. 77–81; Fiechtner J.J., Brodeur R.R., 'Manual and manipulation techniques for rheumatic disease', *The Medical Clinics of North America*, 2002, 88 (1), pp. 91–103.
36. Sainte-Rose M., *La Santé au bout des doigts. L'osteopathie, médecine moderne*, Paris, Robert Laffont, 2000.
37. Giaquinto-Wahl D., 'Craniosacral therapy', in Davis C.M. (ed.) *Complementary Therapies in Rehabilitation: Evidence for Efficacy in Therapy, Prevention and Wellness*, Thorofare NJ, Slack Inc., 2004.
38. Retzlaff E.W., Upledger J.E., Mitchell F., Beggert T., 'Structure of the cranial bone sutures: research report', *Journal of the American Osteopathic Association*, 1976, 75, pp. 607–608; Retzlaff E.W., Upledger J.E., Mitchell F., Beggert T., 'Nerve fibre and endings in cranial sutures', *Journal of the American Osteopathic Association*, 1978, 77, pp. 474–475.
39. Upledger J.E., *Craniosacral Therapy Study Guide*, Palm Beach Gardens FL, Upledger Institute Publishing, 1997; Adams T. *et al.*, 'Parietal bone mobility in the anaesthetised cat', *Journal of the American Osteopathic Association*, 1992, 92 (5).
40. Rogers J.S., Witt P.L., 'The controversy of cranial bone motion', *Journal of Orthopaedic and Sports Physical Therapy*, 1997, 26, pp. 95–103.
41. Upledger J.E., 'The reproducibility of craniosacral examination findings: a statistical analysis', *Journal of the American Osteopathic Association*, 1977, 76, pp. 890–899; Upledger J.E., 'Relationship of craniosacral examination findings in grade school children with developmental problems', *Journal of the American Osteopathic Association*, 1978, 77, pp. 760–776; Green C., Martin C.W., Bassett K., Kazanjian A., 'A systematic review of craniosacral therapy: biological plausibility, assessment,

reliability and clinical effectiveness', *Contemporary Therapies in Medicine*, 1999, 7, pp. 201–207; Rogers J.S., Witt P.L., Gross M.T., Hacke J.D., Genova P.A., 'Simultaneous palpation of the craniosacral rate at the head and the feet: intra-rater and inter-rater reliability and rate comparison', *Physical Therapy*, 1997, 78, pp. 1175–1185; Hartman S.E., Norton J.M., 'Interexaminer reliability and cranial osteopathy', *Scientific Review of Alternative Medicine*, 2002, 6, pp. 23–34.

42. Upledger J.E., 'Craniosacral therapy', in Leskowitz E.D. (ed.) *Complementary and Alternative Medicine in Rehabilitation*, New York, Churchill Livingstone, 2003.
43. Green C., Martin C.W., Bassett K., Kazanjian A., 'A systematic review of craniosacral therapy, biological plausibility, assessment, reliability and clinical effectiveness', *Contemporary Therapies in Medicine*, 1999, 7, pp. 201–207.

CHAPTER 9 BEHIND THE CHINESE THEORIES

1. Phillips D.P., Ruth T.E., Wagner L.M., 'Psychology and survival', *Lancet*, 1993, 342, pp. 1142–1145.
2. Veith I., *The Yellow Emperor's Classic of Internal Medicine*, Berkeley, University of California Press, 1973.
3. Liang T.T., *T'ai Chi Ch'uan for Health and Self-Defense: Philosophy and Practice*, New York, Vintage Books, 1977.
4. Sancier K.M., 'Therapeutic benefits of qigong exercises in combination with drugs', *Journal of Alternative and Complementary Medicine*, 1999, 5, pp. 383–389; Reuther I., Aldridge D., 'Qigong Yangsheng as a complementary therapy in the management of asthma: a single-case appraisal', *Journal of Alternative and Complementary Therapies*, 1998, 4, pp. 173–183; Ernst E., 'Breathing techniques: adjunctive treatment modalities for asthma? A systematic review', *European Respiratory Journal*, 2000, 15, pp. 969–972.
5. Mayer M., 'Qigong and hypertension: a critique of research', *Journal of Alternative and Complementary Medicine*, 1999, 5, pp. 371–382; Mayer M., 'Qigong clinical studies', in Jonas W.B. and Crawford C.C. (eds) *Healing, Intention and Energy Medicine: Science, Research Methods and Clinical Implications*, New York, Churchill Livingstone, 2003.
6. Tsujiuchi T., Kumano H., Yoshiuchi K. et al., 'The effect of Qi-gong relaxation exercise on the control of type 2 diabetes mellitus: a randomized controlled trial', *Diabetes Care*, 2002, 25, pp. 241–242.
7. Lai J.S., Lan C., Wong M.K., Teng S.H., 'Two-year trends in cardio-respiratory function among older T'ai Chi Chuan practitioners and sedentary subjects', *Journal of the American Geriatrics Society*, 1995, 43, pp. 1222–1227; Lee M.S., Kim B.G., Huh H.J., Ryu H., Lee H.S., Chung H.T., 'Effect of Qi-training on blood pressure, heart rate and respiration rate', *Clinical Physiology*, 2000, 20, pp. 173–176.
8. Lee M.S., Kang C.W., Ryu H., Kim J.D., Chung H.T., 'Effects of ChungDoSunBup Qi-training on growth hormone, insulin-like growth factor-I and testosterone in young and elderly subjects', *American Journal of Chinese Medicine*, 1999, 27, pp. 167–175.
9. Lee M.S., Kang C.W., Shin Y.S., Huh H.J., Ryu H., Park J.H., Chung H.T., 'Acute effects of ChungDoSunBup qigong Qi-training on blood concentrations of TSH, calcitonin, PTH and thyroid hormones in elderly subjects', *American Journal of Chinese Medicine*, 1998, 26, pp. 275–281.
10. Hirschberg C., Barasch M.I., '*Remarkable Recovery*, New York, Riverhead Books, 1995.

11. Jin P., 'Changes in heart rate, noradrenaline, cortisol and mood during T'ai Chi', *Journal of Psychosomatic Research*, 1989, 33, pp. 197–206; Ryu H., Lee H.S., Shin Y.S. et al., 'Acute effect of Qigong training on stress hormonal levels in man', *American Journal of Chinese Medicine*, 1996, 24, pp. 193–198.
12. Sun X.S., Xu Y., Xia Y.J., 'Determination of E-rosette forming lymphocytes in aged subjects with T'ai Chi Quan exercise', *International Journal of Sports Medicine*, 1989, 10, pp. 217–219; Ryu H., Mo H.Y., Mo G.D. et al., 'Delayed cutaneous hypersensitivity reaction in Qigong (ChungDoSunBup) trainees by multi-test cell mediated immunity', *American Journal of Chinese Medicine*, 1995, 23, pp. 139–144; Ryu H., Jun C.D., Lee B.S. et al., 'Effects of Qigong training on proportion of lymphocyte subsets in human peripheral blood', *American Journal of Chinese Medicine*, 1995, 23, pp. 27–36; Fukushima M., Kataoka T, Hamada C., Matsumoto M., 'Evidence of Qigong energy and its biological effect on the enhancement of the phagocytic activity of human polymorphonuclear leukocytes', *American Journal of Chinese Medicine*, 2001, 29, pp. 1–16.
13. Quah T.C., 'Alternative and complementary cancer treatments', *Oncologist*, 1996, 1, pp. 324–325; Wu W.H., Bandilla E., Ciccone D.S. et al., 'Effects of Qigong on late-stage complex regional pain syndrome', *Alternative Therapies in Health and Medicine*, 1999, 5, pp. 45–54.
14. Shang C., 'Emerging paradigms in mind–body medicine', *Journal of Alternative and Complementary Medicine*, 1999, 5, pp. 83–91; Xu S.H., 'Psychophysiological reactions associated with qigong therapy', *Chinese Medical Journal*, 1994, 107, pp. 230–233.
15. Li M., Chen K., Mo Z., 'Use of qigong in the detoxification of heroin addicts', *Alternative Therapies in Health and Medicine*, 2002, 8, pp. 50–59.
16. Bottomley J.M., 'T'ai Chi: choreography of body and mind', in Davis C.M. (ed.) *Complementary Therapies in Rehabilitation: Evidence of Efficacy in Therapy, Prevention and Wellness*, Thorofare NJ, Slack Inc., 2004; Chen K.M., Synder M., Krichbaum K., 'Facilitators and barriers to elders' practice of T'ai Chi. A mind–body low-intensity exercise', *Journal of Holistic Nursing*, 2001, 19, pp. 238–255.
17. Jin P., 'Efficacy of Tai Chi, brisk walking, meditation and reading in reducing mental and emotional stress', *Journal of Psychosomatic Research*, 1992, 36, pp. 361–370; Frontana J.A., 'The energy costs of a modified form of Tai Chi exercise', *Nursing Research*, 2000, 49, pp. 91–96.
18. Young D.R., Appeal L.J., Lee S.H. et al., 'The effects of aerobic exercise and Tai Chi on blood pressure in older people: result of a randomized trial', *Journal of the American Geriatrics Society*, 1999, 47, pp. 277–284.
19. Lan C., Chen S.Y., Lai J.S. et al., 'The effects of aerobic exercise and Tai Chi on cardiorespiratory function in patients with coronary artery bypass surgery', *Medicine in Sports and Exercise*, 1999, 47, pp. 634–638.
20. Channer K.S., Barrow D., Barrow R. et al., 'Changes in haemodynamic parameters following Tai Chi Chuan and aerobic exercise in patients recovering from acute myocardial infarction', *Postgraduate Medicine*, 1996, 72, pp. 349–351; Fontana J.A., Colella C., Baas L.S., Ghazi F., 'T'ai Chi Chih as an intervention for heart failure', *Nursing Clinics of North America*, 2000, 35 (4), pp. 1031–1046.
21. Brown D.D., Mucci W.G., Hetzeler R.K. et al., 'Cardiovascular and ventilatory response during formalized T'ai Chi Chuan exercise', *Research Quarterly in Exercise and Sports*, 1989, 60, pp. 246–250.
22. Wolf S.L., Barnhart H.X., Kutner N.G. et al., 'Reducing frailty and falls in older persons: an investigation of Tai Chi and computerized balance training: Atlanta FICSIT group-frailty and injuries: co-operative studies of intervention techniques',

Journal of the American Geriatrics Society, 1996, 44, pp. 489–497; Kessenich C.R., 'Tai Chi as a method of fall prevention in the elderly', *Orthopaedic Nursing*, 1998, 17, pp. 27–29.

23. Chan K.M., Au S.K., Choy W.Y. et al., 'Beneficial effect of one-year Tai Chi in retardation of bone loss in post-menopausal women', *Journal of Bone and Mineral Research*, 2000, 15, p. S444; Lane J.M., Nydick M., 'Osteoporosis: current modes of prevention and treatment', *Journal of the American Academy of Orthopaedic Surgeons*, 1999, 7, pp. 19–31.
24. Shapira M.Y., Chelouche M., Yanai R., Kaner C., Szold A., 'T'ai Chi Ch'uan practice as a tool for rehabilitation of severe head trauma', *Archives of Physical Medicine and Rehabilitation*, 2001, 82, pp. 1283–1285; Husted C., Pham L., Hekking A., Niederman R., 'Improving quality of life for people with conditions: the example of T'ai Chi and multiple sclerosis', *Alternative Therapies in Health and Medicine*, 1999, 5, pp. 70–74.
25. Hartman C.A., Manos T.M., Winter C. et al., 'Effects of Tai Chi training on function and quality of life indicators in older adults with osteoarthritis', *Journal of the American Geriatrics Society*, 2000, 48, pp. 1553–1559; Yocum D.E., Castro W.L., Cornett M., 'Exercise, education and behavioral modification as alternative therapy for pain and stress in rheumatic disease', *Rheumatic Disease Clinics of North America*, 2000, 26, pp. 145–159.
26. Li F., Fisher K.J., Harmer P., Irbe D., Tearse R.G., Weimer C., 'Tai Chi and self-rated quality of sleep and daytime sleepiness in older adults: a randomized controlled trial', *Journal of the American Geriatrics Society*, 2004, 52, pp. 892–900.
27. Cassileth B.R., 'Evaluating complementary and alternative therapies for cancer patients', *CA: A Cancer Journal of Clinicians*, 1999, 49, pp. 362–375.
28. Brown D.R., Wang Y., Ward A. et al., 'Chronic psychological effects on exercise and exercise plus cognitive strategies', *Medicine and Science in Sports and Exercise*, 1995, 27, pp. 765–775.
29. Verity L.S., Czubryt P., Hamilton L. et al., 'Effects of Taichi, meditation and walking on stress and immune responses', *Medicine and Science in Sports and Exercise*, 1999, 31, p. S346.
30. Damas J.C. et al., 'Nuclear medicine investigation of transmission of acupuncture information', *Acupuncture in Medicine*, 1993, 11, pp. 22–28; Damas J.C., 'Isotopic and cytologic assays', in *Acupuncture in Energy Fields Medicine*, Kalamazoo, John E. Feltzer Foundation, 1989, pp. 44–68.
31. Reichmanis M., Marino A.A., Becker R.O., 'DC skin conductance variation at acupuncture loci', *American Journal of Chinese Medicine*, 1976, 4, pp. 69–72; Reichmanis M., Marino A.A., Becker R.O., 'Laplace plane analysis of transient impedance between acupuncture points LI-4 and LI-12', *IEEE Transactions on Biomedical Engineering*, 1977, 24, pp. 402–427.
32. Comunetti A., Laage S., Schiessl N. et al., 'Characterisation of human skin conductance at acupuncture points', *Experientia*, 1995, 51, pp. 328–331; Sullivan S.G., Eggleston W.W., Martinoff J.T., Kroenig R.J., 'Evoked electrical conductivity on the lung acupuncture points in healthy individuals and confirmed cancer patients', *American Journal of Acupuncture*, 1985, 13, pp. 261–266.
33. Bergsman O., Woolley-Hart A., 'Differences in electrical skin conductivity between acupuncture points and adjacent skin areas', *American Journal of Acupuncture*, 1973, 1, pp. 27–32.
34. Oschman J.L., *Energy Medicine. The Scientific Basis*, Edinburgh, Churchill Livingstone, 2000.
35. Szent-Györgyi A., 'Toward a new biochemistry?', *Science*, 1941, 93, pp. 609–611.

36. Shang C., 'Electrophysiology of growth control and acupuncture', *Life Sciences*, 2001, 68, pp. 1333–1342.
37. Reston J., 'Now about my operation in Peking', *The New York Times*, 26 July 1971.
38. NIH Consensus Conference, 'Acupuncture', *Journal of the American Medical Association*, 1998, 280, pp. 1518–1524.
39. British Medical Association Board of Sciences, *Acupuncture: Efficacy, Safety and Practice*, London, Harwood Academic, 2000.
40. Linde K., Vickers A., Hondras M., ter Riet G., Thormahlen J., Berman B., Melchart D., 'Systematic reviews of complementary therapies – an annotated bibliography. Part 1: acupuncture', *BMC Complementary and Alternative Medicine*, 2001, 1, p. 3.
41. Ramey D.W., Rollin B.E., *Complementary and Alternative Veterinary Medicine Considered*, Ames IA, Iowa State Press, 2004.
42. LaRiccia P.J., Galantino M.L., 'Acupuncture theory and acupuncture-like therapeutics in physical therapy', in Davis C.M. (ed.) *Complementary Therapies in Rehabilitation: Evidence for Efficacy in Therapy, Prevention and Wellness*, Thorofare NJ, Slack Inc., 2004, p. 313.
43. Lu G.D., Needham J., *Celestial Lancets: A History and Rationale of Acupuncture and Moxa*, Cambridge, Cambridge University Press, 1980, pp. 225–226.
44. Streitberger K., Witte S., Mansmann U., Knauer C., Krämer J., Sharf H-P., Victor N., 'Efficacy and safety of acupuncture for chronic pain caused by gonarthrosis: a study protocol of an ongoing multi-centre randomised controlled clinical trial [ISRCTN27450856]', *BMC Complementary and Alternative Medicine*, 2004, 4, p. 6.
45. Kaptchuk T.J., 'Acupuncture: theory, efficacy and practice', *Annals of Internal Medicine*, 2002, 136, pp. 374–383.
46. Wu M.T., Hsieh J.C., Xiong J., Yang C.F., Pan H.B., Chen Y.C., Guochuan T., Rosen B.R., Kwong K.K., 'Central nervous pathway for acupuncture stimulation: localisation of processing with functional MR imaging of the brain – preliminary experience', *Radiology*, 1999, 212, pp. 133–141; Hui K.K., Liu J., Makris N., Gollub R.L., Chen A.J., Moore C.I., Kennedy D.N., Rosen B.R., Kwong K.K., 'Acupuncture modulates the limbic system and subcortical gray structures of the human brain: evidence from fMRI studies in normal subjects', *Human Brain Mapping*, 2000, 9, pp. 13–25.
47. Avants S.K., Margolin A., Chang P. *et al.*, 'Acupuncture for treatment of cocaine addiction: investigation of a needle-puncture control', *Journal of Substance Abuse Treatment*, 1995, 12, pp. 195–205; He D., Medbo J.I., Hostmark A.T., 'Effect of acupuncture on smoking cessation or reduction: an 8-month and 5-year follow-up study', *Preventive Medicine*, 2001, 33, pp. 364–372.
48. Alavi A., LaRiccia P.J., Sadek A.H. *et al.*, 'Neuroimaging of acupuncture in patients with chronic pain', *Journal of Alternative and Complementary Medicine*, 1997, 3, pp. 547–553.
49. Lewith G.T., White P.J., Pariente J., 'Investigating acupuncture using brain imaging techniques: the current state of play', eCAM, 2005, 2, pp. 315–319, on-line: http://ecam.oxfordjournals.org/content/vol2/issue3/index.dtl; Pariente J., White P.J., Frackowiak R.S.J., Lewith G.T., 'Expectancy and belief modulate the neuronal substrates of pain treated by acupuncture', *Neuroimage*, 2005, 25, pp. 1161–1167.
50. Wang B.C., Wang E.Z. *et al.*, 'Han's acupoint nerve stimulator (HANS) in combination with enfluran for anaesthesia in cranial operations', *Chinese Journal of Anaesthesiology*, 1994, 14, pp. 427–429; Qu G.L., Zhunag X.L. *et al.*, 'Clinical

observation on combined anesthetics: acupuncture anesthesia in 50 patients undergoing renal transplantation', *Clinical Journal of Pain Medicine*, 1996, 2, pp. 72–77.
51. Sung J.J.Y., 'Acupuncture for gastrointestinal disorders: Myth or magic', *Gut*, 2002, 51, pp. 617–619.
52. Luo H.C., Jia Y.K. et al., 'Electroacupuncture vs Amitryptilene in the treatment of depressive states', *Journal of Traditional Chinese Medicine*, 1985, 5, pp. 3–8; Luo H.C., Shen Y.C. et al., 'A comparative study of the treatment of depression by electroacupuncture', *Acupuncture Scientific International Journal*, 1990, 1, pp. 20–26; Wang S.M., Kain Z.N., 'Auricular acupuncture: a potential treatment for anxiety', *Anaesthesia and Analgesia*, 2001, 92, pp. 548–553.
53. Cho Z.H., Chung S.C., Jones J.P., Park J.B., Park H.J., Lee H.J., Wong E.K., Min B.I., 'New findings of the correlation between acupoints and corresponding brain cortices using functional MRI', *Proceedings of the National Academy of Sciences*, 1998, 95, pp. 2670–2673.
54. Li G., Cheung R.T.F., Ma Q.Y., Yang E.S., 'Visual cortical activations on fMRI upon stimulation of the vision-implicated acupoints', *Neuroreport*, 2003, 14, pp. 669–673; Lee H., Park H.J., Kim S.A., Lee H.J., Kim M.J., Kim C.J., 'Acupuncture stimulation of the vision-related acupoint (BI-67) increases c-Fos expression in the visual cortex in binoculary deprived rat pups', *American Journal of Chinese Medicine*, 2002, 30, pp. 379–385; Siedentopf C., Golaszewski S.M., Mottaghy F.M., Ruff C.C., Felber S., Schlager A., 'Functional magnetic resonance imaging detects activation of the visual association cortex during laser acupuncture of the foot in humans', *Neuroscience Letters*, 2002, 327, pp. 53–56; Litsher G., Rachbauer D., Ropele S., Wang L., Achikora D., Fazekas F., 'Acupuncture using laser needles modulates brain functions: first evidence from functional transcranial Doppler sonography and functional magnetic resonance imaging', *Lasers in Medical Science*, 2004, 19, pp. 6–11.
55. Gareus I.K., Lacour M., Schulte A.C., Hennig J., 'Is there a BOLD response of the visual cortex on stimulation of the vision-related acupoint GB 37?', *Journal of Magnetic Resonance Imaging*, 2002, 15, pp. 227–232; Gareus I.K., Hennig J., Dobos G.J., 'Enhanced efforts to investigate acupuncture by means of functional magnetic resonance imaging (fMRI) – a critical appraisal', *Focus on Alternative and Complementary Therapies*, 2003, 8, p. 4.
56. Cho Z.H., Na C.S., Wang E.K., 'Functional magnetic resonance imaging of the brain in the investigation of acupuncture', in Stux G., Hammerschlag R. (eds) *Clinical Acupuncture: Scientific Basis*, Berlin, Springer, 2001, pp. 83–95.
57. Li G., Liu H.L., Cheung R.T.F., Hung Y.C., Wong K.K.K., Shen G.G.X., Ma Q.Y., Yang E.S., 'An fMRI study comparing brain activation between word generation and electrical stimulation of language-implicated acupoints', *Human Brain Mapping*, 2003, 18, pp. 233–238.
58. Yoo S.S., Teh E.K., Blinder R.A., Jolesz F.A., 'Modulation of cerebellar activities by acupuncture stimulation: evidence from fMRI study', *Neuroimage*, 2004, 22, pp. 932–940.
59. Alimi D., Rubino C., Pichard-Leandri E., Fermand-Brule S., Dubreuil-Lemaire M.L., Hill C., 'Analgesic effect of auricular acupuncture for cancer pain: a randomized, blind controlled trial', *Journal of Clinical Oncology*, 2003, 21, pp. 4120–4126.
60. Oleson T.D., Kroening R.J., Bresler D.E., 'An experimental evaluation of auricular diagnosis: the somatotopic mapping of musculoskeletal pain at ear acupuncture points', *Pain*, 1980, 8, pp. 1347–1360.
61. Talbot M., *The Holographic Universe*, New York, HarperCollins, 1991.

62. Joderkovsky R., 'Hand acupuncture', *Physical Medicine and Rehabilitation Clinics of North America*, 1999, 10, pp. 563–571; Yamamoto T., *New Scalp Acupuncture*, Japan, Alex Springer Publishing, 1998.
63. Field T., *Touch*, Cambridge MA, MIT Press, 2001.
64. Cardini F., Weixin H., 'Moxibustion for correction of breech presentation', *Journal of the American Medical Association*, 1998, 280, pp. 1580–1584.
65. Kawada Y., Karcher S., *Essential Shiatsu*, London, Time Warner Books, 2002.

CHAPTER 10   BEHIND THE INDIAN TRADITIONS

1. Hunt V.V., *Infinite Mind. Science of the Human Vibrations of Consciousness*, Malibu CA, Malibu Publishing Company, 1996; Tiller W.A., *Science and Human Transformation. Subtle Energies, Intentionality and Consciousness*, Walnut Creek CA, Pavior, 1997; Schwartz G.E.R., Russek L.G.S., *The Living Energy Universe*, Charlottesville VA, Hampton Roads, 1999.
2. Oschman J.L., *Energy Medicine. The Scientific Basis*, Edinburgh, Churchill Livingstone, 2000.
3. Tiller, *Science and Human Transformation*.
4. McCraty R., *Science of the Heart: Exploring the Role of the Heart in Human Performance*, Boulder Creek CA, Institute of HeartMath, 2001 (available to order: www.heartmath.org).
5. Wisneski L.A., Anderson L., *The Scientific Basis of Integrative Medicine*, Boca Raton FL, CRC Press, 2005.
6. Keller S., Schleifer S., Bartlett J., Eckholdt H., 'Affective processes and immune dysfunction have health consequences', *Biological Psychiatry*, 1992, 31, p. 236A.
7. Taylor M.J., 'Yoga therapeutics: an ancient practice in a 21st century setting', in Davis C.M. (ed.) *Complementary Therapies in Rehabilitation: Evidence for Efficacy in Therapy, Prevention and Wellness*, Thorofare NJ, Slack Inc., 2004.
8. Ross R., 'Yoga Therapy', in Leskowitz E.D. (ed.) *Complementary and Alternative Medicine in Rehabilitation*, New York, Churchill Livingstone, 2003.
9. Schell F.J., Allolio B., Schonecke O.W., 'Physiological and psychological effects of Hatha-Yoga exercise on healthy women', *International Journal of Psychosomatics*, 1994, 41, pp. 46–52.
10. Malathi A., Damodaran A., 'Stress due to exams in medical students: role of yoga', *Indian Journal of Physiology and Pharmacology*, 1999, 43, pp. 218–224.
11. Cohen L., Warneke C., Fouladi R.T., Rodriguez M.A., Chaoul-Reich A., 'Psychological adjustment and sleep quality in a randomized trial of the effects of a Tibetan yoga intervention in patients with lymphoma', *Cancer*, 2004, 100, pp. 2253–2260; Platania-Scolazzo A. *et al.*, 'Relaxation therapy reduces anxiety in child and adolescent psychiatric patients', *Acta Paedopsychiatrica*, 1992, 55, pp. 115–120; Khumar S.S., Kaur P., Kaur S., 'Effectiveness of Shavasana on depression among university students', *Indian Journal of Clinical Psychology*, 1993, 20, pp. 82–87; Woolery A., Myers H., Sternlieb B., Zeltzer L., 'A yoga intervention for young adults with elevated symptoms of depression', *Alternative Therapies in Health and Medicine*, 2004, 10, pp. 60–63; Schaffer H.J., LaSalvia T.A., Stein J.P., 'Comparing Hatha Yoga with dynamic group psychotherapy for enhancing methadone maintenance treatment: a randomized clinical trial', *Alternative Therapies in Health and Medicine*, 1997, 3, pp. 57–66; Gopinath K.S., Rao R., Raghuram N., Rama Rao N., Shirley T., Vinay C., Chandrashekara S., Srinath B.S. (The Yoga Study Group), 'Evaluation of Yoga therapy as a psychotherapeu-

tic intervention in breast cancer patients on conventional combined modality of treatment', Bangalore, Bangalore Institute of Oncology, 2003.
12. Ornish D., Scherwitz L., Billings J.H., 'Intensive lifestyle changes for reversal of coronary heart disease', *Journal of the American Medical Association*, 1998, 280, p. 23.
13. Manchanda S.C., Narang R., Reddy K.S., Sachdeva U., Prabhakaran D., Dharmanand S., Rajani M., Bijlani R., 'Retardation of coronary atherosclerosis with yoga lifestyle intervention', *Journal of the Association of Physicians of India*, 2000, 48, pp. 687–694; Mahajan A.S., Reddy K.S., Sachdeva U., 'Lipid profile of coronary risk subjects following yogic lifestyle intervention', *Indian Heart Journal*, 1999, 51, pp. 37–40; Jatuporn S., Sangwatanaroj S., Saengsiri A.O., Rattanapruks S., Srimahachota S., Uthayachalerm W., Kuanoon W., Panpakdee O., Tangkijvanich P., Tosukhowong P., 'Short-term effects of an intensive lifestyle modification program on lipid peroxidation and antioxydant systems in patients with coronary heart disease', *Clinical Hemorheology and Microcirculation*, 2003, 29, pp. 429–436.
14. Patal C., North W.R., 'Randomized controlled trial of yoga and biofeedback in management of hypertension', *Lancet*, 1975, 2, pp. 93–95; Murugesan R., Govindarajulu N, Bera T.K., 'Effect of selected yogic practices on the management of hypertension', *Indian Journal of Physiology and Pharmacology*, 2000, 44, pp. 207–210.
15. Nagaranthna R., Nagendra H.R., 'Yoga for bronchial asthma: a controlled study, *British Medical Journal (Clinical Research Ed.)*, 1985, 291, pp. 1077–1079; Nagendra H.R., Nagaranthna R., 'An integrated approach of yoga therapy for bronchial asthma: a 3–54-month prospective study', *Journal of Asthma*, 1986, 23, pp. 123–137; Jain S.C., Rai L., Valecha A., Jha U.K., Bhatnagar S.O., Ram K., 'Effect of yoga training on exercise tolerance in adolescents with childhood asthma', *Journal of Asthma*, 1991, 28, pp. 437–442; Ram F.S., Holloway E.A., Jones P.W., 'Breathing retraining for asthma', *Respiratory Medicine*, 2003, 97, pp. 501–507.
16. Taneja I., Deepak K.K., Poojary G., Acharya I.N., Pnadey R.M., Sharma M.P., 'Yogic versus conventional treatment in diarrhea-predominant irritable bowel syndrome: a randomized control study', *Applied Psychophysiology and Biofeedback*, 2004, 29, pp. 19–33.
17. Ross R., 'Yoga therapy', in Leskowitz E.D. (ed.) *Complementary and Alternative Medicine in Rehabilitation*, New York, Churchill Livingstone, 2003.
18. Bhargava R., Gogate M.G., Mascarenhas J.F., 'Autonomic response to breath holding and its variations following pranayama', *Indian Journal of Physiology and Pharmacology*, 1988, 32, pp. 257–264.
19. Website of Sri Shyam-ji Bhatnagar: www.innertuning.org.
20. Klein R., Armitage R., 'Rhythms in human performances: one-and-a-half-hour oscillations in cognitive style', *Science*, 1979, 204, pp. 1326–1328.
21. Werntz D., Bickford R., Bloom F., Shannahoff-Khalsa D., 'Alternating cerebral hemispheric activity and lateralization of autonomic nervous function', *Human Neurobiology*, 1982, 2, pp. 225–229; Telles S., Nagarathna R., Nagendra H.R., 'Breathing through a particular nostril can alter metabolism and autonomic activities', *Indian Journal of Physiology and Pharmacology*, 1994, 38, pp. 133–137.
22. Shannahoff-Khalsa D., 'Lateralized rhythms of the central and autonomic nervous systems', *International Journal of Psychophysiology*, 1991, 11, pp. 225–251; Werntz D., Bickford R., Shannahoff-Khalsa D., 'Selected hemispheric stimulation by unilateral forced nostril breathing', *Human Neurobiology*, 1982, 6, pp. 165–171; Stancak K., Kuna M., 'EEG changes during forced alternate nostril breathing', *International Journal of Psychophysiology*, 1994, 18, pp. 75–79.

23. Osowiec D., 'Ultradian rhythms in self-actualization, anxiety and stress-related somatic symptoms', unpublished doctorate thesis, California Institute of Integral Studies.
24. Satyananda P., *Swara Yoga*, Chesley, Swam Editions, 2000; Johari H., *Breath, Mind and Consciousness*, Rochester VT, Destiny Books, 1989.
25. Reinberg A., Labrecque G., Smolensky M., *Chronobiologie et chronothérapeutique*, Paris, Flammarion, 1991.
26. Weitzman E.D., Zimmerman J.C., Czeisler C.A., Ronda J., 'Cortisol secretion is inhibited during sleep in normal man', *Journal of Clinical Endocrinology and Metabolism*, 1983, 56, pp. 352–358.
27. Rossi E.L., *The Psychobiology of Mind–Body Healing*, New York, Norton, 1993.
28. Coudron O., *Les Rhythmes du corps. Chronobiologie et santé*, Paris, Nil Editions, 1997, p. 112.

CHAPTER 11 BEHIND THE BELIEFS OF THE 'NEW AGE'

1. Vernette J., *Le XXIe siècle sera mystique ou ne sera pas*, Paris, PUF, 2002, p. 75.
2. Lenoir F., *La Rencontre du bouddhisme et de l'Occident*, Paris, Fayard, 1999.
3. Krieger D., *Accepting Your Power to Heal: The Personal Practice of Therapeutic Touch*, Santa Fe NM, Bear and Company Inc., 1993; Krieger D., *The Therapeutic Touch: How to Use Your Hands to Help or Heal*, New York, Simon & Schuster, 1979.
4. Anderson E.Z., 'Therapeutic touch', in Davis C.M. (ed.) *Complementary Therapies in Rehabilitation: Evidence for Efficacy in Therapy, Prevention and Wellness*, Thorofare, Slack Inc., 2004.
5. Rosa L., Rosa R., Sarner L., Barrett S., 'A close look at therapeutic touch', *Journal of the American Medical Association*, 1998, 279, pp. 1005–1010.
6. Achterberg J., 'Clearing the air in the therapeutic touch controversy', *Alternative Therapies in Health and Medicine*, 1998, 4, p. 100; Leskowitz E.D., 'Undebunking therapeutic touch', *Alternative Therapies in Health and Medicine*, 1998, 4, pp. 101–102.
7. Ireland M., 'Therapeutic touch with HIV-infected children: a pilot study', *Journal of the Association of Nursing in AIDS Care*, 1998, 9, p. 68; Kramer N.A., 'Comparison of therapeutic touch and causal touch in stress reduction of hospitalized children', *Pediatric Nursing*, 1990, 16, pp. 483–485; Quinn J.F., Strelkauskas A.J., 'Psycho-immunologic effects of therapeutic touch on practitioners and recently bereaved recipients: a pilot study', *Advances in Nursing Science*, 1993, 15, pp. 13–26; Heidt P., 'Effect of therapeutic touch on the anxiety level of hospitalized patients', *Nursing Research*, 1981, 30, pp. 32–37; Turner J.G., Clarck A.J., Gauthier D.K., Williams M., 'The effect of therapeutic touch on pain and anxiety in burn patients', *Journal of Advanced Nursing*, 1998, 28, pp. 10–28; Gagne D., Toye R.C., 'The effects of therapeutic touch and relaxation therapy in reducing anxiety', *Archives of Psychiatric Nursing*, 1984, 8, pp. 184–187; Simington J.A., Laing G.P., 'Effects of therapeutic touch on anxiety in the institutionalized elderly', *Clinical Nursing Research*, 1993, 2, pp. 184–187; Lin Y., Taylor A.G., 'Effects of therapeutic touch in reducing pain and anxiety in an elderly population', *Integrative Medicine*, 1998, 1, pp. 155–162; Samarel N, Fawcett J., Davis M.M., Ryan F.M., 'Effects of dialogue and therapeutic touch on preoperative and postoperative experiences of breast cancer surgery: an exploratory study', *Oncology Nursing Forum*, 1998, 25, pp. 1369–1376.

8. Leskowitz E.D., 'Phantom limb pain treated with therapeutic touch: a case report', *Archives of Physical Medicine and Rehabilitation*, 2000, 81, pp. 522–524; Peck S.D., 'The effectiveness of therapeutic touch for decreasing pain in elders with degenerative arthritis', *Journal of Holistic Nursing*, 1997, 15, pp. 176–198; Gordon A., Merenstein J.H., D'Amico F., Hudgen D., 'The effects of therapeutic touch on patients with osteoarthritis of the knee', *The Journal of Family Practice*, 1998, 47, pp. 271–276; Keller E., Bzdek V.M., 'Effects of therapeutic touch on tension headache pain', *Nursing Research*, 1986, 35, pp. 102–106; Meehan T.C., 'Therapeutic touch and postoperative pain: a Rogerian research study', *Nursing Science Quarterly*, 1993, 6, pp. 69–78.
9. Warber S., Kile G., Gillespie B., '"Energy" healing research', in Jonas W.B. and Crawford C.C. (eds) *Healing, Intention and Energy Medicine: Science, Research, Methods and Clinical Implications*, New York, Churchill Livingstone, 2003.
10. Austin J.A., Harkness E., Ernest E., 'The efficacy of "distant healing": a systematic review of randomized trials', *Annals of Internal Medicine*, 2000, 132, pp. 903–910.
11. Mackay N., 'Autonomic nervous system changes during reiki treatment: a preliminary study', *Journal of Alternative and Complementary Medicine*, 2004, 10, pp. 1077–1081.
12. Wardell D.W., Engebreston J., 'Biological correlates of Reiki Touch healing', *Journal of Advanced Nursing*, 2001, 3, pp. 439–445.
13. Wirth D.P., Chang R.J., Eidelman W.S., Paxton J.B., 'Hematological indicators of complementary healing intervention', *Complementary Therapies in Medicine*, 1996, 4, pp. 4–20.
14. Olson K., Hanson J., 'Using Reiki to manage pain: a preliminary report', *Cancer Prevention and Control*, 1997, 1, pp. 108–113; Wirth D.P., Brelan D.R., Levine R.J., Rodriguez C.M., 'The effect of complementary healing therapy on postoperative pain after surgical removal of impacted third molar teeth', *Complementary Therapies in Medicine*, 1993, 1, pp. 113–138; Wirth D.P., Richardson J.T., Eidelman W.S., 'Wound healing and complementary therapies: a review', *Journal of Alternative and Complementary Medicine*, 1996, pp. 493–502; Bullock M., 'Reiki: a complementary therapy for life', *American Journal of Hospice and Palliative Care*, 1997, 14, pp. 31–33.
15. Singg S., 'Reiki: an alternative and complementary healing therapy', in Davis C.M. (ed.) *Complementary Therapies in Rehabilitation: Evidence for Efficacy, in Therapy, Prevention and Wellness'*, Thorofare NJ, Slack Inc., 2004.
16. Dressen L.J., Singg S., 'Effects of Reiki on pain and select affective and personality variables of chronically ill patients', *Subtle Energies & Energy Medicine*, 1998, 9, pp. 51–82; Singg S., Dressen L.J., 'Desirable self-perceived psychophysiological changes in chronically ill patients: an experimental study of Reiki', presented at the 9th Annual Conference of the International Society for the Study of Subtle Energies and Energy Medicine, June 1999, Boulder, Colorado.
17. Mansour A., Beuche M., Laing G., Leis A., Nurse J., 'A study to test the effectiveness of placebo Reiki standardisation procedures, developed for a planned Reiki efficacy study', *Journal of Alternative and Complementary Medicine*, 1999, 5, pp. 153–164.
18. Alandydy P., Alandydy K., 'Using Reiki to support surgical patients', *Journal of Nursing Care Quality*, 1999, 13, pp. 89–91.
19. Rand W.L., 'Reiki news articles: the International Center for Reiki Training. Reiki in hospitals', can be consulted at http://www.reiki.org/reikinews/reiki_in_hospitals.html; Barnett L., Chambers M., *Reiki Energy Medicine: Bringing Healing Touch into Home, Hospital and Hospice*, Rochester VT, Healing Arts Press, 1996; Sawyer J., 'The first Reiki practitioners in our OR', *Association of Operating Room Nurses*

Journal, 1998, 67, pp. 674–677; Wing J., Wolf A., 'How we got Reiki into the hospital', *Reiki News*, 28–29 September 2000; Miles P., True G., 'Reiki – review of a biofield therapy. History, theory, practice and research', *Alternative Therapies*, 2003, 9, pp. 62–72.
20. Motz J., *Hands of Life*, New York, Bantam, 1998; Oz M., *Healing from the Heart*, New York, Dutton, 1999.
21. Brennan A.B., *Hands of Light*, New York, Bantam, 1987; Brennan A.B., *Light Emerging*, New York, Bantam, 1993.
22. Williams H., Pembroke A., 'Sniffer dogs in the melanoma clinic?', *Lancet*, 1989, 1, p. 734; Church J., Williams H., 'Another sniffer dog for the clinic?', *Lancet*, 2001, 358, p. 930; Phillips M., Gleeson K., Hughes J.M., Greenberg J., Cataneo R.N., Baker L., 'Volatile compounds in breath as a marker of lung cancer: a cross-sectional study', *Lancet*, 1999, 353, pp. 2897–2898; Phillips M., Cataneo R.N., Ditkoff B.A., Fisher P., Greenberg J., Gunawardena R., 'Volatile markers of breast cancer in the breath', *Breast Journal*, 2003, 9, pp. 184–191.
23. Willis C.M., Church S.M., Guest C.M., Cook W.A., McCrathy N., Bransbury A.J., Church M.R.T., Church J.C.T., 'Olfactory detection of human bladder cancer by dogs: proof of principle study', *British Medical Journal*, 2004, 329, pp. 712–715.
24. Benor D.J., *Spiritual Healing: Scientific Validation of a Healing Revolution (Healing Research Vol. I)*, Southfield, Vision Publication, 2001.
25. Wirth D.P., 'The effect of non-contact therapeutic touch on the healing rate of full thickness dermal wounds', *Subtle Energies*, 1992, 1, p. 1; Wirth D.P., Richardson J.T., Eidelman W.S., O'Malley A.C., 'Full thickness dermal wounds treated with non-contact therapeutic touch: a replication and extension', *Complementary Therapies in Medicine*, 1993, 1, pp. 127–132; Wirth D.P., Barrett M.J., Eidelman W.S., 'Non-contact therapeutic touch and wound re-epithelialization: an extension of previous research', *Complementary Therapies in Medicine*, 1994, 2, pp. 187–192; Wirth D.P., Richardson J.T., Martinez R.D., Eidelman W.S., Lopez M.E., 'Non-contact therapeutic touch intervention and full-thickness cutaneous wounds: a replication', *Complementary Therapies in Medicine*, 1996, 4, pp. 237–240.
26. Ginandes C.S., Rosenthal D.I., 'Using hypnosis to accelerate the healing of bone fractures: a randomized controlled pilot study', *Alternative Therapies*, 1999, 5 (2), pp. 67–75.
27. Ginandes C., Brooks P., Sando W., Jones C., Aker J., 'Can medical hypnosis accelerate post-surgical wound healing: result of a clinical trial', *American Journal of Clinical Hypnosis*, 2003, 45, pp. 333–351.
28. Cha K.Y., Wirth D.P., Lobo R.A., 'Does prayer influence the success of *in vitro* fertilization-embryo transfer?', *Journal of Reproductive Medicine*, 2001, 46, pp. 781–787.
29. Flamm B.L., 'Faith healing by prayer: review of Cha K.Y., Wirth D.P., Lobo R.A., "Does prayer influence the success of *in vitro* fertilization-embryo transfer?"', *Scientific Review of Alternative Medicine*, 2002, 6, pp. 47–50; Flamm B.L., 'Faith healing confronts modern medicine', *Scientific Review of Alternative Medicine*, 2004, 8, pp. 9–14.
30. Cohen D., 'Magnetic fields around the torso: production by electrical activity of the human heart', *Science*, 1967, 156, pp. 652–654.
31. Cohen D., 'Magnetoencephalography: detection of the brain's electrical activity with a superconducting magnetometer', *Science*, 1972, 175, pp. 664–666.
32. Oschman J.L., *Energy Medicine: The Scientific Basis*, Edinburgh, Churchill Livingstone, 2000.

33. Bassett C.A.L., Mitchell S.N., Gaston S.R., 'Pulsing electromagnetic field treatment in ununited fractures and failed arthrodeses', *Journal of the American Medical Association*, 1982, 247, pp. 623–628; Bassett C.A.L., 'Bioelectromagnetics in the service of medicine', *Electromagnetic Fields: Biological Interactions and Mechanisms. Advances in Chemistry Series 250*, American Chemical Society, Washington DC, 1995, pp. 261–275.
34. Sisken B.F., Walter J., 'Therapeutic aspects of electromagnetic fields for soft tissue healing', *Electromagnetic Fields: Biological Interactions and Mechanisms. Advances in Chemistry Series 250*, American Chemical Society, Washington DC, 1995, pp. 277–285.
35. Zimmerman J., 'Laying-on-of-hands healing and therapeutic touch: a testable theory', *BEMI Currents, Journal of the Bio-Electro-Magnetics Institute*, 1990, 2, pp. 8–17, (available from Dr John Zimmermann, 2490 West Moana Lane, Reno, Nevada, 89509-3936 USA; see also an article by him published in 1985, 'New technologies detect effects of healing hands', *Brain/Mind Bulletin*, 30 September, 10, p. 3).
36. Seto A., Kusaka C., Nakazato S. et al., 'Detection of extraordinary large biomagnetic field strength from human hand', *Acupuncture and Electro-Therapeutics Research International Journal*, 1992, 17, pp. 75–94.
37. Beck R., 'Mood modification with ELF magnetic fields: a preliminary exploration', *Archaeus*, 1986, 4, p. 48.
38. Galejs J., *Terrestrial Propagation of Long Electromagnetic Waves*, Oxford, Pergamon Press, 1972; Balser M., Wagner C.A., 'Observation of earth: ionosphere cavity resonances, *Nature*, 1960, 188, p. 4751.
39. Direnfeld L.K., 'The genesis of the EEG and its relation to electromagnetic radiation', *Journal of Bioelectricity*, 1983, 2, pp. 111–121; Gould J.L., 'Magnetic field sensitivity in animals', *Annual Review of Physiology*, 1984, 46, pp. 585–598; Gaugelin M., *The Cosmic Clock*, New York, Avon Books, 1984.
40. Oschman J.L., *Energy Medicine: The Scientific Basis*, Edinburgh, Churchill Livingstone, 2000.
41. Friedenberg R., Reese W., Reading W.H., 'Detector device and process for detecting ovulation', United States Patent 3 924 609, 9 December 1975.
42. McCraty R., Atkinson M., Tomasino D., Tiller W., 'The electricity of touch: detection and measurement of cardiac energy exchange between people', in Pribram K. (ed.) *Brain and Values: Is a Biological Science of Values Possible?*, Mahwah NJ, Lawrence Erlbaum Associates, 1998, pp. 359–379.
43. Russek L.G., Schwartz G.E., 'Interpersonal heart–brain registration and the perception of parental love: a 42-year follow-up of the Harvard Mastery of Stress Study', *Subtle Energies*, 1994, 5, pp. 195–208; Russek L.G., Schwartz G.E., 'Energy cardiology: a dynamical energy systems approach for integrating conventional and alternative medicine', *The Journal of Mind–Body Health*, 1996, 12, pp. 4–24.
44. Tiller W., McCraty R., Atkinson M., 'Cardiac coherence: a new non-invasive measure of autonomic nervous system order', *Alternative Therapies in Health and Medicine*, 1996, 2, pp. 52–65; McCraty R., *The Energetic Heart. Bioelectromagnetic Interactions Within and Between People*, Boulder Creek CA, Institute of HeartMath, 2003 (available to order: www.heartmath.org).
45. Hatfield E., *Emotional Contagion*, New York, Cambridge University Press, 1994; Levenson R.W., Ruef A.M., 'Physiological aspects of emotional knowledge and rapport', in Ickes W. (ed.) *Empathic Accuracy*, New York, Guilford Press, 1997; Reidborg S.P., Redington D.J., 'Non-linear analysis of autonomic responses in a therapist during psychotherapy', *Journal of Nervous and Mental Disease*, 1993, 181,

pp. 428–435; Robinson J., Herman A., Kaplan B., 'Autonomic responses correlate with counsellor–client empathy', *Journal of Counselling Psychology*, 1982, 29, pp. 195–198.
46. Jonas W.B., Crawford C.C. (eds), *Healing, Intention and Energy Medicine: Science, Research Methods and Clinical Implications*, New York, Churchill Livingstone, 2003, p. 107; Lee M.S., Huh H.J., Jang H.S. *et al.*, 'Effects of emitted Qi on in vitro natural killer cell cytotoxicity activity', *American Journal of Chinese Medicine*, 2001, 29, pp. 17–22.
47. Lu Z., *Scientific Qigong Exploration: The Wonders and Mysteries of Qi*, Malvern PA, Amber Leaf Press, 1997.
48. Jonas W.B., Crawford C.C. (eds), *Healing, Intention and Energy Medicine: Science, Research Methods and Clinical Implications*, New York, Churchill Livingstone, 2003, pp. 39–57.

CONCLUSION

1. Million Women Study Collaborators, 'Breast cancer and hormone replacement therapy in the million women study', *Lancet*, 2003, 362, pp. 419–427.
2. Servan-Schreiber D., *Guérir le stress, l'anxiété et la dépression sans médicaments ni psychanalyse*, Paris, Robert Laffont, 2003.
3. Johnson P., *The Birth of the Modern*, New York, Harper Perennial, 1991; Randall J.H., *The Making of the Modern Mind*, Cambridge MA, Houghton Mifflin, 1940.
4. Mokdad A.H., Marks J.S., Stroup D.F., Gerberding J.L., 'Actual causes of death in the United States, 2000', *Journal of the American Medical Association*, 2004, 291, pp. 1238–1241.
5. Rifkin J., *The European Dream: How Europe's Vision of the Future is Quietly Eclipsing the American Dream*, New York, Penguin, 2004.
6. Ray P.H., Anderson S.R., *The Cultural Creatives: How Fifty Million People are Changing the World*, New York, Harmony Books, 2000.
7. Ibid.
8. Luyckx Ghisi M., *Au-delà de la modernité, du patriarcat et du capitalisme*, Paris, L'Harmattan, 2001, p. 84.
9. Rosnay J. de, *L'Homme symbiotique*, Paris, Seuil, 1995, p. 370. (American translation: *The Symbiotic Man*, New York, McGraw-Hill, 2000.)
10. Weil A., *Spontaneous Healing*, New York, Alfred Knopf Inc., 1995.
11. *La Recherche*, June 2004, n° 376, p. 32.
12. Kitano H., 'Systems biology: a brief overview', *Science*, 2002, 295, p. 1662.
13. Fields D.R., 'The other half of the brain', *Scientific American*, 2004, 290 (4), pp. 27–33.
14. Holmes M.D., Chen W.Y., Feskanich D., Kroenke C.H., Colditz G.A., 'Physical activity and survival after breast cancer diagnosis', *Journal of the American Medical Association*, 2005, 293, pp. 2479–2486.
15. Strauss L., *Natural Right and History*, Chicago, University of Chicago Press, 1950, p. 315.

BIBLIOGRAPHY

ABRAHAM, Nicholas, TORÖK, Maria, *L'Écorce et le noyau*, Paris, Aubier-Flammarion, 1987.
ACHTERBERG, Jeanne, *Imagery in Healing: Shamanism and Modern Medicine*, Boston, Shambhala, 1985.
ALEXANDER, Frederick Matthias, *The Use of the Self and Conscious Constructive Control of the Individual*, Long Beach, Centerline Press, 1984.
—— *Man's Supreme Inheritance*, Long Beach, Centerline Press, 1984.
ANCELIN SHÜTZENBERGER, Anne, *Aïe, mes aïeux*, Paris, Desclée de Brouwer, 1993.
ANCELIN SHÜTZENBERGER, Anne, DEVROEDE, Ghislaine, *Ces enfants malades de leurs parents*, Paris, Payot, 2003.
ANSERMET, François, MAGISTRETTI, Pierre, *A chacun son cerveau: plasticité neuronale et inconscient*, Paris, Odile Jacob, 2004.
APOSHYAN, Susan, *Natural Intelligence: Body–Mind Integration and Human Development*, Baltimore MD, Williams and Wilkins, 1999.
AUSTIN, James H., *Zen and the Brain*, Cambridge MA, MIT Press, 1998.
BARNETT, Libby, CHAMBERS, Maggie, *Reiki Energy Medicine: Bringing Healing Touch into Home, Hospital and Hospice*, Rochester VT, Healing Arts Press, 1996.
BECKER, Robert O., SELDEN, Garry, *The Body Electric: Electromagnetism and the Foundation of Life*, New York, William Morrow and Company, 1985.
BEINFIELD, Harriet, KORNGOLD, Efrem, *Between Heaven and Earth: A Guide to Chinese Medicine*, New York, Ballantyne, 1991.
BENSON, Herbert, *The Relaxation Response*, New York, Morrow, 1975.
BERTHERAT, Thérèse, *Le Corps a ses raisons: autoguérison et anti-gymnastique*, Paris, Seuil, 1976.
—— *Les Saisons du corps: garder et regarder la forme*, Paris, Albin Michel, 1985.
BRELET, Claudine, *Médecines du monde: histoire et pratiques des médecines traditionelles*, Paris, Robert Laffont, 2002.
BRENNAN, Barbara Ann, *Hands of Light*, New York, Bantam, 1987.
—— *Light Emerging*, New York, Bantam, 1993.
BUCHANAN, Gregory McLellan, SELIGMAN, Martin E.P., *Explanatory Style*, Hillsdale NJ, Lawrence Erlbaum Associates, 1995.
CALLAHAN, Daniel, *The Role of Complementary and Alternative Medicine: Accommodating Pluralism*, Washington DC, Georgetown University Press, 2002.
CHILDRE, Doc, MARTIN, Howard, *The HeartMath Solution*, New York, HarperCollins, 1999.
COUDRON, Olivier, *Les Rhythmes du corps: chronobiologie et santé*, Paris, Nil Editions, 1997.
CSIKSZENTMIHALYI, Mihaly, *Flow: The Psychology of Optimal Experience*, New York, Harper and Row, 1990.
DAMASIO, Antonio R., *Descarte's Error: Emotion, Reason and the Human Brain*, New York, Avon Books, 1994.
DAVIS, Carol M. (ed.), *Complementary Therapies in Rehabilitation: Evidence for Efficacy in Therapy, Prevention and Wellness*, Thorofare NJ, Slack Inc., 2004.
DEVROEDE, Ghislain, *Ce que les maux de ventre disent de notre passé*, Paris, Payot, 2003.

DRANSART, Philippe, *La Maladie cherche à me guérir*, Grenoble, Le Mercure dauphinois, 1999.
ERICKSON, Milton, ROSSI, Ernest L., *Experiencing Hypnosis: Therapeutic Approaches to Altered States*, New York, Irvington, 1981.
FELDENKRAIS, Moshe, *The Potent Self. A Guide to Spontaneity*, San Francisco, Harper and Row, 1985.
—— *Body Awareness as Healing Therapy: The Case of Nora*, Berkeley Frog Ltd, 1993.
FERRAGUT, Eliane, *Emotion et memoire. Le corps et la souffrance*, Paris, Masson, 2004.
FIELD, Tiffany (ed.), *Touch in Early Development*, Mahwah NJ, Lawrence Erlbaum Associates, 1995.
FIELD, Tiffany, *Touch therapy*, Edinburgh, Churchill Livingstone, 2000.
—— *Touch*, Cambridge MA, MIT Press, 2001.
FLÊCHE, Christian, *Mon corps pour me guérir: décodage psychobiologique des maladies*, Barret le Bas, Le Souffle d'Or, 2000.
FRAWLEY, David, *Ayurveda and the Mind*, Twin Lakes WI, Lotus Press, 1997.
FREUD, Sigmund, *Studies on Hysteria*, (1895), in *Penguin Freud Library*, vol. 3, Harmondsworth, Penguin, 1974.
FRIEDMAN, Meyer, ROSENMAN, Ray, *Type A Behavior and your Heart*, New York, Knopf, 1974.
GAMPEL, Yolanda, *Ces parents qui vivent à travers moi*, Paris, Fayard, 2005.
GAUGELIN, Michel, *The Cosmic Clock*, New York, Avon Books, 1984.
GAZZANIGA, Michael, *The Social Brain: Discovering the Networks of the Mind*, New York, Basic Books, 1985.
GOLDMAN, Daniel, *Emotional Intelligence*, New York, Bantam Books, 1995.
—— *Destructive Emotions*, New York, Bantam Books, 2003.
GOLDTHWAIT, Joel E., BROWN, Lloyd T., SWAIN, Loring T., KUHNS, John G., *Body Mechanics in the Study and Treatment of Disease*, Philadelphia, J.B.Lippincott, 1934.
GROOPMAN, Jerome, *The Anatomy of Hope: How People Prevail in the Face of Illness*, New York, Random House, 2004.
HAMMOND, Pierre, *La Guérison à portée de la main*, Paris, Presses de la Rénaissance, 2001.
—— *La Mémoire du corps: l'approche ostéopathique*, Paris, Presses de la Rénaissance, 2004.
HARRINGTON, Anne (ed.), *The Placebo Effect. An Interdisciplinary Exploration*, Cambridge MA, Harvard University Press, 1997.
HATFIELD, Elaine, *Emotional Contagion*, New York, Cambridge University Press, 1994.
HILL, Leonard Erskine, *Philosophy of a Biologist*, London, Arnold, 1930.
HIRSHBERG, Caryle, BARASCH, Marc Ian, *Remarkable Recovery*, New York, Riverhead Books, 1995.
HUNT, Valerie V., *Infinite Mind. Science of the Human Vibrations of Consciousness*, Malibu CA, Malibu Publishing Company, 1996.
ICKES, William (ed.), *Empathic Accuracy*, New York, Guilford Press, 1997.
JAMES, William, *The Priciples of Psychology*, Cambridge MA, Harvard University Press, 1981.
JANOV, Arthur, *Why You Get Sick and How You Get Well*, West Hollywood CA, Dove Books, 1996.
—— *The Biology of Love*, New York, Prometheus Books, 2000.
JOHARI, Harish, *Breath, Mind and Consciousness*, Rochester VT, Destiny Books, 1989.
JOHNSON, Paul, *The Birth of the Modern*, New York, Harper Perennial, 1991.

JONAS, Wayne B., CRAWFORD Cindy C. (eds), *Healing, Intention and Energy Medicine: Science, Research Methods and Clinical Implications*, New York, Churchill Livingstone, 2003.
JUHAN, Deane, *Job's Body: A Handbook for Bodywork*, New York, Station Hill Press, 1987.
JUNG, Carl Gustav, *Collected Works of C.G. Jung*, 2nd edition, Vol. 2, Princeton NJ, Princeton University Press, 1972.
KAWADA, Yuichi, KARCHER, Stephen, *Essential Shiatsu*, London, Time Warner Books, 2002.
KRIEGER, Dolores, *The Therapeutic Touch: How to Use Your Hands to Help or Heal*, New York, Simon and Shuster, 1979.
—— *Accepting Your Power to Heal: The Personal Practice of Therapeutic Touch*, Santa Fe NM, Bear and Company Inc., 1993.
LEDOUX, Joseph, *The Emotional Brain*, New York, Simon and Schuster, 1996.
LENOIR, Frédéric, *La Rencontre du bouddhisme et de l'Occident*, Paris, Fayard, 1999.
LERNER, Michael, *Choices in Healing: Integrating the Best of Conventional and Complementary Approaches to Cancer*, London, MIT Press, 1996.
LESKOWITZ, Eric D. (ed.), *Complementary and Alternative Medicine in Rehabilitation*, New York, Churchill Livingstone, 2003.
LEVI-STRAUSS, Claude, *Structural Anthropology*, Garden City, New York, Anchor Books, 1967. (American translation).
LEWIS, Dennis, *The Tao of Natural Breathing*, San Francisco, Mountain Wind Publishing, 1998.
LIANG, T.T., *T'ai Chi Ch'uan for Health and Self-Defense: Philosophy and Practice*, New York, Vintage Books, 1977.
LOWEN, Alexander, *The Language of the Body*, New York, Macmillan, 1971.
—— *Bioenergetics*, New York, Penguin Books, 1975.
—— *The Vibrant Way to Health: A Manual of Exercises*, New York, Harper and Row, 1977.
LU, Gwei-Djen, NEEDHAM, Joseph, *Celestial Lancets: A History and Rationale of Acupuncture and Moxa*, Cambridge, Cambridge University Press, 1980.
LU, Zuyin, *Scientific Qigong Exploration: The Wonders and Mysteries of Qi*, Malvern PA, Amber Leaf Press, 1997.
LUYCKX GHISI, Marc, *Audelà de la modernité, du patriarcat et du capitalisme*, Paris, L'Harmattan, 2001.
MARTEL, Jacques, *Le Grand Dictionaire des malaises et des maladies*, Aubagne, Éditions Quintessence, 1998.
MASSON, J. (ed.), *The Complete Letters of Sigmund Freud to Wilhelm Fliess*, Harvard MA, Belknap, 1985.
MATTINGLY, Cheryl, GARROW, Linda C. (eds), *Narrative and the Cultural Construction of Illness and Healing*, Berkeley CA, University of California Press, 2000.
MICOZZI, Marc S. (ed.), *Fundamentals of Complementary and Alternative Medicine*, New York, Churchill Livingstone, 1996.
MOERMAN, Daniel, *Meaning, Medicine, and the 'Placebo Effect'*, Cambridge, Cambridge University Press, 2002.
MONTAGU, Ashley, *Touching. The Human Significance of the Skin*, New York, Harper and Row, 1986.
MOTZ, Julie, *Hands of Life*, New York, Bantam, 1998.
NATHAN, Bevis, *Touch and Emotion in Manual Therapy*, Edinburgh, Churchill Livingstone, 1999.

NATHAN, Tobie, STENGERS, Isabelle, *Médecins et sorciers*, Paris, Les Empêcheurs de penser en rond, 1999.
NOGIER, Paul, *De l'auriculotherapie à l'auriculomédecine*, Paris, Maisonneuve et Larose, 1998.
ODOUL, Michel, *Dis-moi où tu as mal, je te dirai pourqoi*, Paris, Albin Michel, 2002.
ORNISH, Dean, *Love and Survival: 8 Pathways to Intimacy and Health*, New York, Harper Perennial, 1998.
OSCHMAN, James L., *Energy Medicine: The Scientific Basis*, Edinburgh, Churchill Livingstone, 2000.
—— *Energy Medicine in Therapeutics and Human Performance*, Philadelphia, Butterworth Heinemann, 2003.
OZ, Mehmet, *Healing from the Heart*, New York, Dutton, 1999.
PAYER, Lynn, *Medicine and Culture*, New York, Holt, 1988.
PENNEBAKER, James W., *Opening Up. The Healing Power of Confiding in Others*, New York, W.M. Morrox & Co., 1990.
PERLMAN, Adam (ed.), *Complementary and Alternative Medicine*, Philadelphia, W.B. Saunders Company, 2002.
PERRIN, Luis, *Le Psychisme, le stress et l'immunité. La santé est en nous*, Paris, Odile Jacob, 2003.
PERT, Candace B., *Molecules of Emotion. The Science Behind Mind–Body Medicine*, New York, Touchstone, 1997.
PETERS, David (ed.), *Understanding the Placebo Effect in Complementary Medicine: Theory, Practice and Research*, Edinburgh, Churchill Livingstone, 2001.
PHILLIPS, Maggie, *Finding the Energy to Heal: How EMDR, Hypnosis, TFT, Imagery and Body-Focused Therapy Can Help Restore Mind–Body Health*, New York, Norton, 2000.
PILATES, Joseph H., *Return to Life Through Contrology*, New York, J.J. Augustin, 1945.
PRIBRAM, Karl (ed.), *Brain and Values: Is a Biological Science of Values Possible*, Mahwah NJ, Lawrence Erlbaum Associates, 1998.
RAMEY, David W., ROLLIN, Bernard E., *Complementary and Alternative Veterinary Medicine Considered*, Ames IA, Iowa State Press, 2004.
RANDALL, John Herman Jr., *The Making of the Modern Mind*, Cambridge MA, Houghton Mifflin, 1940.
RAY, Paul H., ANDERSON, Sherry Ruth, *The Cultural Creatives: How 50 Million People are Changing the World*, New York, Harmony Books, 2000.
REICH, Wilhelm, *Character Analysis*, New York, Touchstone, 1972.
REINBERG, Alain, LABRECQUE, Gaston, SMOLENSKY, Michael, *Chronobiologie et chronothérapeutique*, Paris, Flammarion, 1991.
REUTER, Liliane, *Votre esprit est votre meilleur médecin*, Paris, Robert Laffont, 1999.
RICARD, Matthieu, *Le Moine et le Philosophe*, Paris, Nil Éditions 1997.
—— *Plaidoyer pour le bonheur*, Paris, Nil Éditions, 2003.
RICH, Grant Jewell (ed.), *Massage Therapy: The Evidence for Practice*, St Louis, Mosby, 2002.
RIFKIN, Jeremy, *The European Dream: How Europe's Vision of the Future is Quietly Eclipsing the American Dream*, New York, Penguin, 2004.
ROLF, Ida P., *Rolfing: The Integration of Human Structures*, Santa Monica CA, Dennis-Landman, 1977.
ROSENBERG, Jack Lee, *Body, Self, and Soul: Sustaining Integration*, Atlanta, Humanics Ltd Partners, 1985.
ROSENBERG, Marshall, *Nonviolent Communication: A Language of Compassion*, Del Mar CA, PuddleDancer Press, 1999.

ROSNAY, Joël de, *The Symbiotic Man*, New York, McGraw-Hill, 2000. (American translation).
ROSSI, Ernest L., *The Psychobiology of Mind–Body Healing: New Concepts of Therapeutic Hypnosis*, New York, Norton, 1993.
—— *The Psychobiology of Gene Expression: Neuroscience and Neurogenesis in Hypnosis and the Healing Arts*, New York, Norton, 2002.
SAINTE-ROSE, Maurice, *La Santé au bout des doigts. L'Osteopathie médecine moderne*, Paris, Robert Laffont, 2000.
SANDOZ, Thomas, *Histoires parallèles de la médecine*, Paris, Seuil, 2005.
SATYANANDA, Paramahamsa, *Swara Yoga*, Chesley, Swam Editions, 1998.
SCHLITZ, Marilyn, AMOROK, Tina, MICOZZI, Marc (eds), *Consciousness and Healing: An Integral Approach to Mind–Body Medicine*, St Louis MO, Elsevier Churchill Livingstone, 2005.
SCHWARTZ, Gary E.R., RUSSEK, Linda G.S., *The Living Energy Universe*, Charlottesville VA, Hampton Roads, 1999.
SELIGMAN, Martin E.P., *Authentic Happiness. Using the New Positive Psyhchology to Realize Your Potential for Lasting Fulfilment*, New York, The Free Press, Simon and Schuster, 2002.
SELLAM, Salomon, *Origine et prévention des maladies*, Aubagne Éditions Quintessence, 2000.
SELYE, Hans, *The Stress of Life*, New York, McGraw-Hill, 1978.
SERVAN-SCHREIBER, David, *Guérir le stress, l'anxieté et la dépression sans medicaments ni psychanalyse*, Paris, Robert Laffont, 2003.
SHAPIRO, Debbie, *Your Body Speaks Your Mind*, London, Judy Piatkus Pub., 1996.
SHELDON, William H., *The Varieties of Temperament*, New York, Harper and Brothers Publishers, 1942.
SIEGEL, Bernie S., *Peace, Love, and Healing*, New York, Harper and Row, 1989.
SIMONTON, Carl O., MATTHEWS-SIMONTON, Stephanie, CREIGHTON, James, *Getting Well Again*, New York, Bantam, 1978.
SMITH, Edward W.L., *The Body in Psychotherapy*, Jefferson NC, McFarland & Company, 1985.
SOUZENELLE, Annic de, *Le Symbolisme du corps humain*, Paris, Albin Michel, 1991.
SPIEGEL, Herbert, SPIEGEL, David, *Trance and Treatment: Clinical Uses of Hypnotism*, Washington DC, American Psychiatric Press Inc., 1978.
STAUNTON, Tree (ed.), *Body Psychotherapy*, Hove UK, Brunner-Routledge, 2002.
STILL, Andrew Taylor, *Autobiography with a History of the Discovery and Development of the Science of Osteopathy*, New York, Arno Press, 1972.
STONIER, Tom, *Information and the Internal Structure of the Universe*, New York, Springer-Verlag, 1990.
STRAUSS, Leo, *Natural Right and History*, Chicago, University of Chicago Press, 1950.
STUX, Gabriel, HAMMERSCHLAG, Richard (eds), *Clinical Acupuncture: Scientific Basis*, Berlin, Springer, 2001.
SVOBODA, R., LADE, A., *Tao and Dharma: Chinese Medicine and Ayurveda*, Twin Lakes WI, Lotus Press, 1995.
TALBOT, Michael, *The Holographic Universe*, New York, HarperCollins, 1991.
TILLER, William A., *Science and Human Transformation. Subtle Energies, Intentionality, and Consciousness*, Walnut Creek CA., Pavior, 1997.
TONNAC, Jean-Philippe de, LENOIR, Frédéric (eds), *La Mort et l'immortalité. Encyclopédie des savoirs et des croyances*, Paris, Bayard, 2004.
VAN EERSEL, Patrice, MAILLARD, Catherine, *J'ai mal à mes ancêtres. La psychogénéalogie aujourd'hui*, Paris, Albin Michel, 2002.

VEITH, I., *The Yellow Emperor's Classic of Internal Medicine*, Berkeley, University of California Press, 1973.
VELDMAN, Frans, *Haptonomie, amour, et raison*, Paris, PUF, 2004.
VERNETTE, Jean, *Le XXIe siècle sera mystique ou ne sera pas*, Paris, PUF, 2002.
WAINAPEL, Stanley F., FAST, Avital (eds), *Alternative Medicine and Rehabilitation: A Guide for Practitioners*, New York, Demos Medical Publishing, 2003.
WATKINS, Alan, *Mind Body Medicine: A Clinician's Guide to Psychoneuroimmunology*, New York, Churchill Livingstone, 1997.
WEIL, Andrew, *Spontaneous Healing*, New York, Alfred Knopf Inc., 1995.
WISNESKI, Leonard A., ANDERSON, Lucy, *The Scientific Basis of Integrative Medicine*, Boca Raton FL, CRC Press, 2005.
ZAJDE, Nathalie, *Souffle sur tous ces morts et qu'ils vivent!*, Grenoble, La Pensée sauvage, 1993.

INDEX

Compiled by Sue Carlton

Abraham, Nicolas 103
acupuncture 145–53
    effect on brain 148–9
    and embryology 149–51
    energy channels 145–6
    meridians 145, 146, 151–3, 157
    microsystems of 151
    and placebo effect 147–8
    Western style of 146–8
Ader, Robert 25, 26
adrenal glands 27, 36, 38, 148, 158, 167
    see also hypothalamic-pituitary-adrenal axis
adrenaline 36, 37, 44, 49, 158
adreno-cortico-trophic-hormone (ACTH) 36, 148
Alexander, Frederick Matthias 96, 124–5
Alexander technique 124–5, 127, 162
alexithymy 93–4, 100, 107
Allen, Paul 77
alpha rhythm 65, 66, 70, 182
alternative and complementary therapies
    classification of 7
    definition 2–3
    lack of information about 4–5
    and modern scientific culture 6–7, 8
    see also integrated medicine
Alzheimer's disease 116, 167
    in spouse 41, 179
American Association of Ayurvedic Medicine 154
American Medical Association 73
American Psychological Association 53
amygdala 30, 31, 53, 58, 59
Ancelin Schützenberger, Anne 102, 103, 104
Andersen, Barbara 63
anger 30, 37, 87, 95, 152–3
    expressing 91, 92–3, 98–9, 101, 160
    and rage to live 59–61
anti-gymnastic approach 127
asthma 24–5, 57, 70, 114, 119, 141, 163
    and placebo effect 15–16
attention-deficit hyperactivity disorders 50, 115
attitudes, changing 195–201
auriculotherapy 150, 151

auto-immune diseases 37–8, 42, 101, 106, 152
autogenic training 73
autonomic nervous system 13, 27, 30, 90, 99, 149, 157, 165, 166
    sympathetic/parasympathetic balance 35–6, 71, 90, 121, 138, 149, 152, 159, 160, 163
    see also Ida and *Pingala*; parasympathetic system; sympathetic system; *yin* and *yang*
autosuggestion 20, 73, 74, 104, 132, 178
ayurvedic medicine 84–5, 86, 88, 154, 156, 159, 161, 166

babies and children
    and massage 117, 119
    and stress 40
    and touch 111, 113–15, 116, 117
Bakke, Antony 68–9
Barasch, Mark Ian 58
Barbara Brennan School of Healing 175–6
Beecher, Henry 14
behavioural patterns (Type A and Type) B 49, 50, 83
    changing 50–1
Benedetti, Fabrizio 14
Benson, Herbert 15, 65, 66
Berk, Lee 55–6
Bernard, Claude 9
Bertherat, Thérèse 127
Bhatnagar, Sri Shyam-ji 164
bioenergetic analysis and therapy 91–2
biofeedback 70–1, 101
biological clocks 166
biomagnetism 180–2, 183
Blavatsky, Helena 170, 171, 176
body 120–34
    alignment 97, 121–2, 128, 162
        see also Alexander technique; chiropractic method; Rolfing technique
    bodily symbolism 105–8, 161
    bodily unconscious 85
    cells 122–4
    concentric segments (Reich) 86
    equilibrium 128–34

as hologram 150–1
listening to 94–6, 100–1
and magnetic fields 180
  see also biomagnetism
movement 124–8
muscular contractions 86, 96, 121, 161
rhythms of 166–8
as self-stabilising structure 120–4, 133
touching 111–15
body–mind relationship 23, 24–8
disequilibrium 43–4
equilibrium 3, 4, 19, 28, 154
and information 27–8, 35
mind–body unity 26–7, 159–60, 161–2, 169–70
and muscle training 69–71
see also qi
bony subluxation 128
Boszormenyi-Nagy, Ivan 103
brain 27, 28–32
and the *chakras* 157–9
effect of acupuncture 148–9
effect of breathing techniques 165
effect of hypnosis 76–7
effect of massage 116, 119
effect of meditation 182
effect of relaxation 64–5, 66
three layers of 28–9
two hemispheres 29–30
breathing 141, 162
nasal alternation 164–6, 167
and yoga 163–4
Brennan, Barbara Ann 75, 175–6
British Medical Association 147
Buddhism 52, 65
Buitelaar, Jan 49
Burr, Harold Saxton 183

cancer 33–4, 45–8, 167
detected by dogs 176–7
and psychotherapy 62–4
and *qigong* 142
and stress 45–6, 47–8
and *tai-chi* 145
and visualisation 68–9
Cannon, Walter 13, 14, 65
cardiac problems, and personality types 49, 50
carers, stress and health 41–2
catharsis 96, 101
cells 122–4
centring, by practitioner 171, 173, 176, 177
Chaitow, Leon 7–8
chakras 86, 154, 156, 157–61, 184, 190
as psychosomatic tool 159–61
chemotherapy 21, 63, 69, 147, 151, 190–1

Chinese medicine 137–53, 196
and diet 137, 154, 155–6
chiropractic method 128–9
Chopra, Deepak 154
circadian rhythms 167
Clark, Mary Ellen 133
Clow, Angela 34–5
Cohen, Nicholas 25
Cohen, Sheldon 39
Cole, Steven 61
communication/connections, unseen 183–5
coronary illness 44–5, 163
corticotrophin releasing hormone (CRH) 36, 38
cortisol 30, 36–8, 41, 42, 44, 49, 148, 158
reducing levels of 53, 117, 118, 142
and rhythms of body 166–7
Coué, Emile 73
Cousins, Norman 55
cranial bones, mobility of 131–2
craniosacral therapy 132–3
Crawford, Cindy 184
Crawford, Helen 76
creativity
ectomorphs and 83
and meditation 66
and positive emotions 31, 53, 54, 91
Csikszentmihalyi, Mihaly 54
cytokins 26, 33, 34
cytoskeleton 122–3, 124

Dale, Ralph Alan 151
Damasio, Antonio 100, 127
Davidson, Richard 32, 34, 52–3, 67
depression 32, 54, 167
and cancer 46–7, 48
and deep breathing 142
and inflammation 41–3, 44, 59
and massage 118, 119
Descartes, René 3
Devroed, Ghislain 100–1, 104
diet 137, 154, 155–6, 163, 193
distress (negative stress) 31, 32, 40
DNA 46, 47, 120, 123, 181, 184
doctors
and art of communication 199
and nocebo effect 20–2, 60
referrals to alternative practitioners 5
dogs, recognising cancer 176–7
dopamine 19, 32, 58, 118, 119
doshas 84, 154, 155
Dressen, Linda 174

ear, cartography of 150
ectomorphs 82, 83
Einstein, Albert 195
Eisen, Alice 31

embryology 81–2
  and acupuncture 149–51
emotions
  and the brain 28–32
  expressing 91–3, 97, 101
  function of 30–2
  and meridians 151–3
  physical experience of 91
  positive 31–2, 130
    and biofeedback 71
    and creativity 31, 53, 54, 91
    effect on health 9, 52
    and immune system 34–5, 47, 67, 68, 69, 91, 140, 160
    and massage 119
    and meditation 67
    and pychotherapy 64
    and *qigong* 142
  repression of 85–8, 99
  transforming negative emotions into positive 52–3, 91
  see also alexithymy; stress response
endocrine system 27, 158, 159
endomorphs 82–4
endorphins 26, 58, 118, 127, 144, 148
energy 9, 27, 36–7, 38, 68, 84, 139–40, 154–5, 171–5
  and diet 155–6
  'energy cysts' 132–3
  energy therapies 175–6, 177, 185
  exercises 137, 141–5, 163–4
  freeing 90–3, 132–3, 171, 173
  healing 181–6
  see also chakras; *prana*; *qi*
Epel, Elissa 83–4
Erickson, Milton 73
Esdaile, James 72
eustress (positive stress) 40

faith 58, 142
Fawzy, Fawzy 62
Faymonville, Marie-Elisabeth 76–7
fear 22, 30–1, 53, 58, 87, 88, 126, 194
Feldenkrais Method 126–7, 162
Feldenkrais, Moshe 96, 126
Felten, David 25–6, 55–6
Field, Tiffany 114, 117, 151
fields, electrical and magnetic 180–3
five elements theory (Chinese medicine) 137, 138, 143
Flamm, Bruce 179
flight or fight 13, 35, 36, 38, 65, 85, 157, 158
Franklin, Benjamin 178
Fredrickson, Barbara 31, 54
Freud, Sigmund 73, 82, 90, 105–6, 111
Friedman, Meyer 48–9, 50

Fuller, Richard Buckminster 120, 125
functional Magnetic Resonance Imaging (fMRI) 15, 67, 76–8, 93, 148–9

Galen 46, 115, 128
Gampel, Yolanda 103
Gareus, Isabel 149
Ginandes, Carol 179
glial cells 200
Goldthwait, Joel 121
Goodwin, Pamela 62
gravity 120–2, 143
Groopman, Jerome 20
group therapy 92–3, 94
Gruzelier, John 34
Guo Ling 142

Hahn, Robert 22–3
Hamer, Ryke Geerd 106–7
happiness 31, 52, 53–4, 163, 194, 201
haptonomy 116
Harlow, Harry 114
Harrington, Anne 108
Havel, Vaclav 58
heart, and communication 183–4
Heisenberg, Werner 168
Helicobacter pylori 44
Hilgard, Josephine 103
Hinduism 65, 161, 173
Hippocrates 115
Hirshberg, Caryle 58
HIV/AIDS 22, 34, 59, 60, 61, 118
Hoffman, Hunter 77
holistic approach 3, 6, 154–5, 170, 196
Holocaust victims, descendants of 103–4, 105
Holt, Luther Emmett 111
homoeostasis (self-regulation of biological systems) 13, 28–9, 30, 138, 157, 162
homosexuals, and acceptance of own sexuality 61
hope 58–9, 60
Huang Ti Nei Ching (Chinese medical text) 140
Huizink, Anja 49
Huxley, Aldous 115
hypertension 16, 20, 65, 66
hypnosis 71–8, 179
  components of hypnotic trance 74
  and experience of pain 62, 72–3, 75–8
  personality types and 74–5
  self-hypnosis 74
  and surgical procedures 72
hypothalamic-pituitary-adrenal axis 27, 30, 36–7, 49
hypothalamus 38, 53, 116, 148, 157, 159, 165, 182

Ida and *Pingala* 157, 164, 166
illness, as multifactorial process 43–5, 46
imagination
    power of 13–14, 20, 68, 178–9
    see also autosuggestion; suggestion;
        visualisation
immune system 33–5, 90–1, 189
    and cancer 46–7
    and *chakras* 157–61
    emotional writing and 56–7
    hope and 58
    influence of healers 172, 184
    laughter and 55–6
    massage and touch and 114, 117, 118
    meditation and 67, 145
    and nervous system 25–7, 55, 99
    positive emotions and 34–5, 68, 140
    qigong and 142
    and stress 36, 37–8, 40, 41–3
    visualisation and 68–9
    yoga and 162
    see also psycho-neuro-endocrino-
        immunology; psycho-neuro-
        immunology
immunoglobulins/antibodies 34, 57
    IgA 35, 40, 55, 174
Indian medicine 154–68, 196
    and diet 155–6
    see also *ayurvedic* medicine; breathing;
        chakras; yoga
inflammation 33, 37–8, 101, 109
    and depression 41–3, 44–5, 59
infradian rhythms 167
Ingber, Donald 123
Ingham, Eunice 151
inner resources 126, 130, 188, 191–2, 196, 201
integrated medicine 4, 5, 7–9, 139, 141, 175, 196, 197–200
International Society of Complementary Medicine Research 6
intuition 8, 84–5, 95, 133, 152, 159, 176, 177
Irwin, Michael 47

James, William 91
Janov, Arthur 29, 98, 99, 100
Jonas, Wayne 184
Juhan, Deane 113
Jung, Carl Gustav 24, 82
Jung, Waymond 47

Kaivalyadhama Institute (Lonavla) 161
kapha 84, 154
Kataria, Dr Madan 56
Kiecolt-Glaser, Janice 41, 179
Krieger, Dolores 171

Kübler-Ross, Elisabeth 91
Kunz, Dora 171

Lang, Elvira 72, 74
Lao Tseu 141
laughter 32, 55–6
Lavoisier, Antoine Laurent de 178
LeDoux, Joseph 31, 95
Leskowitz, Eric 172
Levenstein, Susan 44
Lévi-Strauss, Claude 18, 64
Li, Geng 149
life-style, changing 193, 195
limbic system 28, 30, 31, 53, 74, 93, 116, 148–9
    see also amygdala
Ling, Henrik 115
living matrix 122–4, 129, 130, 146, 157, 181
Locke, John 201
Lowen, Alexander 90–1, 160
lymphocytes 33–4, 41, 119, 159
    see also NK (natural killer) cells

Maccari, Stefania 49
McCraty, Rolin 183
magnetic fluid 72, 178–9
Maharishi Mahesh Yogi 65–6, 154
marital relationships, stress and immune system 41
masochistic personalities (Reich's classification) 87
massage 115–16, 117–19
    and premature babies 117
    see also Rolfing; touching
Mazarin, Cardinal 54
meaning 19–20, 29, 56–8, 64, 96, 100, 107–9, 130, 190
    and alexithymy 93–4
    'meaning effect' 14–17, 18, 20, 108, 139, 187
media, effect on public health 22–3
medicines see remedies, external
meditation 65–8, 141, 142, 144, 162, 181, 182
    effect on immune system 67, 145
    mantras 66
    reshaping of brain 67–8
memories 98–105
    expressed by physical symptoms 98–103, 106–7
    inherited 101–2
    recovered/reawakened 97–100
    transgenerational 103–5, 107
meridians 145, 146, 157
    effect on emotions 151–3
Mesmer, Franz Anton 72, 178, 180

mesmerism 178–9
mesomorphs 82, 83, 84
metaphors 7, 9, 29, 75, 99, 137, 138, 139, 145, 177
Mézières, Françoise 127
Miller, Gregory 44
Moerman, Daniel 16
Molière 8
Montagu, Ashley 114
morphology
   connection with psychology 82–9
   major types 82–3, 84–5
   observing/reading the body 88–9, 91
   and reaction to stress 83–4, 121
   see also ayervedic medicine; emotions, repression of; Reich, Wilhelm
Mosely, Bruce 18
Motz, Julie 175
Murphy, Michael 115
muscle training, through mental activity 69–71
myths and legends 57

nadis 154, 157
naloxone 14
Nathan, Tobie 17
negativity, and depression 53–4
neocortex 28, 29, 158
nervous system
   and immune system 25–7
   and stress 85
   see also autonomic nervous system
neuropeptides 26
neuroplasticity 50–1, 53, 68, 71, 86, 100, 143, 200
neurotransmitters 26, 32
New Age 169–85
NK (natural killer) cells 5, 33, 34, 40, 46–7, 62, 69, 118, 119, 184
Noble, Denis 200
nocebo effect 20–3, 108–10, 161, 199
Nogier, Paul 150
noradrenaline 32

odours 34–5
Oleson, Terence 150
Olivares, Arnulfo 20, 107, 185
optimism 23, 52, 54
   see also emotions, positive
oral personalities (Reich's classification) 87
Ornish, Dean 162–3
Oschman, James 146, 157, 182
Osowiec, Dorlene 165
osteopathy 130–1
oxytocin 117, 159
Oz, Mehmet 175

pain 58, 62, 72–3, 75–8, 83, 96–7
Palmer, Daniel David 128
parasympathetic system 27, 35–6, 130, 145, 157, 174
   and breathing 162, 164, 165
   and massage 116, 117, 119
   reparatory processes of 35, 43, 65, 86, 142
   see also autonomic nervous system, sympathetic/parasympathetic balance
Parkinson's disease 125, 167
Pasteur, Louis 39
Patterson, David 77
Pavlov, Ivan 25
personality types 49, 50, 86–8
Pert, Candace 26
pessimism 23, 52–4
pharmaceutical industry 3, 17, 196
Phillips, David 139
Pierrakos, John 90–1
Pilates, Joseph 127
Pilates Method 127
pitta 84, 154
pituitary gland 36, 38, 157, 158, 159
   see also hypothalamic-pituitary-adrenal axis
placebo effect 14–20, 106, 130, 147–8, 174–5, 199
Poggi Davis, Elysia 50
postmodern medicine 198–201
   see also integrated medicine
posture 124–5
   see also Alexander technique; body, alignment
prana 154, 156–7
pregnancy, and transmission of information to foetus 102–3
Price, Richard 115
Prigogine, Ilya 168
Primal Therapy 29, 98–100
'primary respiratory mechanism' (PRM) 131
prolactin 38
Protheroe, David 45
Proust, Marcel 25
Prozac® 32
psycho-neuro-endocrino-immunology 104, 157–61, 187
psycho-neuro-immunology 26, 52, 55, 73, 138
psychocorporal therapies 90–7
   see also Qigong; *tai-chi*
psychogenealogy 105
psychology, positive 52–6
psychopathic/narcissistic personalities (Reich's classification) 87
'psychosomatic' pathologies 100

psychotherapy
  health benefits of 62–4
  and relationship with patient 191–2
  and touching 111, 112–13

qi 137, 139–41, 145, 146
qigong 141–3, 181
Quesalid 18

Rainville, Pierre 75–6, 77
Rampa, Lobsang (Cyril Hoskin) 170
Ray, Paul 197
Redfield, James 170
reductionism 3, 6, 8, 26, 107, 180, 199, 200
reflexology 151
Reich, Wilhelm 85–8, 90, 97, 111, 121, 127, 160, 161
reiki 172–5
relaxation 64–8
  and acupuncture 152
  and brain activity 119
  exercises 64–5
    see also breathing; yoga
  and massage and touch 110, 116–17, 151
  and power of mind 58, 70, 71, 73
  and psychocorporal therapies 90–1, 94, 95, 96
  'relaxation response' 65, 66
  and *tai-chi* 143–5
  see also parasympathetic system
remedies, external 192–5
responsibility 201
  and guilt 188–9, 190
  and omnipotence 189–91
Reston, James 147
revelation 178
Ricard, Matthieu 67–8
Rifkin, Jeremy 195
rigid personalities (Reich's classification) 87–8
Rolf, Ida 97, 122
Rolfing technique (Structural Integration) 97, 122
Rosenberg, Marshall 91
Rosenman, Ray 48–9
Rosnay, Joël de 198
Ross, Robyn 163
Rossi, Ernest 167
Russek, Linda 183

San hunter-gatherers 113–14
Sangh, Raghubir 156, 159–60, 185
schizoid personalities (Reich's classification) 87
Schultz, Johannes 73

Schwartz, Gary 183
self-awareness 29, 66, 95, 124–5, 127, 144, 158, 162
self-confidence 54, 125, 126, 163, 191
Seligman, Martin 52, 54
Selye, Hans 36, 37, 65
serotonin 32, 118, 119
Servan-Schreiber, David 193
shamanism 2, 18, 64, 68, 137, 147
Sheldon, William 82–4, 88
shiatsu 151–2, 190
Siegel, Bernie 108
Simonton, Carl 68
Singg, Sangeeta 174
skin 113, 116, 118, 172
smoking 47
Snelson, Kenneth 120, 123
Spiegel, David 57, 62, 74–5
Spiegel, Herbert 74–5
Spitz, René 114
SQUID (Superconducting Quantum Interference Device) 180, 181
Stengers, Isabelle 17
Still, Andrew Taylor 129–30
stress
  antenatal 49–50, 102–3
  as danger to health 37–8, 39–51, 53
  and efficacy of medical treatments 61–2, 63
  and inflammatory diseases 41–3
  positive and negative 39–40
  and repression of emotions 85–6
  'stress response' 36–8, 49
  and yoga 162
Strupp, Hans 64
suggestion 14, 21, 71–8, 106, 108, 139, 178–9
  see also auto-suggestion; hypnosis; noccebo effect; placebo effect
surgery
  and hypnosis 72
  and placebo effect 18–19
Sushumna 157
Sutherland, William 131–2
swara yoga 164–6, 167
sympathetic system 27, 35–6, 37, 44, 85–6, 157, 164
  see also autonomic nervous system, sympathetic/parasympathetic balance
Szent-Györgyi, Albert 146

tai-chi 143–5
Takata, Hawayo 173
tan tien 143
tang-kis healers (Taiwan) 19
Taoism 35, 139, 141
telomeres 47

tensegrity 120–1, 123, 125, 129, 130
Theosophical Society 170, 171
Theosophy 171, 176
Therapeutic Touch 171–2, 179, 181
Tinbergen, Nikolaas 125
tomographic positron scanner (PETscan) 15
Török, Maria 103
touching 111–15
   and healing 115–17
   and prohibitions 111–13, 115
   see also massage
Transcendental Meditation 65–6
transgenerational psychology 189–90
tritherapy 61

ultradian rhythms 167
Upledger, John 132, 133
Usui, Mikao 173

vata 84, 154
vegetotherapy 90
Veldman, Frans 116
vibrations 182–3
visualisation 68–71, 141, 142

vitalists
   versus mechanists 178–82
   vital force 180

Watson, John 111
Weil, Andrew 4, 198
Weitzman, Elliott 166
Western medicine
   costs of 3–4
   and medical training 198–9
   and reductionism 3, 6, 8, 26, 107, 180, 199
Wirth, Daniel 179
witch-doctors 13–14, 17–18
writing, emotional 56–7

yin and *yang* 35–6, 137, 138, 144, 149, 157
yoga 97, 161–3, 181
   swara yoga 164–6, 167

Zajde, Nathalie 105
Zang-Hee Cho 149
Zimmerman, John 181